CEREBROVASCULAR
DISEASE

CEREBROVASCULAR DISEASE

by

JAMES PETER MURPHY, M. D.

Assistant Clinical Professor of Neurological Surgery,
George Washington University School of Medicine

FOREWORD BY
PERCIVAL BAILEY, M. D.

THE YEAR BOOK PUBLISHERS   •   INC.

200 EAST ILLINOIS STREET   •   CHICAGO

To

BARBARA

in appreciation

Foreword

I HAVE BEEN asked to write a foreword to this book. In my opinion it is quite unnecessary. If a book is good (and this one is), it will make its own way; if it is not, no introduction will make it succeed. Yet, when asked by a pupil and friend, it is difficult to refuse, even though one is conscious of having no expert knowledge or experience in the field with which the book deals. But, I reflected, I was not asked to write a critical review.

I know very well that the book is timely. In these past years a great deal of work has been done on the cerebral circulation and its regulation. The functioning of the brain is acutely dependent on its well-being, and the steady increase in the average age of the population makes the study of the circulation of ever-increasing importance to the practicing physician who needs to know what bearing these studies have on the management of his increasing number of elderly patients. The author of this book, a neurological surgeon with an extensive basic training in the anatomy, physiology and pathology of the brain, is eminently fitted to bring all these dispersed studies together in a compact volume which the practitioner can utilize.

Much of the information in this book is of recent acquisition; much is old but forgotten or neglected. The carotid sinus syndrome was known to Rufus of Ephesus. The syndrome of "little strokes" of which we hear so much these days was well known to the French neurologists; I heard much of it from my master, Pierre Marie. There used to be a chapter on cerebral anemia in all the treatises on neurology, recently ignored but now restored to importance.

The book is comprehensive and judicious but not pedantic. No aspect of the subject is neglected and the bibliography is adequate to enable the reader who wishes more details concerning any aspect to find them quickly. I believe that Dr. Murphy has written a scholarly and useful book which will have a well merited success.

—PERCIVAL BAILEY

Preface

CEREBROVASCULAR DISEASE is of growing concern to the general practitioner, internist, geriatrician and pediatrician as well as to the neurologist and neurosurgeon. Disorders of the intracranial circulation constitute the paramount problem in clinical neurology today; there are more patients with cerebrovascular accidents admitted to the neurologic wards of large general hospitals in a year than with any other type of disorder of the nervous system. Major brain stroke is the third most frequent cause of death in the United States, outranked only by heart disease and malignancy. It is estimated that one-half million persons in this country sustain strokes each year, and that one and one-fourth million hemiplegic patients are surviving in the hospital or at home.

The progressive aging of the population as a whole is largely responsible for the increasing incidence of cerebrovascular accidents. Deaths from cerebral hemorrhage and infarction are concentrated in the later years of life even more than cardiac fatalities. The introduction, perfection and widening application of new diagnostic technics are revealing more and more cases of previously mysterious or vaguely classified neurologic syndromes, especially in the young, to be of cerebrovascular origin. The term stroke is no longer restricted to hemiplegia but may apply to any focal cerebral dysfunction, and strokes are recognized to be as varied in their manifestation as are the activities of the brain.

Thus, the field of cerebrovascular disease is ever-widening, and in this volume I have attempted to include its many aspects. A summary is given of present knowledge in the basic sciences as applied to the circulation of the brain. Then, proceeding from the examination of the patient and the differential diagnosis of the types of cerebrovascular accident, the specific pathologic conditions affecting the intracranial blood vessels are discussed individually. The paradoxical lack of interest in the treatment of cerebrovascular accidents is at last being overcome by repeated and successful

9

demonstration that medical, neurosurgical and physical therapy offer a great deal to the patient with a stroke or other disability from disease of the intracranial circulatory system. Therefore, special chapters are devoted to the general care of these patients and to applicable diagnostic and therapeutic technics.

I received valuable criticism and assistance from many sources in the preparation of the manuscript. In particular, I wish to thank Drs. Paul Chodoff, Arthur Ecker, Walter Freeman, John F. Fulton, Webb Haymaker, Seymour S. Kety, Oscar Legault, F. L. McNaughton, Fred A. Mettler, Oscar Sugar, A. Earl Walker, Charles S. Wise, Harold G. Wolff and Mrs. Dorcas H. Padget, and the Hutchins Fund of the George Washington University School of Medicine, direction of Dr. Walter Freeman, under whose auspices this book was prepared. For secretarial help, I am indebted to my wife and to Miss Norma Kethcart, Miss Ceceile Murphy and Mrs. Elizabeth Braum. Miss Phyllis Anderson prepared the drawings, in which we have attempted to present the consensus of anatomic investigations by many authorities. To the Year Book Publishers I also wish to express my thanks.

—J.P.M.

ACKNOWLEDGMENTS

Acknowledgment is made to the following individuals and publishers whose illustrations have been used in this volume.

Figure 1: D. H. Padget, in W. E. Dandy, *Intracranial Arterial Aneurysms* (Ithaca, N.Y.: Comstock Publishing Co., Inc., 1944).

Figure 2: E. L. Potter, Arch. Path. 48:87-96, 1948.

Figure 3: F. B. Walsh, *Clinical Neuro-ophthalmology* (Baltimore: Williams & Wilkins Company, 1947).

Figures 6, 11, 22, 74, *D* and *J*: O. Sugar, J. Neurosurg. 8:3-22, 1951.

Figures 9 and 16: A. Kristenson, Acta med. scandinav. (supp. 196) 128:200-211, 1947.

Figure 17: H. A. Shenkin and S. S. Kety, Arch. Neurol. & Psychiat. 60:240-252, 1948.

Figure 19: B. Schlesinger, Brain 62:274-291, 1938.

Figure 20: J. A. Gius and D. H. Grier, Surgery 28:305-321, 1950.

Figure 23: D. E. Hale, Anesthesiology 9:498-505, 1948.

Figure 24: Dr. J. Huertas.

Figure 27: R. D. Adams and M. E. Cohen, Bull. New England M. Center 9:261, 1947.

Figure 30: E. W. Amyes and S. M. Perry, J.A.M.A. 142:15-20, 1950.

Figure 31: H. Krayenbühl, Schweiz. med. Wchnschr. 75:1025-1029, 1945.

Figure 32: I. M. Scheinker, Arch. Neurol. & Psychiat. 55:216-231, 1946.

Figures 34, 35, 40, 55, 57, 61, 67, *A*, 68, 98 and 103: Armed Forces Institute of Pathology.

Figures 36, 44, 52, 56, 60, 62, 67, *B*, 72, 74, *I*, 81, 104 and 115: George Washington University Laboratory of Neurology.

Figure 37: J. P. Murphy and M. S. Neumann, Arch. Neurol. & Psychiat. 49: 724-731, 1943.

Figure 38: M. Fisher, A.M.A. Arch. Neurol. & Psychiat. 65:346-377, 1951.

Figure 41: F. P. Moersch and J. W. Kernohan, Arch. Neurol. & Psychiat. 41: 365-372, 1939.

Figure 42: J. C. Richardson and H. H. Hyland, Medicine 20: 1-83, 1941.

Figure 43: Dr. W. Freeman.

Figure 47: A. B. King, J. Neurosurg. 8:536-539, 1951.

Figure 48: J. P. Murphy and J. S. Garvin, Arch. Neurol. & Psychiat. 58:436-446, 1947.

Figure 49: H. C. Johnson and A. E. Walker, J. Neurosurg. 8:631-659, 1951.

Figure 63, *A*: Dr. S. W. Gross.

Figure 65: P. M. Levin, A.M.A. Arch. Neurol. & Psychiat. 67:771-787, 1952.

Figure 70: C. A. McDonald and M. Korb, Arch. Neurol. & Psychiat. 42:298-328, 1939.

Figure 71: J. T. B. Carmody, J. Neurosurg. 3:81-85, 1946.

Figure 74, *B*: V. A. Hospital, Washington, D.C.

Figure 74, *K*: M. Bushard, E. Yuhl and R. W. Barris, Neurology 2:356-359, 1952.

11

Figure 75, *A*: D. Oscherwitz and L. M. Davidoff, J. Neurosurg. 4:539-541, 1947.

Figure 75, *B*: D. H. Echols and H. D. Kirgis, Surgery 27:260-267, 1950.

Figure 77: A. Ecker and P. A. Riemenschneider, J. Neurosurg. 8:348-353, 1951.

Figure 78: W. E. Dandy, Ann. Surg. 107:654-659, 1938.

Figure 80: Dr. G. M. Swain.

Figure 83: H. O. Tonning, R. F. Warren and H. J. Barrie, J. Neurosurg. 9:124-132, 1952.

Figure 84: N. Antoni, Acta chir. scandinav. 85:7-24, 1941.

Figure 86: J. R. Jaeger, J. Neurosurg. 8:335-340, 1951.

Figure 87: A. D. McCoy and H. C. Voris, Arch. Neurol. & Psychiat. 59:504-510, 1948.

Figures 88 and 92: J. R. Green, J. Foster and D. L. Berens, Am. J. Roentgenol. 64:391-398, 1950.

Figure 89: P. Danis, Acta neurol. et psychiat. belg. 50:615-679, 1950.

Figure 95: Dr. J. W. Watts.

Figures 96 and 107: Dr. J. M. Williams.

Figure 97: G. Norlén, J. Neurosurg. 6:475-494, 1949.

Figure 100: B. S. Ray, H. S. Dunbar and C. T. Dotter, J. Neurosurg. 8:23-37, 1951.

Figure 111: N. W. Winkelman and M. T. Moore, J. Neuropath. & Exper. Neurol. 9:60-77, 1950.

Figure 114: R. K. Thompson, J. A. Wagner and C. M. MacLeod, Ann. Int. Med. 29:921-928, 1948.

Figure 119: *Medical Horizons,* Sandoz Pharmaceuticals Co.

Figure 120: L. N. Rudin, Current M. Dig. 19:21-25, 1952.

Figure 121: S. W. Gross, S. Clin. North America 28:405-411, 1948.

Figure 126: F. A. D. Alexander and B. K. Lovell, J.A.M.A. 148:885-886, 1952.

Figure 128: R. C. Bassett, J. Neurosurg. 8:132-133, 1951.

Table of Contents

1. Embryology of the Intracranial Vessels 17

2. Anatomy of the Arteries of the Brain 24
   Circle of Willis 24
   Carotid System 26
   Vertebral-Basilar System 36
   Arteries of the Intracranial Dura Mater 44
   Choroid Plexuses 44
   Arterial Anomalies 45
   Anastomoses and Collateral Circulation 45
   Microscopic Anatomy 47

3. The Veins and Dural Venous Sinuses 50
   Veins of the Brain 50
   Dural Venous Sinuses 56
   Jugular Veins 62
   Accessory Venous Drainage of Brain 62
   Microscopic Anatomy 64

4. Nerve Supply of the Intracranial Vessels 65
   Vasosensory Nerves 65
   Vasomotor Nerves 67

5. Physiology of the Intracranial Circulation 73
   Cerebral Blood Flow 73

Cerebrovascular Resistance 83

Intracranial Pressure and Cerebral Blood Flow 92

Cerebral Metabolism 94

Electroencephalography 99

Cerebrospinal Fluid 101

6. The Acute Cerebrovascular Accident: Examination 106

    General Physical Examination 106

    Neurologic Examination 111

    Laboratory Examinations 119

    Differential Diagnosis 121

7. Cerebral Vasospasm 122
      Etiology, Pathogenesis, Pathology; Symptoms and Signs;
      Laboratory Studies; Diagnosis; Treatment; Prognosis

8. Cerebral Thrombosis; Infarction 131

    Arterial Thrombosis 131

    Infarction without Thrombosis 138

    Specific Arterial Syndromes 142

    Laboratory Studies 156

    Diagnosis 162

    Treatment 163

    Prognosis 167

9. Cerebral Embolism 171
      Etiology, Pathogenesis; Pathology; Symptoms and Signs;
      Laboratory Studies; Diagnosis; Treatment; Prognosis

10. Cerebral Hemorrhage 180
      Etiology, Pathogenesis; Pathology; Symptoms and Signs;
      Laboratory Studies; Diagnosis; Treatment; Prognosis

11. Subarachnoid Hemorrhage; Intracranial Aneurysm 199
      Etiology, Pathogenesis; Pathology; Symptoms and Signs;
      Laboratory Studies; Diagnosis; Treatment; Prognosis

The Acute Episode 209

Aneurysmal Syndromes 212

Carotid-Cavernous Aneurysm (Fistula) 235

12. Vascular Tumors; Arteriovenous Malformations of the Brain . . . 242
Etiology, Pathogenesis; Pathology; Symptoms and Signs;
Laboratory Studies; Diagnosis; Treatment; Prognosis

13. Intracranial Venous Disease; Venous Sinus Disease 263
Etiology, Pathogenesis; Pathology; Symptoms and Signs;
Laboratory Studies; Diagnosis; Treatment; Prognosis

14. Hypertensive Brain Disease 275
Etiology, Pathogenesis; Pathology; Symptoms and Signs;
Laboratory Studies; Diagnosis; Treatment; Prognosis

15. Cerebral Arteriosclerosis 287
Etiology, Pathogenesis; Pathology; Symptoms and Signs;
Laboratory Studies; Diagnosis; Treatment; Prognosis

16. Inflammatory and Collagenous Diseases 305

Inflammatory Vascular Disease 305

Collagenous Vascular Disease 310

17. Blood Dyscrasias; Vitamin Deficiencies; Poisons 319

Blood Dyscrasias 319

Vitamin Deficiencies 324

Cerebrovascular Poisons 326

18. Headache 330

19. General Management of the Patient 345

Home or Hospital? 345

Increased Intracranial Pressure 346

Heart and Circulation 348

Lungs and Respiration 348

Urinary Tract 351

Gastrointestinal Tract 352

Skin: Decubitus Ulcers 353

Fever 354

Nutrition 355

Restraints 357

Control of Pain and Convulsive Seizures 357

Physical Therapy 359

Psychiatric Treatment 364

20. Diagnostic Technics 368

Lumbar Spinal Puncture 368

Pneumoencephalography 370

Ventriculography 370

Angiography 370

Electroencephalography 378

21. Therapeutic Technics 380

Stellate Block 380

Ligation of the Cervical Carotid Artery 383

Subtemporal Decompression 389

Craniotomy 390

CHAPTER 1

Embryology of the
Intracranial Vessels

TO BEGIN A discussion of the cerebral vascular system, its various aspects and diseases with some embryologic considerations not only satisfies tradition but is a matter of practical interest. In the study of development of intracranial blood vessels the explanation of the appearance, constitution and location of congenital aneurysms and angiomas is found, and variation in the arrangement of the components of the circle of Willis is understood (Fig. 1). Increasing interest in the operative treatment of cerebral vascular anomalies is actually leading to an applied or surgical embryology. Moreover, from embryology comes anatomy, and knowledge of one assures remembrance of the other.

The progressive development and differentiation of the circulation of the brain passes through several distinct embryologic stages (Streeter).

Angioblasts arranged into plexus

The most primitive type of intracranial vasculature results from the differentiation of angioblasts from mesoderm (Sabin). Angioblastic cells which are to form vessels rather than erythrocytes are first arranged into a primordial plexus of channels which are neither arteries nor veins. Persistence of the angioblastic syncytium may be recognized in hemangioblastoma of the cerebellum and hemangioma of the fourth ventricle.

Arteries, veins, capillaries appear

In the embryo the plexus further differentiates into capillaries, arteries and veins which are recognizable as such only by their connections. Developmental arrest at this stage is undoubtedly responsible for per-

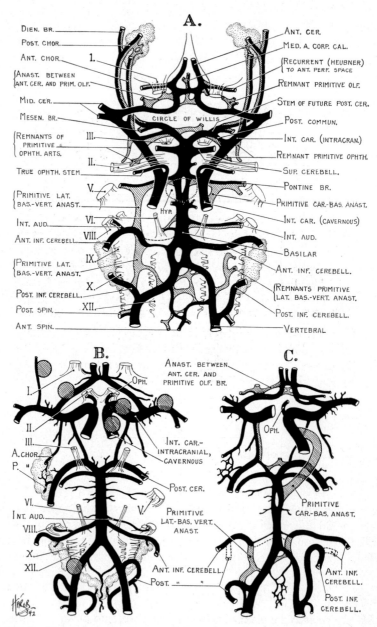

FIG. 1.—Embryologic development of the arteries of the brain. *A*, formation of the circle of Willis and major vessels; *B*, sites of congenital aneurysms (shaded circles); *C*, other developmental arterial anomalies (shaded). (Courtesy of D. H. Padget.)

18

sistence of diffuse pial telangiectasia, a rare cerebral malformation of the newborn which is associated with congenital cardiac disease (Fig. 2). Persistence of irregular connections between poorly differentiated arteries and veins in arteriovenous aneurysm or malformation, a not uncommon

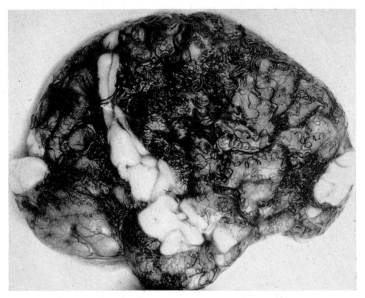

FIG. 2.—Telangiectasia of the brain. (Courtesy of E. L. Potter.)

vascular anomaly in the adult, is explained in part by failure of islands of the primordial plexus to progress in maturity.

Separation into three layers

The network of differentiated but unarranged vessels of the embryonic head is split or cleft, in the 15 mm. embryo, into three superimposed layers by the intrusion of the dura and cranium. Thus individual but interconnected circulations in the scalp, dura and pia result. When such cleavage does not take place at all, cirsoid aneurysm of the brain extends to and through the skull and involves the scalp. Van Bogaert attributes the preferential occurrence of large wedge-shaped arteriovenous anomalies in the middle cerebral distribution to the fact that inward growth of the meninges is most likely to be incomplete laterally. Angiomas or varices of the scalp, epidural space, dura and pia may also be residuals of arrest at this stage. Virchow described racemose hemangiomas of the cranial soft tissues ("pulsating earthworms") which penetrated the skull and involved meningeal or cerebral vessels.

Development of circle of Willis and branches

The congeries of newly formed arteries and veins, now truly cerebral and cerebellar, undergoes a tedious and seemingly aimless but actually purposeful arrangement and rearrangement which eventuate in the pattern of blood supply characteristic of the adult. In this stage of development "ontogeny recapitulates phylogeny," many vascular connections which are anatomic in lower forms of animal life persisting for some time in the expanding head of the human fetus only to be replaced ultimately by the typical artery or vein. The vessels also adjust themselves to pronounced changes in surrounding structures of the head. Final arrangement of the circle of Willis and fusion of the posterior portion to the anterior circulation through the posterior communicating arteries have been completed by the 40 mm. stage (human embryo of 2 months' age). The anterior communicating artery is the last component of the circle to form, just after the vertebral arteries have appeared.

It is with this phase of cerebral vascular embryology that the studies of Padget have been principally concerned. She has carefully traced the trials, errors and formation by natural selection of the adult circle of Willis and its divisions and branches from the relatively unintelligible pattern shown in Figure 1, A. From these investigations Padget concluded that most of the recorded variations and anomalies of the cerebral arteries are readily explained by persistence of definite but transitory anastomoses found in the fetus, that faulty union of immature connections leaves persistent defects and that incomplete involution of temporary vessels is related to the formation of congenital arterial aneurysms.

Many varieties of congenital aneurysms and supernumerary vessels found in patients with neurologic complaints represent examples of embryologic failure. Sacculations of the basilar artery occur in the midline, owing to the mode of formation of this vessel by fusion of two longitudinal neural arteries. Persistence of at least a part of the primitive trigeminal artery (for a time, the connection between carotid and basilar systems) accounts for spontaneous rupture of the adult carotid artery into the cavernous sinus. Finger- or saclike aneurysms depending from the internal carotid stem are retained fragments of primitive ventral and dorsal ophthalmic arteries, extra hypophyseal branches of the carotid or recurrent striate derivatives of the anterior cerebral artery. These vestigial pre-arterioles are usually devoid of media and elastica and apt to rupture.

Persistence of the connections of the hyoid-stapedial artery may lead in adult man to a strong anastomosis between the internal and external carotid arteries via ophthalmic and meningeal branches, which is the rule in lower animals. The human ophthalmic artery may be supplied entirely from the middle meningeal artery.

After the primitive internal carotid first divides into two trunks (4 mm. stage), the anterior cerebral, middle cerebral and anterior choroidal arteries grow out from the anterior primary branch, and the posterior communicating, posterior choroidal and posterior cerebral arteries are derived from the posterior division. All of the brain, supra- and infra-tentorial, is supplied up to the 14 mm. stage by carotid blood (Padget). Further evidence that the posterior cerebral artery is really a branch of the internal carotid is given in the finding that the carotid sympathetic plexus extends along the posterior cerebral artery and that carotid arteri-ography in the adult succeeds in filling this artery. Persistence of the carotid-basilar anastomosis has been demonstrated by angiography on occasion (Harrison and Luttrell).

The posterior half of the circle of Willis has a greater tendency to be anomalous than has the anterior circulation, although these variations are in size only because the posterior communicating and basilar arteries are completed early. Anywhere in or on the circle, primitive channels which normally are replaced may persist. One or both cervical carotid arteries may be found wanting when the basilar system has increased in importance. Conversely, the basilar artery may not join with the carotids at all, and the two circulations can be entirely independent in the adult.

As the brain matures, it changes in shape from a long, hollow tube to a complex and variably enlarged and chambered organ, in which pre-viously neighboring areas may be found widely separated. Such spatial alterations permit arteriovenous malformations of ophthalmic and mesen-cephalic vessels, which are closely associated at the 4 mm. stage, to be found in the retina and midbrain in later life. Ocular, facial and occipital cerebral angiomas coexist in the Sturge-Weber syndrome (Figs. 87, 88 and 92) and recall the anterior vascular plexus which drains the fore-brain and eye in very early existence.

Differentiation of veins and dural sinuses

The intracranial veins and dural sinuses are formed *pari passu* with the growth of the arterial circulation. In general, the venous drainage of the embryonic cerebrum is directed inferiorly and laterally toward the conjunction of the developing sigmoid, transverse and inferior petrosal sinuses. The cavernous sinus receives blood from the eye only during intrauterine life, and even in the adult midline flow into the cavernous sinus is of late and inconstant appearance (Padget).

From the manifold venous channels passing upward to the superior sagittal sinus, three or four major veins are eventually selected on each side to connect with the sinus proper, a pattern which persists anatomically. These superior cerebral veins run through the dura before terminating in the sagittal sinus in the fetus, the newborn infant and to some extent in the adult. Great venous channels conducting blood from the rhombencephalon (brain stem and cerebellum) also fill the immature tentorium cerebelli, which is extremely vascular during intrauterine life.

Aberrancy of the dural sinuses is not uncommon. The superior petrosal sinus may not develop at all, and its anatomic connection with the cavernous sinus is often absent. The sphenoparietal sinus, which is really a confluence of middle cerebral veins in the dura covering the lesser wing of the sphenoid bone, will not be present if a midline route to the cavernous sinus does not become sufficiently dominant. The occipital sinus is an unimportant remnant of the posterior dural plexus and is of inconstant presence.

More importantly, one transverse sinus is lacking in some adult brains (Woodhall), and a major disproportion in the cross-sectional diameters of the two transverse sinuses is not infrequent. The superior sagittal sinus is rarely absent, but variations in size of the venous lacunae are not uncommon. Although these pockets usually enlarge only during adult life, vestigial lateral extensions of the sagittal sinus into the dura may be wide and long.

Late histologic changes; completion of vessels

During the final period of development, the arteries and veins acquire medial and adventitial coats and the peculiarly strong internal elastic membrane which characterizes cerebral vessels. Now, again, histologic differentiation may go wrong. Forbus found that medial tissue condenses separately around a parent artery and branch, and it is his contention that the junctional gap or cleft is primarily responsible for aneurysm formation in later life. Bremer relates such medial defects to a failure of growth of muscle where an endothelial tube is well supported and to a change in the angle of branching vessels as the enlarging brain, which they supply, pulls them apart. The formerly abutting vascular walls, which are devoid of media because they were supporting each other, thus become areas of decreased resistance and potential sites of aneurysm formation. How the elastic membrane, especially prominent in arteries, develops has not been adequately described. The only adventitia surrounding cerebral arteries and veins is condensed arachnoid and therefore flimsy.

Further changes occur in the vascularity of the brain after birth. Multiplication of capillaries proceeds in the newborn rat from the tenth to the twenty-first day post partum (Craigie). The posterior communicating artery is much larger in the human infant than in the adult, and the number of venous anastomoses increases with progressing age (Padget).

BIBLIOGRAPHY

Bremer, J. L.: Congenital aneurysms of the cerebral arteries: An embryologic study, Arch. Path. 35:819-831, 1943.

Craigie, E. H.: Postnatal changes in vascularity in the cerebral cortex of the male albino rat, J. Comp. Neurol. 39:301-324, 1925.

Forbus, W. D.: On the origin of military aneurysms of the superficial cerebral arteries, Bull. Johns Hopkins Hosp. 47:239-284, 1930.

Harrison, C. R., and Luttrell, C.: Persistent carotid-basilar anastomosis, J. Neurosurg. 10:205-215, 1953.

Padget, D. H.: The development of the cranial arteries in the human embryo, Contrib. Embryol. 32:205-262, 1948.

Padget, D. H.: Unpublished data.

Sabin, F. R.: Preliminary note on the differentiation of angioblasts and the method by which they produce blood vessels, blood plasma and red blood cells as seen in the living chick, Anat. Rec. 13:199-205, 1917.

Streeter, G. L.: The developmental alterations in the vascular system of the brain of the human embryo, Contrib. Embryol. 8:7-38, 1918.

Van Bogaert, L.: Pathology of angiomatosis, Acta neurol. et psychiat. belg. 50:525-620, 1950.

Woodhall, B.: Variations of the cranial venous sinuses in the region of the torcular Herophilii, Arch. Surg. 33:297-314, 1936.

CHAPTER 2

Anatomy of the
Arteries of the Brain

CIRCLE OF WILLIS

STRUCTURE OF THE CIRCLE.—Blood from the heart is carried to the brain by two sets of vessels, the right and left carotid and the right and left vertebral arteries. The anterior three fifths of the brain—the cerebrum, with the exception of a part of the temporal and occipital lobes—is irrigated by the carotid circulation. The posterior two fifths of the brain—the brain stem, cerebellum and part of the temporal and occipital lobes of the cerebrum—is supplied by arterial blood from the vertebral-basilar system.

Branches derived from the carotid and basilar arteries join at the base of the brain to form the anastomotic circle or polygon of Willis, a nine-sided ring of vessels which underlies the hypothalamus and third ventricle and surrounds the optic chiasm and pituitary stalk (Fig. 3). It is composed of the two anterior cerebral arteries, the anterior communicating artery, the carotids, the two posterior communicating arteries and both posterior cerebral arteries. Each terminal carotid artery at the circle is equal in cross-section to the basilar artery and is one-fourth the caliber of the cervical carotid at its origin.

STREAM OF FLOW.—Although potentially anastomotic and redistributing, the arterial circle does not function in the manner of a gas ring under normal conditions. The circle of Willis may be compared to a traffic circle, to which automobiles come on a certain avenue and from which they leave via the continuation of the same thoroughfare. Maintenance of the original stream of flow is similarly evident in the basal arterial polygon in health (Rogers).

IRRIGATION OF BRAIN.—In lower animals, the circle of Willis functions as a true hilus, from which penetrating blood vessels enter the cerebrum. In man, six main branches or divisions course outward on the surface of the brain to varying distances and then break up into smaller and smaller vessels. These minute blood plexuses are contained in the pia

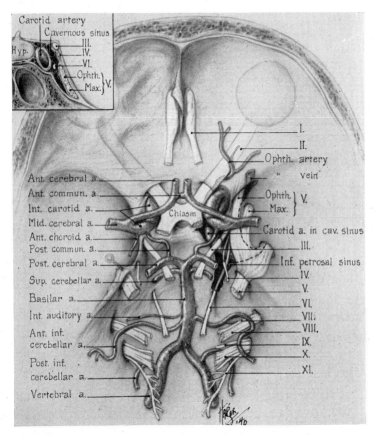

FIG. 3.—The circle of Willis and relations to the cranial nerves. (Courtesy of F. B. Walsh.)

mater, a fine membrane of mesothelial cells. From the pia, blood returns through the cerebral parenchyma toward the base in centripetal fashion, a pattern apparently associated with the development of cortical dominance. The actual nutrient arteries and arterioles are either *ganglionic* branches, which supply the interior nuclear masses, or *cortical* branches which penetrate and enter the cortex perpendicularly.

SUPPORT OF BRAIN.—Another, minor function of the circle of Willis is that of support. The brain almost, but not quite, floats in the cerebrospinal fluid with which it is surrounded; it hangs from suspending veins which run to the intracranial sinuses and is buoyed up by the brain stem and the main arteries at the base as a flower is held up by its stalk.

CAROTID SYSTEM

Common carotid artery

The common carotid arteries arise in the root of the neck as primary branches of the aorta. The right arises indirectly, springing from the innominate trunk with the subclavian, while the left comes directly from the aortic arch just within the thoracic inlet. The common carotids are large, muscular arteries with thick walls and a vigorous pulse. Each runs upward, slightly backward and laterally toward the head. In its cervical portion the carotid is one of the most easily palpable and accessible major arteries in the body.

The common carotid arteries lie within the anterior cervical triangles, at first medial to and then somewhat underneath the sternocleidomastoid muscles. At their origin they are separated by the trachea alone, but higher up the thyroid gland, larynx and pharynx project forward between them. Structures which are in principal relation to the cervical course of the carotid are the vagus nerve and the internal jugular vein. The vein lies externally and in front and covers the artery to a considerable degree; the nerve runs between and slightly behind both. The three structures are contained in separate compartments of the carotid sheath, a fibrous envelope derived from the deep cervical fascia and continuous with the vascular adventitia and vagus epineurium. Behind all, from the upper thorax to the base of the skull runs the cervical sympathetic chain. The descendens hypoglossi nerve is also found in the carotid sheath (Fig. 127).

At the upper border of the thyroid cartilage, or thereabouts, the common carotid artery divides into external and internal branches. The point of division is an expansion of the vessel lumen, the *carotid sinus,* in the wall of which is found the carotid body. The ascending pharyngeal artery arises between the external and internal carotid arteries.

Internal carotid artery

At its origin, the internal carotid artery is actually lateral and anterior to its external counterpart, but it quickly becomes internal as it turns medially. This confusing external-internal relationship necessitates care in ligating one or the other vessel. The internal and external carotid arteries are equal in size in the adult. A chief distinguishing feature is that there are no branching arteries from the cervical portion of the internal carotid, whereas the external carotid gives off many vessels.

As the internal carotid ascends toward the floor of the cranium, it immediately overlies the long, fusiform superior cervical sympathetic

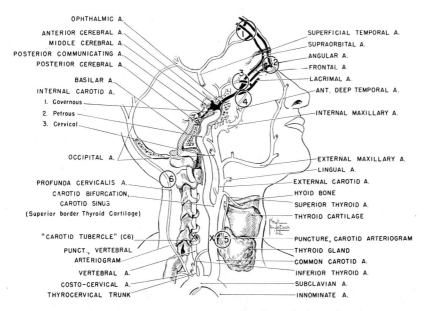

OPHTHALMIC A.
ANTERIOR CEREBRAL A.
MIDDLE CEREBRAL A.
POSTERIOR COMMUNICATING A.
POSTERIOR CEREBRAL A.
BASILAR A.
INTERNAL CAROTID A.
  1. Cavernous
  2. Petrous
  3. Cervical

OCCIPITAL A.

PROFUNDA CERVICALIS A.
CAROTID BIFURCATION,
CAROTID SINUS
(Superior border Thyroid Cartilage)

"CAROTID TUBERCLE" (C6)

PUNCT., VERTEBRAL
ARTERIOGRAM

VERTEBRAL A.
COSTO-CERVICAL A.
THYROCERVICAL TRUNK

SUPERFICIAL TEMPORAL A.
SUPRAORBITAL A.
ANGULAR A.
FRONTAL A.
LACRIMAL A.
ANT. DEEP TEMPORAL A.
INTERNAL MAXILLARY A.

EXTERNAL MAXILLARY A.
LINGUAL A.
EXTERNAL CAROTID A.
HYOID BONE
SUPERIOR THYROID A.
THYROID CARTILAGE

PUNCTURE, CAROTID ARTERIOGRAM
THYROID GLAND
COMMON CAROTID A.
INFERIOR THYROID A.
SUBCLAVIAN A.
INNOMINATE A.

FIG. 4.—The cervical and intracranial carotid and vertebral arteries. Anastomoses between branches of the external and internal carotid arteries are circled. X, sites of puncture for carotid and vertebral angiography. (Modified from Netter.)

ganglion. At the base of the skull, the artery is separated from the internal jugular vein by the glossopharyngeal, vagus, accessory and hypoglossal nerves. The internal carotid enters a channel (carotid canal) in the petrous portion of the temporal bone (Fig. 4), ascends in a forward and medialward direction and becomes intracranial after it passes through the foramen lacerum. Still extradural, or rather within the layers of the dura, it continues to ascend and curves upon itself, backward and forward, as it runs through the cavernous sinus alongside the body of the sphenoid bone and against the clinoid processes. The S-shaped curvature is called the carotid siphon. In its cavernous portion the internal carotid is unique in being the only artery in the body which lies within a vein.

The carotid then pierces the dura on the medial side of the anterior clinoid process, gives off its first significant branch, the ophthalmic artery, and soon breaks up into the important arteries which form the anterior part of the circle of Willis and supply the greater part of the brain with blood.

Minor twigs from the bony and cavernous carotid are important only as potential anastomoses. The anterior meningeal artery, a somewhat larger branch, runs to the dura of the floor of the anterior fossa. Direct, anteromedial ganglionic branches from the terminal portion of the carotid supply the genu of the internal capsule and adjacent basal ganglions, the hypothalamus and the anterior lobe of the hypophysis.

Ophthalmic artery

This vessel arises just inside the dura, runs forward and slightly downward, enters the orbit just below and lateral to the optic nerve and supplies the orbit, eye, upper nose and forehead (Fig. 4). The *central artery* of the retina is a direct continuation of the ophthalmic artery and represents a clearly visible (ophthalmoscopy) branch of the internal carotid. Some of the lesser derivatives of the ophthalmic artery become important when collateral circulation is necessary from the external to the internal carotid. Rarely, blood in the ophthalmic artery comes entirely from a persistent connection with the middle meningeal artery and not from the carotid.

MAJOR CEREBRAL ARTERIES OF CAROTID SYSTEM

These four arteries, the result of final subdivision of the internal carotid, are the anterior cerebral, middle cerebral, anterior choroidal and posterior communicating arteries. Embryologically, the carotid ends in a bifurcation into anterior and middle cerebral arteries, the anterior choroidal and posterior communicating vessels being preterminal branches.

Anterior cerebral artery

This artery runs horizontally and medially from the carotid bifurcation, coursing between the olfactory and optic tracts toward the inferior (ventral) part of the fissure which separates the two cerebral hemispheres (Fig. 5) and joins with its mate from the opposite side through the *anterior communicating artery*. This meeting may take the form of a letter X or H, may be affected by multiple channels or, rarely, may be

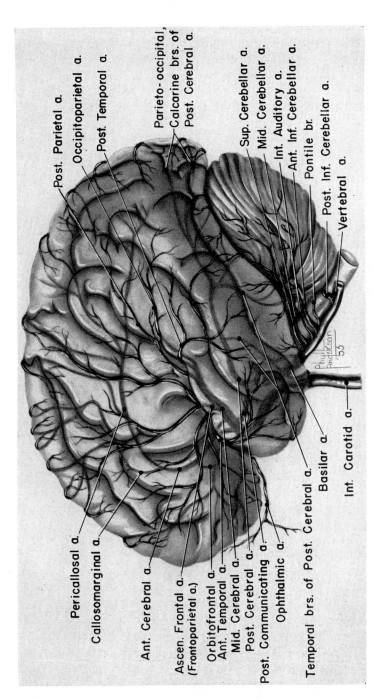

Post. Parietal a.

Occipitoparietal a.

Post. Temporal a.

Parieto-occipital,

Calcarine brs. of

Post. Cerebral a.

Sup. Cerebellar a.

Mid. Cerebellar a.

Int. Auditory a.

Ant. Inf. Cerebellar a.

Pontile br.

Post. Inf. Cerebellar a.

Vertebral a.

Int. Carotid a.

Basilar a.

Temporal brs. of Post. Cerebral a.

Ophthalmic a.

Post. Communicating a.

Post. Cerebral a.

Mid. Cerebral a.

Ant. Temporal a.

Orbitofrontal a.

Ascen. Frontal a.
(Frontoparietal a.)

Ant. Cerebral a.

Callosomarginal a.

Pericallosal a.

Fig. 5.—The major surface arteries of the brain.

29

absent. The anterior communicating artery completes the circle of Willis.

GANGLIONIC BRANCHES (Figs. 7, 8, and 10).—At this point, or just before, Heubner's *medial striate* artery may be given off. When present, this vessel which is a retained primitive olfactory channel may run with or replace the lenticulostriate artery of Charcot or the anterior choroidal artery and therefore can be quite important in the nutrition of the basal ganglions and internal capsule. Other *anteromedial* ganglionic branches

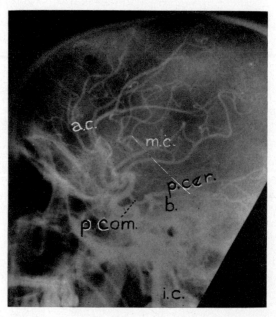

FIG. 6.—Cerebral arteries as seen in a lateral view of the carotid arteriogram. Compare with Figure 5. (Courtesy of O. Sugar.)

of the anterior cerebral and anterior communicating arteries supply the anterior hypothalamus, the forward part of the basal ganglions and the anterior limb of the internal capsule, entering through the anterior perforated space.

CORTICAL BRANCHES.—Just beyond the anterior communicating artery arises the *orbitofrontal* (frontopolar or prefrontal) artery, which runs to the medial and undersurfaces of the frontal lobe and olfactory complex. Continuing forward, the anterior cerebral then furnishes tiny vessels to the septum pellucidum, fornix and rostral corpus callosum, the callosal arteries.

The anterior cerebral artery now ascends rapidly, curving around the genu of the corpus callosum, where it is known as the *pericallosal* artery. Here is given off the *callosomarginal* artery, which is clearly visible in a lateral arteriogram, running backward parallel with the anterior cerebral, one gyrus (cingulate) higher (Fig. 6). This vessel supplies the anterior part of the superior frontal gyrus as well as the cingulum. It may terminate on the paracentral lobule (mesial representation of the sensorimotor area), after having run backward in the cingulate sulcus, and is then spoken of as the central artery.

On the medial aspect of the separated hemisphere, the anterior cerebral artery looks like a long grasshook or scythe, the blade following the surface of the corpus callosum from a short handle. The tip of the blade ends at the internal parieto-occipital fissure or 2–3 cm. in front of it. En route, *anterior, middle* and *posterior frontal* branches are given off; they supply corresponding parts of the superior frontal gyrus. Finally, the anterior cerebral artery breaks up into *paracentral* or central, *precuneal* and *parieto-occipital* branches.

Cortical twigs from the anterior cerebral artery course over the superior edge of the hemisphere and supply the cortex on the lateral surface to a distance of 2–3 cm. from the falx. Below is the middle cerebral zone.

Middle cerebral artery

This most important branch of the carotid is called the "arterial axis of the brain" by Moniz. The middle cerebral artery arises from the upper surface of the internal carotid at its terminus, crosses the anterior perforated space and lateral olfactory striae to enter the lateral cerebral or sylvian fissure, in which it breaks up into terminal rami (sylvian arteries) on the surface of the island of Reil (Fig. 5). It carries arterial blood to the bulk of the cerebral hemisphere, and infarction of the brain in the middle cerebral distribution and hemorrhage from one of its branches are the most common causes of hemiplegic stroke. Since the middle cerebral artery is closely invested with cerebral tissue, rupture of the vessel results in intracerebral hematoma.

GANGLIONIC (STRIATE) BRANCHES (Figs. 7, 8 and 10).—After a few tiny vessels are given off to the pituitary and the anterior hypothalamus, the principal basal branches—the anterolateral ganglionic arteries—flow inward toward the internal capsule, basal ganglions and thalamus, penetrating brain tissue in the area of the anterior perforated space. These vessels are in two groups, the *internal striate* and *external striate* arteries.

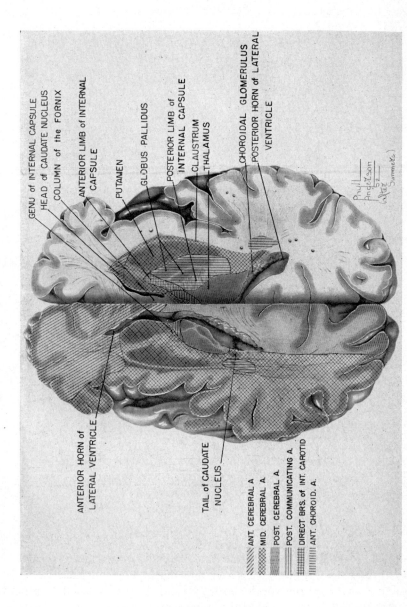

GENU of INTERNAL CAPSULE
HEAD of CAUDATE NUCLEUS
COLUMN of the FORNIX
ANTERIOR LIMB of INTERNAL CAPSULE
PUTAMEN
GLOBUS PALLIDUS
POSTERIOR LIMB of INTERNAL CAPSULE
CLAUSTRUM
THALAMUS
CHOROIDAL GLOMERULUS
POSTERIOR HORN of LATERAL VENTRICLE

ANTERIOR HORN of LATERAL VENTRICLE

TAIL of CAUDATE NUCLEUS

ANT. CEREBRAL A
MID. CEREBRAL A.
POST. CEREBRAL A.
POST. COMMUNICATING A.
DIRECT BRS. of INT. CAROTID
ANT. CHOROID. A.

FIG. 7.—Arterial blood supply of the interior of the cerebrum. Horizontal section on left through the dorsal internal capsule and on right through the ventral striate area. (Modified from Beevor, Mettler.)

32

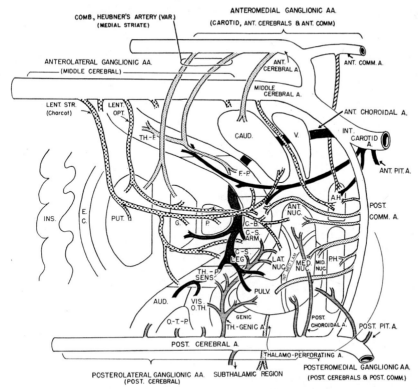

FIG. 8.—The complex distribution of ganglionic arteries to the internal capsule and basal forebrain nuclei. *Lent. str.,* lenticulostriate artery; *Lent. opt.,* lenticulo-optic artery; *Caud.,* caudate nucleus; *V,* lateral ventricle; *TH-F,* thalamofrontal radiation; *F-P,* fronto-pontile tract; *C-B,* corticobulbar fibers of internal capsule; *C-S arm (leg),* corticospinal fibers to arm (leg); *TH-P sens.,* thalamoparietal sensory projection; *Aud.,* geniculotemporal auditory projection; *Vis.O.Th.,* visual projection to optic thalamus; *O-T-P,* occipito-temporopontile tract; *Ins.,* insula; *EC,* external capsule; *Put.,* putamen; *G.P.,* globus pallidus; *Ant. nuc., lat. nuc., pulv., genic.,* etc., thalamic and geniculate nuclei; *AH, PH,* anterior and posterior hypothalamus; *Th-genic. a.,* thalamogeniculate artery; *Ant., post. pit. aa.,* arteries to hypophysis.

The most prominent internal striate vessels are the *lenticulo-optic* arteries, which supply the putamen of the lenticular nucleus, push medially through the globus pallidus and capsular knee (corticobulbar fibers) and end in the anterior and lateral nuclei of the (optic) thalamus.

The great French neurologist Charcot named the largest of the external striate branches, the *lenticulostriates,* the "arteries of cerebral hemorrhage," because he believed they were the most frequent source of cerebral apoplexy. These vessels pierce and nourish the putamen and globus pallidus, send prominent divisions to the anterior part of the posterior limb of the internal capsule (corticospinal fibers to the arm and leg) and to its knee (corticobulbar fibers), then terminate in the caudate nucleus. This capsular supply holds true dorsally. More ventrally, the important posterior limb is fed by the anterior choroidal artery. A few anterolateral ganglionic arteries run forward from the middle cerebral artery to the lateral part of the supraorbital frontal lobe.

Kristenson has shown in dissections that the flow of blood in the

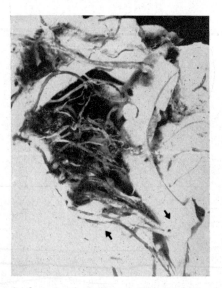

FIG. 9.—Retrograde flow (arrows) from middle cerebral artery into ganglionic branches. (Courtesy of A. Kristenson.)

anterolateral ganglionic branches of the internal carotid and middle cerebral arteries is turned back against the stream in retrograde fashion (Fig. 9). This anatomic peculiarity and the terminal nature of small ganglionic arterioles render the capsular region, a critical area of the brain, especially vulnerable to thrombotic injury.

CORTICAL BRANCHES.—In an arteriogram, the middle cerebral artery may be seen running outward in the sylvian fissure on a plane inclined slightly upward (Fig. 10). For the first half of its length it remains in the fissure, but shortly after giving off the penetrating ganglionic vessels it divides around the insula in a spray of arteries which then extend out from the fissure as ribs of a fan to supply various and important cortical areas.

Chief among these surface arteries are the *anterior temporal,* distributed to the forward one third of the temporal cortex; the *ascending frontal* (frontoparietal or "candelabra"), which again divides on the surface of the island of Reil into numerous branches distributed to the premotor, motor and primary sensory gyri; the *posterior parietal,* supplying the inferior part of the parietal lobe; the *posterior temporal,* supplying the posterior two thirds of the outer surface of the temporal lobe, and the

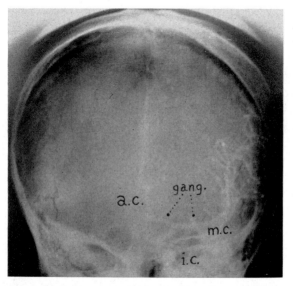

FIG. 10.—Internal carotid artery and its major branches as seen in anteroposterior view of the carotid arteriogram. *Gang.,* ganglionic arteries.

occipitoparietal (angular or "terminal"), distributed to the supramarginal and angular gyri.

Anterior choroidal artery

This artery arises from the carotid artery medial to the optic tract, which it nourishes, then enters the descending or temporal horn of the lateral ventricle to end in the glomus of the choroid plexus. En route, the anterior choroidal is the main arterial supply of the ventral posterior limb of the internal capsule. Branches are also given to the optic and auditory radiations, the globus pallidus, the lateral aspect of the lateral geniculate body, the lateral and pulvinar nuclei of the thalamus and the middle third of the cerebral peduncle and midbrain (Figs. 7 and 8).

Posterior communicating artery

Derived from the internal carotid, this connection between the anterior (carotid) and posterior (vertebral-basilar) portions of the circle of Willis is a principal means of carrying blood to the cerebral hemisphere when the carotid is obstructed. In a vertebral arteriogram the middle cerebral artery may often be visualized if the homolateral carotid artery is occluded at the time of injection. Passage of blood from the carotid to the posterior cerebral artery through the posterior communicating artery is more physiologic, however. Rapid serial x-ray photography during carotid angiography reveals constant filling of the posterior cerebral at some time during the series.

From the posterior communicating artery come *posteromedial ganglionic* twigs to the anterior and posterior hypothalamus and to the midline, medial and pulvinar thalamic nuclei (Fig. 8). A particularly prominent, *thalamoperforating* arterial branch eventually attains the subthalamic body of Luys. The posterior communicating artery is reduced in size with advancing age.

VERTEBRAL-BASILAR SYSTEM

Vertebral artery

The two vertebral arteries arise as first branches of the respective subclavian arteries from the upper and posterior aspect of these vessels, just medial to the anterior scalene muscle. The *first* part of the cervical vertebral artery ascends up and back to the transverse process of the sixth cervical vertebra, which it enters through a special foramen. The *second* part runs higher toward the base of the skull, directed superiorly in a bony tunnel through contiguous transverse processes of the upper six cervical vertebrae. This vertebral passage gives the artery its name. Insertion of a needle into the vessel to perform vertebral arteriography is usually made between the processes of the fifth and sixth cervical vertebrae (Fig. 4).

The *third* or *suboccipital* part of the extracranial vertebral artery runs through the suboccipital triangle from the foramen of the atlas to the foramen magnum and is covered by muscles and accompanied by cervical nerves. This part of the artery forms a complete loop which permits extreme forward flexion and rotation of the head on the neck without avulsion of the vessel or its branches. Where the artery changes from its true vertebral to an intracranial course it is often seen in suboccipital craniectomy (Fig. 11).

Passing through the inlet of the skull and piercing the dura, both vertebral arteries run upward and medially, underneath the medulla oblongata. They join at an angle of about 50 degrees at the junction of

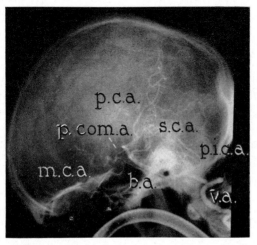

FIG. 11.—Intracranial arteries of the vertebral circulation, seen in lateral view of the vertebral arteriogram. Compare with Figure 5. (Courtesy of O. Sugar.)

the pons and bulb to form the basilar artery. The left terminal vertebral artery is larger than the right in one half of specimens.

Basilar artery

This large, thick-walled, essential vessel inclines upward beneath the pons, lying in a midline furrow, the basilar sulcus. In a lateral vertebral angiogram (Fig. 11), the artery is seen to run almost parallel and internal to the clivus blumenbachii (posterior sphenoid bone) and ends just posterior to and on a plane with the posterior clinoid processes.

From the vertebral and basilar arteries comes the blood supply of the posterior cerebrum, midbrain, pons, medulla and cerebellum, as well as a few small posterior meningeal twigs (Fig. 5).

Posterior cerebral artery

The two posterior cerebral arteries are the largest and longest divisions of the posterior vertebral-basilar circulation. They take origin from the basilar artery as two primary branches of the trunk of a tree, so that the three vessels form the letter T. Rarely, reflecting their embryologic origin as a part of the carotid system, one or both arteries may arise from the internal carotid. Despite the common parenthood of the posterior cerebral arteries, stream of flow principles hold in the posterior as well as in the anterior part of the circle of Willis, and radiopaque material injected in one vertebral artery ordinarily fills only its own arterial derivatives, including the homolateral posterior cerebral artery.

Shortly after its origin below the tentorium, in the posterior fossa, each posterior cerebral artery ascends in curvilinear fashion around the respective half of the mesencephalon. Seen together in an anteroposterior vertebral arteriogram, the two arteries form the inverted Greek letter Ω. Each artery then hooks around the edge of the tentorium, passing through a dural notch, and ascends at an angle of 45 degrees (brain upright) toward the occipital pole, running on the medial surface of temporal and occipital lobes to end in the calcarine fissure (Fig. 5). Where the artery winds around the cerebral peduncle, it lies in the subarachnoid cisterna ambiens. As it passes through the tentorial notch it is particularly susceptible to compression during herniation of the temporal lobe.

GANGLIONIC BRANCHES (Figs. 7 and 8).—*Posteromedial* ganglionic arterioles from the first part of the posterior cerebral artery run in two directions: forward to supply the posterior lobe of the pituitary gland, the posterior hypothalamus, the midline and medial nuclei of the thalamus and the optic tract, and medially to end in the central gray, collicular bodies and cerebral peduncles of the midbrain. One well marked member of this group is the *posterior choroidal* artery which ends in the choroid plexus of the third ventricle and supplies the anterior thalamic nucleus and the medial part of the lateral geniculate body.

Posterolateral ganglionic branches are the next set of perforating derivatives. They are distributed to the posterior thalamus, subthalamus and posterior extremity of the internal capsule. The *thalamogeniculate* artery, supplying the pulvinar, geniculate bodies and capsule is particularly well known, since thrombosis of this vessel results in the hyperpathic thalamic syndrome of Déjerine-Roussy.

CORTICAL BRANCHES.—Cortical arterial branches of the posterior cerebral include the *anterior temporal,* to the anterior one half of the inferior surface of the temporal lobe; the *posterior temporal,* to the posterior inferior temporal and inferior occipital lobes; the *parieto-occipital,* to the cuneus and quadratus of the occipital lobe, and the *calcarine,* to the lips of the calcarine fissure, the primary visual cortex. These vessels curve over the mesial edge of the hemisphere, as do the highest branches of the

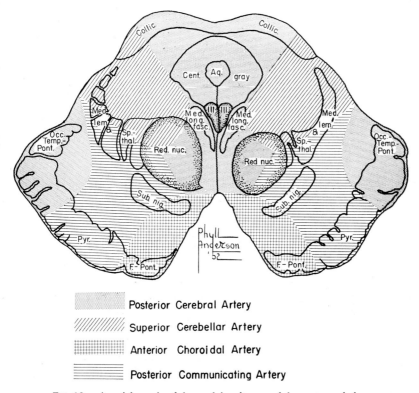

Posterior Cerebral Artery

Superior Cerebellar Artery

Anterior Choroidal Artery

Posterior Communicating Artery

FIG. 12.—Arterial supply of the nuclei and tracts of the mesencephalon.

anterior cerebral, to nourish a strip of cortex forming the local superior border of the middle cerebral arterial distribution. The corpus callosum is irrigated by serial derivatives of the cortical branches.

In at least 5–10 per cent of brains the calcarine visual cortex has a dual blood supply from the posterior and middle cerebral arteries. This is one possible explanation for macular-sparing hemianopsia, characteristic of lesions of the occipital lobe.

Superior cerebellar artery

Next below the posterior cerebral arteries, the right and left superior cerebellar arteries are well developed components of the posterior circulation, coming directly off the basilar artery. Each vessel is separated from the adjacent posterior cerebral artery by the edge of the tentorium and the oculomotor and trochlear cranial nerves.

The superior cerebellar divides on the surface of the pons into *medial* and *lateral* branches, just in front of the trigeminal nerve (Figs. 5 and 11). The medial division supplies the mesencephalon, the contiguous pons, the medial surface of the cerebellum and the deep cerebellar nuclei, of which it is the chief arterial supply (Fig. 12). Lateral branches go to the lateral part of the superior cerebellar cortex.

Pontile arteries

Two sets of these, the *median* pontile and the *lateral* pontile arteries spring from the basilar trunk below the superior cerebellar arteries (Figs. 5 and 13). A vascular ring is formed around the pons, and penetrating vessels supply the tracts and nuclei of the upper brain stem. There are no anastomoses across the midline.

Middle cerebellar artery (Foix)

This vessel, fairly constant in presence, runs laterally from the basilar artery to the pons and to the medial hemisphere and vermis of the cerebellum, winding around the fifth (trigeminal) cranial nerve (Fig. 5).

Internal auditory artery

Lying next inferiorly on the surface of the pons, the internal auditory artery (Fig. 5) really takes origin from a still lower parent vessel, the anterior inferior cerebellar artery, in 83 per cent of cases and from the basilar proper in only 17 per cent (Sunderland). It is in intimate apposition to the facial and acoustic nerves, which it supplies as it does the internal ear. Hemorrhage from the internal or middle ear in chronic mastoiditis may be due to rupture of the internal auditory artery.

Anterior inferior cerebellar artery

The anterior inferior cerebellar artery, also called the "artery of the lateral fissure" (Foix), arises from the basilar trunk just above the junc-

tion of the vertebral arteries. It runs along the pontomedullary border, at
the upper end of the bulb, and supplies the brain stem, the superior
(brachium conjunctivum) and middle (brachium pontis) cerebellar

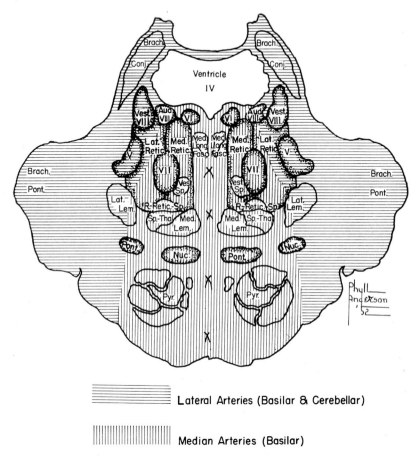

Lateral Arteries (Basilar & Cerebellar)

Median Arteries (Basilar)

FIG. 13.—Arterial supply of the nuclei and tracts of the pons.

peduncles and the anterior portion of the undersurface of the cerebellar
vermis and hemisphere (Figs. 5 and 14). It often gives rise to the internal auditory artery. Foix considers occlusion of this vessel to be the most
common cause of the Wallenberg syndrome, usually attributed to posterior inferior cerebellar thrombosis. Inconsistencies in number and size of
cerebellar arteries may account for seeming clinicoanatomic discrepancies.

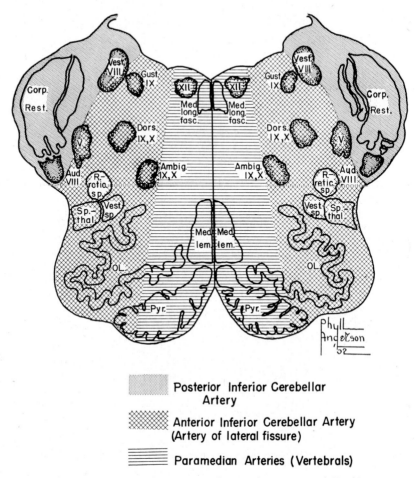

	Posterior Inferior Cerebellar Artery
	Anterior Inferior Cerebellar Artery (Artery of lateral fissure)
	Paramedian Arteries (Vertebrals)

FIG. 14.—Arterial supply of the nuclei and tracts of the upper medulla oblongata.

Posterior inferior cerebellar artery

The posterior inferior cerebellar artery springs from the vertebral artery immediately after the vertebral enters the skull. It runs back and down along the lateral medulla, loops on the cerebellar tonsils and then returns vertically forward, spreading over the inferior aspect of the posterior cerebellum (Figs. 5 and 44). It sends a large branch to the choroid plexus of the fourth ventricle. The artery lies entirely above the foramen magnum unless increased intracranial pressure forces the cerebellar tonsils down into the spinal canal. The posterior inferior cerebellar artery

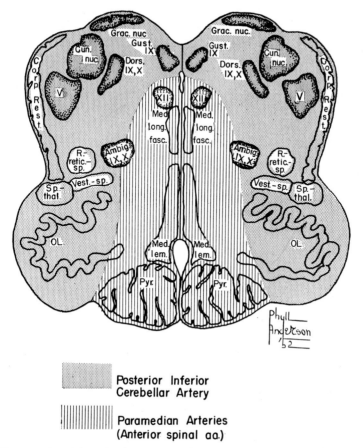

Posterior Inferior
Cerebellar Artery

Paramedian Arteries
(Anterior spinal aa.)

FIG. 15.—Arterial supply of the nuclei and tracts of the lower medulla oblongata.

supplies the lateral medulla, inferior (restiform body) cerebellar peduncle
and cerebellum (Fig. 15).

Paramedian arteries (Foix)

Derived from the vertebral and anterior spinal arteries, the paramedian arteries of the bulb penetrate and irrigate the nuclei and tracts of the
medulla oblongata (Fig. 15). They are tiny and very numerous.

Spinal arteries

The *anterior* spinal artery is formed by the junction of two derivatives
of the terminal portions of the vertebral arteries just above the foramen

magnum. The main artery so constituted descends in the midline on the anterior aspect of the medulla oblongata and continues inferiorly in the anterior median sulcus to supply the upper spinal cord.

Another small vessel arises from the lateral aspect of each vertebral artery and courses posteriorly along the side of the medulla oblongata to join its mate from the other side and form the *posterior* spinal artery. This artery continues downward as a common vessel in the posterior median sulcus of the cervical spinal cord.

ARTERIES OF THE INTRACRANIAL DURA MATER

The chief blood supply of the cerebral dural membrane comes from the *middle meningeal artery,* which arises from the internal maxillary artery, enters the skull through the foramen spinosum of the sphenoid bone and is distributed to the dura over the convexity of the cerebral hemisphere. The bony groove in which this vessel runs is clearly visible in a lateral roentgenogram of the skull.

The *accessory* meningeal artery is sometimes derived from the middle meningeal artery and courses upward through the foramen ovale to reach the gasserian ganglion and the dura of the middle fossa. The *anterior* meningeal artery, supplying the dura of the anterior fossa is a direct branch of the internal carotid artery or is a derivative of the ethmoidal arteries. The *posterior* meningeal artery, a branch of the occipital artery, runs through the jugular foramen to the dura of the posterior fossa.

The arteries of the dura are of clinical importance as a source of head pain in migraine and of extradural hemorrhage after head injury.

CHOROID PLEXUSES

The glomerular vascular tissue present in the roof of the midline ventricular system is the *tela choroidea* of the third and fourth ventricles. The tela choroidea represents a central invagination of the interior of the brain by the pial vessels covering the medial aspects of the cerebral and cerebellar hemispheres. The *anterior choroidal artery* derived from the internal carotid artery supplies the glomus of the choroid plexus of the ipsilateral lateral ventricle. The *posterior* choroidal artery arises from the posterior cerebral artery and terminates with its mate in the choroid plexus of the third ventricle.

The combined surface area of the tela choroidea and the choroid plexuses is over 1 sq. m. Through this vascular tissue fluid diffuses into the ventricular system.

ARTERIAL ANOMALIES

Many anatomic irregularities may involve the cerebral circulation. In the cervical region, one and even both carotids have been reported to be absent; the other carotid or the basilar artery makes up the deficiency. Variations in the size of external-internal carotid anastomoses (Fig. 4) are common. Inequality in size of the two vertebral arteries is almost the rule, the left usually being the larger. Their first intracranial branches, the posterior inferior cerebellars, are often anomalous. These arteries can fill the cisterna magna with redundant coils, making cisternal puncture dangerous.

Variations are numerous in the circle of Willis, a "normal" configuration being found in only 50 per cent of cases. However, most circles examined possess all their component arteries, abnormalities consisting principally in differences in size of individual vessels. The posterior communicating artery is the most variable artery in the circle and is sometimes absent, more often threadlike. When it is insufficient, however, the primitive carotid-basilar anastomosis may serve to carry blood across the gap. The posterior cerebral artery was found by Sunderland to come from one of the internal carotids in 26 of 100 cases and from both sides in six.

ANASTOMOSES AND COLLATERAL CIRCULATION

EXTRINSIC ANASTOMOSES.—The circle or polygon of Willis is the most important source of collateral arterial supply to the brain through the anterior and posterior communicating arteries, permitting occlusion of one or even both carotids without consequent cerebral infarction. The anterior anastomosis is more reliable than the posterior cross-connection. Since pressures are normally equalized in the circle, it is only when one pressure source is eliminated that anastomotic properties become evident. Carotid angiography visualizes only the ipsilateral anterior and middle cerebral arteries until the opposite carotid is compressed, when both sides of the brain fill from a unilateral injection. Naturally, such collateral flow is necessary only when one artery is closed by ligature or disease.

Anastomoses between *external* and *internal* carotid arteries are shown in Figure 4. There are many of these, most of them minute. The four most important are connections between the superficial temporal and supraorbital frontal branches of the ophthalmic, the angular branch of the external maxillary to the frontal ophthalmic, the middle meningeal to the lacrimal branch of the ophthalmic, and the anterior deep temporal

to the lacrimal. These anastomotic channels probably help little to maintain cerebral blood flow in the face of acute obstruction, but with slow
occlusion of the carotid sinus or internal carotid, arteriography has been
successful in visualizing the circulation of the brain by injection of the
external carotid only. Walsh and King have demonstrated collateral flow
in the cadaver by tying off the internal carotid in the neck and skull, after
which colored fluid injected in the external carotid of one side flowed
forth from the cut ends of both ophthalmic arteries.

Cross-channels between the external carotids are abundant and large;
they consist of the midline junction of the right and left superior thyroids,
linguals, external maxillaries and temporal arteries. When the common
carotid is obstructed, blood flow is therefore continued from the opposite
external vessel into the internal carotid above the point of thrombosis
or ligation.

INTRINSIC ANASTOMOSES.—Although Cobb has stated that a single
erythrocyte could wander the entire length of the brain, from olfactory
bulb to occipital pole, the practical question is whether or not intrinsic
anastomoses are of significance. The most reasonable answer is that in the
strict anatomic sense there are few cerebral end-arteries, but from the
functional point of view there are a great many. A well known and
undeniable example of an anatomically terminal artery in the brain is
that supplying Sommer's sector of the hippocampus.

Experimental investigations.—Beevor saw passage of injection fluid
from one of the three major cerebral arteries (anterior, middle and posterior) into the territory of another where their superficial cortical twigs
intermingled. Fay, after clamping off all but one artery, was able to inject
mercury into the entire brain of a cadaver through this single vessel.
Vander Eecken and co-workers found numerous surface anastomoses in
the pia, between and among the anterior cerebral, middle cerebral and
posterior cerebral arterioles of the same side and traversing trunks which
bridge the interhemispheral fissure to link the anterior cerebrals even
beyond the anterior communicating artery. Similar cross-connections exist
between and among cortical branches of the cerebellar arteries and even
across the vermis to connect the superior and inferior cerebellar distribu-
tions. These investigators found no cerebral-cerebellar arterial ties and no
arteriovenous shunts. From histologic researches, Alexander and Putnam
classified all cerebral vessels into seven descending orders, anastomoses
characterizing the second (major artery) and fifth (precapillary) stages.

No such collaterality has been discovered among the penetrating
branches of the major cerebral arteries. This confirms the older observa-

tions of Cohnheim that the ganglionic derivatives of the circle of Willis and adjacent extensions are truly terminal arteries, neither supplying nor receiving anastomoses from origin to termination. The independent nature of these same perforating arteries has been confirmed by Young and Karnosh. Despite numerous superficial connections, therefore, the brain arterial tree is most lacking in anastomoses where they are most needed— in the numerous but not necessarily overlapping areas fed by the ganglionic derivatives of the circle of Willis, the critical field of the internal capsule, basal ganglions and thalamus.

MICROSCOPIC ANATOMY

Pial arteries give off branches which penetrate the brain cortex perpendicularly and are of two types. *Long* medullary vessels traverse the gray mantle, supplying the inner three cortical layers, and run into the white matter to a depth of 3–4 cm., intercommunicating one with another only at the precapillary stage. *Short* vessels are confined to the outer three layers of the isocortex, and they form with the long arterioles a compact network in the middle zone of the gray substance. Outer and inner laminae of the cortex are thus sparingly supplied with blood. The appearance of a penetrating artery has been compared to an elm tree, with long branches leaving the trunk at narrow, graceful angles.

Exposed surface arteries are seen to throb only where they turn. Not only is the angle of bifurcation of major vessels from the circle of Willis severe, but arterioles also leave their parent supply at 90 degrees from the perforating branch. Moreover, there is an annular constriction at the point of arteriolar departure, with slight dilatation just beyond (Fig. 16). All of this means that a rapidly moving volume of blood is forced through a highly resistant system of arteries under high pressure. Splitting of the elastica at arterial angulations is considered to predispose to arteriosclerosis in these loci.

ARTERIAL TISSUE LAYERS.—Apparently as an induced response to a high stress-load, cerebral arteries are characterized by a well developed *internal elastic membrane,* which Wolff believes succeeds in damping the pressure effectively until pathologic changes occur. Increase in elastica and transition to a thick internal membrane begin just as soon as extracranial vessels become intracranial, as in the passage of the vertebral into the basilar artery.

Muscular tissue in the *media* is decreased, however, when extracranial-intracranial transition occurs, a principal microscopic feature distinguishing cerebral arteries from those elsewhere in the body. Baker notes that, in examining arteries of the brain, what would be considered to be fibrosis in other vessels may be normal here.

The *adventitia* of the intracranial arteries is quite deficient, a structural defect which permits easy expansion of aneurysms and may account, in part, for the high incidence of cerebral arterial hemorrhage compared with that of spontaneous hemorrhage into other viscera.

CAPILLARIES.—The capillary bed in gray matter (1,000 mm./cu. mm. of tissue) is about three times as dense as it is in white matter (300 mm./cu. mm.) (Cobb and Talbott). Laminae II to V are particularly vascular in the cerebral cortex. The richness of the small vessel net in any part of the brain parallels the local concentration of nerve cells. There is

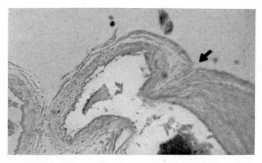

FIG. 16.—Annular constriction (arrow) at origin of ganglionic arteriole. (Courtesy of A. Kristenson.)

also a positive correlation between oxidase content and capillary count (Campbell). The paraventricular nucleus of the hypothalamus is the most highly vascularized area in the brain. Cerebellar cortex is well supplied by vessel loops between adjacent folia. The capillary bed of no organ is ever entirely open, and thus in the brain as in other viscera there exists a considerable potential reservoir.

PERIVASCULAR TISSUES.—Surrounding the small vessels is a *pia-glial membrane,* composed of inward prolongations of fibrous tissue from the arachnoid and footlike terminations of astrocytes and oligodendroglia. This membrane forms the adventitia of arterioles, capillaries and venules and within its loose layers is found the *Virchow-Robin space,* more potential than real and best seen when distended. Tissue fluid from the brain washes upward to the subarachnoid pathways through the perivascular spaces. On the parenchymal side, the pia-glial membrane acts as 'a blood-brain barrier, permitting the ingress of some substances into cerebral tissues and preventing the transmission of others.

BIBLIOGRAPHY

Alexander, L., and Putnam, T. J.: Pathologic alterations of cerebral vascular patterns, A. Res. Nerv. & Ment. Dis., Proc. 18:471-543, 1938.

Baker, A. B.: Structure of the small cerebral arteries and their changes with age, Am. J. Path. 13:453-461, 1937.

Beevor, C. E.: The cerebral arterial supply, Brain 30:403-425, 1907.

Campbell, A. C. P.: Variation in vascularity and oxidase content in different regions of the brain of the cat, Arch. Neurol. & Psychiat. 41:223-242, 1939.

Cobb, S.: The cerebral circulation: The question of "end arteries" of the brain and the mechanism of infarction, Arch. Neurol. & Psychiat. 25:273-280, 1931.

Cobb, S., and Talbott, G. H.: Studies in cerebral circulation: II. Quantitative study of cerebral capillaries, Tr. A. Am. Physicians 42:255, 1923.

Fay, T.: The cerebral vasculature: Preliminary report of study by means of roentgen ray, J.A.M.A. 84:1727, 1925.

Foix, Ch.; Hillemand, P., and Schalit, I.: Sur le syndrome latéral du bulbe et l'irrigation du bulbe superieur, Rev. neurol. 1:160-179, 1925.

Ford, F. R.: *Diseases of the Nervous System in Infancy, Childhood, and Adolescence* (Springfield, Ill.: Charles C Thomas, Publisher, 1937).

Kristenson, A.: The question of pathogenesis of cerebral insultus, Acta med. scandinav. (supp. 196) 128:200-211, 1947.

Mettler, F. A.: *Neuroanatomy* (St. Louis: C. V. Mosby Company, 1948).

Moniz, E.: *L'Angiographie Cérébrale* (Paris: Masson & Cie, 1934).

Rogers, L.: The function of the circulus arteriosus of Willis, Brain 70:171-178, 1947.

Sunderland, S.: The arterial relations of the internal auditory meatus, Brain 68:23-27, 1945.

Sunderland, S.: Neurovascular relations and anomalies at the base of the brain, J. Neurol., Neurosurg. & Psychiat. 11:243-257, 1948.

Vander Eecken, H. M.; Fisher, M., and Adams, R. D.: The arterial anastomoses of the human brain and their importance in the delimitation of human brain infarction, J. Neuropath. & Exper. Neurol. 11:91-94, 1952.

Walsh, F. B., and King, A. B.: Ocular signs of intracranial saccular aneurysms, Arch. Ophth. 27:1-33, 1942.

Wolff, H. J.: The cerebral blood vessels: Anatomical principles, A. Res. Nerv. & Ment. Dis., Proc. 18:29-63, 1938.

Young, A. F., and Karnosh, L. J.: The anterior perforating arterioles and their relation to the internal capsule, Dis. Nerv. System 10:99-103, 1949.

CHAPTER 3

The Veins and
Dural Venous Sinuses

VEINS OF THE BRAIN

THE COLLECTION OF blood from the brain for return to the heart is accomplished by two primary sets of veins, external and internal, which drain into the dural sinuses, thence into the internal jugular veins and eventually into the innominate veins and superior vena cava (Fig. 17). A secondary accessory route via emissary channels to the external jugular veins and vertebral venous plexus is relatively little used normally but can be very important after ligation of the internal jugulars or occlusion of the superior vena cava (Fig. 20).

Having attained the capillary stage only by being forced through angulated arteries under high pressure, the postcapillary cerebral blood flow descends through various stages almost without obstruction, there being no valves on the venous side. Among other factors, tortuosity of the collecting sinuses prevents an absolutely precipitate drop of blood in the upright position. Wolff compares venous return from the cranial cavity to fluid flowing from a flask with a gradually tapering neck.

EXTERNAL CEREBRAL VEINS

Following the anatomic rule, veins of the brain are more numerous than arteries, two or more accompanying each major arterial channel. On the surface, associated venous groups resemble cascades or sea anemones in pattern. The superficial or external cerebral group is divided into superior, middle, inferior and occipital veins and drains the outer portion of the cerebral hemispheres (Fig. 17).

Superior cerebral veins

The superior vessels carry blood from the dorsal, dorsolateral and medial two thirds of each half of the cerebrum. Eight to 12 on each side join to form three or four large trunks, which enter the dura near the

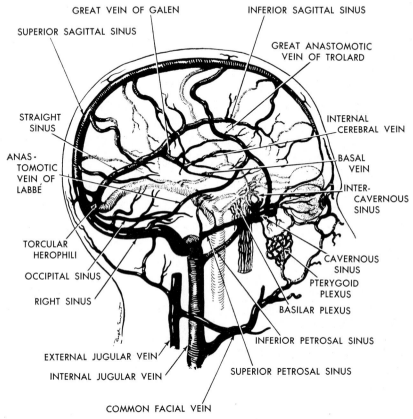

FIG. 17.—The major veins of the brain and the dural venous sinuses. (Courtesy of H. A. Shenkin and S. S. Kety.)

midline of the vertex and empty into the superior sagittal or longitudinal sinus through large venous lacunae which erode the overlying skull. A cuff of arachnoid surrounds these vessels as they lie free in the subdural space. Here and at the base, unprotected and thin-walled channels are easily torn by arrested motion of the brain, as in head injury, and leakage can result in the formation of subdural hematoma. Anterior superior veins point toward the occiput, a result of anteroposterior growth of the cerebrum.

The *great anastomotic vein of Trolard* is the most easily visible member of the superior cerebral group on the exposed surface of the cerebrum or in a late phase of the carotid angiogram (Fig. 18). It runs from a middle (sylvian) cerebral vein upward to the superior sagittal sinus, often marks the central rolandic fissure but as frequently lies in front or behind it, and is a direct connection between the sinuses of the base and

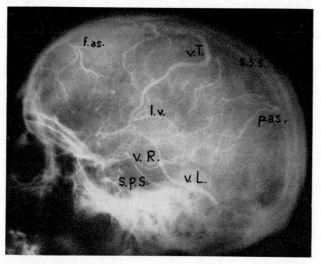

FIG. 18.—The cerebral veins as seen in the venous phase of the carotid angiogram, lateral view. *f.as., p.as.,* frontal, parietal ascending veins; *v.T., v.R., v.L.,* veins of Trolard, Rosenthal, Labbé; *s.s.s., s.p.s.,* superior sagittal and superior petrosal sinuses; *l.v.,* lesser vein of Galen.

vault. So important is the vein of Trolard that ligation or thrombosis of it will produce contralateral hemiplegia due to infarction of the cortical motor area.

Middle cerebral veins

The middle cerebral superficial drainage may be carried by one or several vessels running in the sylvian fissure external to the terminating middle cerebral artery. These veins arise in the center of the hemisphere over the insula, are connected above with the vein of Trolard and below with the lesser anastomotic vein of Labbé and empty inferiorly into the cavernous, sphenoparietal or sigmoid sinuses, particularly the last. Where the veins of Trolard and Labbé and the middle cerebral vessels join, in a tripod, is a point which has been designated by Moniz as the "venous crossroads of the brain." The superficial middle cerebral group must be protected in an operative approach to the optic chiasm and pituitary gland.

Inferior cerebral veins

Inferior external veins include the *lesser anastomotic* vein (Labbé), which courses posteroinferiorly from the lateral cerebrum to the lateral sinus, and the orbital veins which run from the supraorbital cortex to the origin of the superior sagittal sinus just above the crista galli.

Occipital veins

The occipital group comes from the basal occipital lobe. The five or six medial members join the superior petrosal sinus or turn toward the internal cerebral veins instead. The two lateral occipital veins communicate with the horizontal part of the transverse sinus. Lateral thrombosis may result in aphasia and medial occlusion in hemianopsia.

INTERNAL CEREBRAL VEINS

Internal or deep cerebral veins are those of the galenic system (lesser and great veins of Galen), the deep middle cerebral veins and the basal veins of Rosenthal (Figs. 17 and 18).

Galenic venous system

The lesser vein of Galen, or *internal cerebral* vein, arises from three roots and drains the ventricular system and surrounding tissues, the fornix, the corpus callosum and the quadrigeminal plate. The *terminal* vein runs in the hypothalamic sulcus, divides the caudate nucleus and the hypothalamus from the thalamus, acquires the *superior choroidal* and *septal* veins and is the prominent contributor to the lesser vein of Galen. Both lesser galenic veins join below the splenium (posterior end) of the corpus callosum, surrounding the pineal gland as they do so to form the great vein of Galen. Immediately before the junction, each internal cerebral vein receives the ipsilateral basal vein.

The *great vein of Galen,* short and thick, is less than 1 cm. in length and consists largely of a bulbous ampulla. It meets the inferior longitudinal sinus and continues into the straight sinus.

Deep middle cerebral veins

The deep middle cerebral veins lie just outside the lesser galenics and originate in a confluence of tributaries draining the insula and adjacent external basal ganglions. They run in the depths of the sylvian fissure and go outward to their superficial namesakes or turn deep, toward the basal veins.

Basal veins

The rest of the forebrain nuclei and the upper brain stem are served by the basal veins of Rosenthal. These important channels originate at the anterior perforated space, near the anterior ganglionic arteries, by the merger of the veins accompanying the anterior cerebral artery, the deep middle cerebral veins and twigs from the basal ganglions. Each basal vein, right and left, runs backward, curves upward and around the midbrain (cerebral peduncle) with the posterior cerebral artery, receives the inferior choroidal vessel and terminates in the lesser vein of Galen, the great galenic vein or straight sinus. En route it is joined by branches from the medial pallidum, preoptic region, hypothalamus, pituitary gland, subthalamus, midbrain and pons. Where it rounds the mesencephalon, the basal vein is even more subject to compressive injury than the posterior cerebral artery which it accompanies. A common mechanism of death due to increased intracranial pressure is strangulation of the vein of Rosenthal against the edge of the tentorial notch, with consequent edema and hemorrhage in the midbrain or pons.

VENOUS ANASTOMOSES

EXTERNAL COLLATERALS.—Cross-connections among the veins on the surface of the brain are numerous and effective. The number of anastomotic channels increases with advancing age, as plexiform vessels enlarge and transmit more blood (Padget).

INTERNAL ANASTOMOSES.—Intracerebral vessels pass through the white matter and connect the superficial venous channels with the tributaries of the galenic system (Fig. 19). These anastomoses are numerous and overlap widely; for example, the pons, frontal and occipital lobes can be injected through a single surface connection of the vein of Galen.

The principal area in which such collaterals are absent is the zone of the basal ganglions and internal capsule.

The transverse caudate vein is the main intracerebral anastomotic vein, passing from the lateral angle of the lateral ventricle to the venous crossroads of the brain over the island of Reil. It has ties at one end with the terminal vein and at the other with channels draining superiorly to

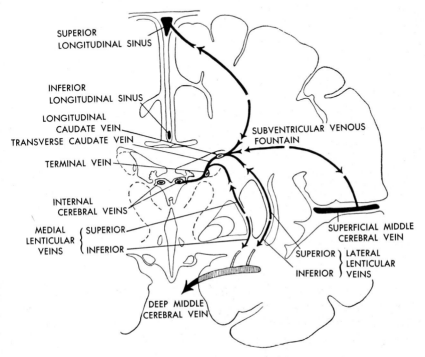

FIG. 19.—The transcerebral venous anastomotic connections. (Courtesy of B. Schlesinger.)

the sagittal sinus. Other vessels traversing the hemisphere in cross-sectional fashion are the septal and anterior terminal veins. They also connect superficial and deep circulations, shunting blood from the superior sagittal and petrosal sinuses to the straight sinus, or vice versa, as necessary.

Schlesinger was unable to reproduce the hydrocephalus reported by Dandy to occur after occlusion of the great vein of Galen and attributed this failure to the presence of venous anastomoses just described. He did note hemorrhages in the caudate nuclei subsequent to ligation of the great vein of Galen in monkeys, a pathologic finding similar to that in human birth injury.

CEREBELLAR VEINS

The veins of the cerebellum correspond to the arteries but drain larger areas than the arteries supply. They are formed by a merging of a subpial net and the cortical capillary plexus and all are interconnected by anastomoses.

The *superior cerebellar* drainage from the upper vermis empties into the greater or lesser veins of Galen. *Anterior inferior* tributaries join with vessels from the interior of the cerebellum and twigs from the pons to make a well defined trunk, the *petrosal* vein, which connects with the superior petrosal sinus and is frequently injured in explorations of the cerebellopontile angle. The important dentate nucleus of the cerebellum is drained by the petrosal vein. *Middle inferior* veins pass to the torcular Herophili, and vessels from the *posterior inferior* surface of the cerebellar hemisphere make immediate connection with the nearby transverse sinus.

A short, stout vein which often enters the transverse sinus near its midline origin has been named by the Gibbs the *tentorial sinus.* This venous trunk, when present, is a confluence of three vessels coming from the superior cerebellar hemisphere, the inferior cerebellar hemisphere and the vermis.

VEINS OF THE BRAIN STEM

The central and lateral veins of the *mesencephalon* drain into the basal vein of Rosenthal. The vein of the trigeminal ganglion, which goes to the superior petrosal or cavernous sinus, may be lacerated in the temporal operation for trigeminal neuralgia.

The *pons* also has central and lateral veins; the former fuse to create a prominent channel accompanying the basilar artery, which longitudinal vein joins that of Rosenthal. Lateral pontile veins run to the cerebellar veins.

The venous drainage of the *medulla oblongata* is effected by vessels less numerous and larger than bulbar arteries. All pass either to neighboring cerebellar veins or directly into the transverse sinus of the side.

DURAL VENOUS SINUSES

Veins from all parts of the brain empty into nearby sinuses which are situated between the two layers of the dura mater. The dural venous sinuses are large vessels with rigid, fibrous walls applied intimately to the skull, which supports each sinus externally. The sinuses have great width compared with the relatively small size of the veins emptying into them. The current in many veins enters these larger channels against the stream of flow. The course of the basal sinuses as they wind toward the jugular foramens is tortuous. There is marked narrowing at the points of exit of most blood from the brain, the jugular bulbs. All these anatomic peculiarities tend to compensate for the lack of restraining valves in the sinuses, and the return flow of blood is thus retarded so that the brain is spared the full brunt of sudden and extreme changes in relative vascular pressures.

Most of the sinuses are interconnected, and the blood from all normally drains into the internal jugular veins except for a moderate fraction reaching other routes via emissary connections.

Superior sagittal (longitudinal) sinus

This large channel occupies the line of attachment of the cerebral falx to the dura of the vault and is therefore triangular in cross-section. The superior sagittal sinus runs from the crista galli, just above the nose, back of the internal occipital protuberance, exactly in the midline of the internal aspect of the skull, becoming larger as it passes backward (Fig. 17). It is virtually bloodless from its origin at the foramen cecum half way up to the coronal suture, a fact which facilitates removal of frontal tumors. Farther back the sinus can represent a formidable surgical problem.

Several large venous lakes extend outward from the sinus into the adjacent dura, and it is into these that most of the superficial lateral cerebral veins open. The lacunae may push outward for some distance, especially just anterior to the rolandic fissure, and this must be remembered in incising the superior cerebral dura near the midline. They enlarge during life, are often clearly visible in x-ray films of the skull and should not be confused with pathologic erosions. Pacchionian granulations or bodies project into the lakes or side pockets of the sinus from below. Fibrosis is natural around these arachnoid granulations with increasing age and does not constitute "adhesions." The arachnoid villi (granulations) are mesothelial derivatives of the leptomeninges and serve as a pathway for diffusion of cerebrospinal fluid into the superior sagittal and transverse sinuses.

The interior of the superior sagittal sinus is rough in appearance, although it is lined with endothelium as are all the sinuses. It is crisscrossed internally with fibrous bands (the chordae willisii) which impede blood flow to some extent. The orifices of entering superior cerebral veins point forward for the most part and are concealed by fibrous folds.

The superior sagittal sinus receives the superior cerebral veins, the most important being the vein of Trolard; veins from the diploë and dura mater, and vessels from the scalp, pericranium and nose which come in through tiny foramens in the skull and are potential routes for extracranial infection to invade the brain. Injection of the anterior part of the superior sinus with Diodrast in health visualizes only the large channel itself and the lower connections with the torcular and transverse sinus; however, if there is occlusion beyond the site of injection, entering veins and their collaterals may be demonstrated (Fig. 100).

At the posterior termination of the superior sagittal sinus is the dilated junction or confluence of the sinuses called the torcular Herophili ("winepress of Herophilus"). This is an ampullary formation producing a concavity on the inner aspect of the occipital protuberance. Blood from here is conveyed to the jugular veins by the transverse sinuses. There is a slight predominance of flow to the right, but the Gibbs in examining 24 autopsy specimens estimated that 95 per cent of the blood draining into the right transverse sinus and 84 per cent of that in the left transverse sinus comes from the superior sagittal sinus.

Inferior sagittal sinus

This rather insignificant channel runs backward in the posterior one half of the inferior, free margin of the falx. It is directly continuous with the straight sinus and acquires a few medial veins from the cerebrum and corpus callosum in passage (Fig. 17). It is often the first sinus to fill and the first to empty in the venous angiogram and, if seen to be displaced upward, may reveal pressure on one side of the falx.

Straight sinus

The straight sinus, a directly posterior continuation of the inferior sagittal sinus, is joined by the great vein of Galen, runs in the line of junction of the cerebral falx and tentorium and is triangular when cut across (Fig. 17). In a lateral angiogram the straight sinus may be seen to be elevated with tumor of the posterior fossa. It ends where the transverse sinuses arise from the torcular and is said to flow principally into that transverse vessel which does not receive the superior sagittal sinus. Since the latter sends blood laterally to right and left in about equal amounts, the same is probably true of the sinus rectus.

The straight sinus has five roots: the two internal cerebral veins (lesser galenic veins) which form the great vein of Galen, the two basal veins of Rosenthal and the inferior sagittal sinus. Thus, it drains the interior of the cerebrum. Tentorial tears in birth injury may cause hemorrhage from the galenic system or sinus rectus and produce lethal clots in the posterior fossa or chronic damage to the basal ganglions (choreoathetosis).

Occipital sinus

The occipital sinus, the smallest of the intracranial sinuses, is situated in the attached margin of the falx cerebelli and drains upward from a ring of vessels around the foramen magnum into the torcular confluence, acquiring veins from the falx and medial cerebellum en route (Fig. 17). It communicates with the vertebral plexus beneath the skull. The occipital sinus is often absent, may be single, double, laterally placed or so wide (2–3 cm.) as to almost preclude surgical exposure of the cerebellar vermis. It is ligated routinely in bilateral surgical exploration of the posterior fossa.

Sphenoparietal sinus

The smallest of the anteroinferior group of paired basal sinuses is the sphenoparietal sinus which runs along the lesser wing of the sphenoid bone to end in the cavernous sinus. It receives vessels running downward from the superficial middle cerebral plexus and upward from the temporal tip. Since motion of the temporal lobe invariably occurs with severe head injury, tearing of vessels at this otherwise unimportant venosinal connection can result in subdural hematoma in the middle (temporal) fossa.

Cavernous sinus

The cavernous sinuses are so named because they are bridged internally by many interlacing fibrous filaments. The largest and most important of the anteroinferior, paired basal group, they hug the sides of the body of the sphenoid bone in special shallow fossae and drain the eye as well as the undersurface of the cerebrum and upper brain stem (Fig. 17). The internal carotid artery turns upward toward the circle of Willis through this sinus (carotid siphon).

Lateral to the artery and just inside the external wall of the sinus run the nerves of ocular motion and sensation of the head above the lower jaw. Listed from above downward, these nerves are the oculomotor, trochlear, ophthalmic division of trigeminal, abducens and maxillary trigeminal. The carotid sympathetic plexus surrounds the artery in passage. Immediately posteriorly, the sinus is in direct relation to the trigeminal (gasserian) ganglion, from which it receives a prominent vein. Medially, the pituitary gland is situated in the sphenoid fossa of the sella turcica.

Into each cavernous sinus pour the ophthalmic veins from the globe of the eye and other contents of the orbit, the sphenoparietal sinus, the superior petrosal sinus, vessels from the basilar plexus on the clivus of the sphenoid bone, veins from adjacent tissues of the cerebrum and upper brain stem, particularly the superficial cerebrals, and tiny channels accompanying the carotid artery. The cavernous sinus communicates posterolaterally with the superior petrosal sinus and posteroinferiorly with the internal jugular vein via the inferior petrosal sinus. Extracranial anastomoses are numerous: they occur to the vertebral veins through the basilar plexus, by junction of the ophthalmic and angular veins at the corner of the eye and by passage of emissaries down through the foramens in the middle fossa of the skull to the pterygoid plexus. The cavernous sinus is particularly vulnerable to extension of infection from the eye, nose, face, paranasal sinuses and teeth. The two cavernous sinuses also are connected across the midline by anterior and posterior intercavernous vessels which run in the diaphragma sellae, encircle the pituitary stalk and form the *circular sinus.*

Superior petrosal sinus

The superior petrosal sinus, small and narrow, functions chiefly as a link between the cavernous sinus and the transverse sinus into which it empties (Figs. 17 and 18). This sinus is often absent. It courses downward, backward and laterally, crosses the gasserian ganglion and then lies in the attachment of the tentorium along the crest of the petrous bone. It acquires some inferior occipital veins and some veins from the cerebellum and drains the middle ear.

Inferior petrosal sinus

Where the petrous bone unites with the basiocciput there is a shallow sulcus in which runs the inferior petrosal sinus, another paired basal sinus which joins the cavernous sinus with the internal jugular vein (superior bulb). Into it come vessels from the inner ear, pons, medulla and undersurface of the cerebellum. The inferior petrosal sinus is constantly present (Fig. 17).

Transverse sinus

The transverse (lateral) sinuses are large, well developed and begin at the internal occipital protuberance at the torcular confluence. Each extends laterally and forward, curving slightly, in the external attached margin of the tentorium to the base of the petrous bone. From here downward it occupies the groove on the inner aspect of the mastoid bone and is called the *sigmoid sinus,* familiar to otologists. The transverse sinus ends in, or rather is the beginning of, the internal jugular vein, and together the transverse sinuses conduct the major portion of the cerebral blood flow from the brain toward the heart.

Where the sinus is situated in the posterior attached border of the tentorium, the skull is thickened and this serves as an upper landmark in the performance of suboccipital craniectomy. Grooving of the inner table by the transverse portion of the lateral (suprasigmoid) sinus is often clearly seen in anteroposterior roentgenograms of the head and is an accurate indication of the true size of the vessel. Woodhall in a study of 100 brains post mortem found the right lateral sinus to be the chief mode of drainage in 29, whereas the left was dominant in 13; a significant disproportion existed between the two sides in 24. Cross-circulation was inadequate through the torcular in 10, and one transverse sinus was absent in four.

The main input to each transverse sinus comes from the superior sagittal sinus (external cerebral drainage) and the straight sinus (internal cerebral drainage). In addition, however, a considerable fraction of the blood returning from the lateral exterior surface of the cerebrum passes directly through the inferior cerebral veins into the sigmoid sinus instead of up to the sagittal or medially to the cavernous sinuses. When the superior petrosal sinus is present, it joins the sigmoid at its bend. A large tributary on either side of the torcular Herophili, the tentorial sinus, transmits blood from one half of the cerebellum to each transverse sinus at its origin. Mastoid and condyloid emissary veins communicate between the transverse sinuses and the small vessels of the pericranium.

Basilar plexus

The basilar plexus is a network of sinusoidal veins which lie in the dura covering the clivus of the sphenoid bone. These small venous channels communicate with the two inferior petrosal sinuses and receive blood from the anterior vertebral venous plexus.

JUGULAR VEINS

The internal jugular veins receive over 75 per cent of the blood from the brain and through them the cerebral venous return reaches the innominate veins, the superior vena cava and the right atrium of the heart. Each jugular vein begins in the floor of the skull in the posterior compartment of the jugular foramen (Fig. 20), the glossopharyngeal, vagus and accessory nerves passing just in front. The jugular foramen is lateral to and slightly forward from the foramen magnum and lies just behind and somewhat lateral to the entrance of the carotid artery into the petrous bone.

The jugular vein is dilated at its origin; this part, called the superior bulb, receives the inferior petrosal sinus. As the jugular vein runs down the side of the neck it is lateral to and partially overlies the internal and later the common carotid artery. The vagus nerve descends between the artery and vein. At the root of the neck, each internal jugular vein unites with the subclavian to form the innominate vein. In its course it accepts blood from the superficial parts of the face (facial vein) and neck (thyroid veins).

ACCESSORY VENOUS DRAINAGE OF BRAIN

By means of emissary channels, the intracranial venous return may reach one of two accessory routes, the *external jugular* veins or the *vertebral* venous system (Fig. 20). Likewise, extracranial infection may extend within by retrograde thrombophlebitis.

The chief *emissary veins* are nine in number (Fig. 20): (1) parietal, from the superior sagittal sinus to the scalp veins via parietal foramens; (2) diploic, from the superior sagittal sinus to bone marrow, a not inconsiderable mode of drainage; (3) occipital, from the torcular confluence to the occipital plexus; (4) mastoid, from the transverse sinus to the occipital plexus (a prominent landmark for lateral bone removal in suboccipital surgery; this emissary may become formidably large with chronically increased intracranial pressure); (5) condyloid, from the sigmoid sinus through the condyloid canal to the deep veins of the neck; (6) hypoglossal, from the sigmoid sinus to the vertebral veins, passing out the hypoglossal canal; (7) pharyngeal, from the cavernous and petrosal sinuses to the pterygoid plexus via the foramens in the base of the middle fossa of the skull; (8) ophthalmic, from the inferior ophthalmic vein to the pterygoid plexus, and (9) ethmoidal, from the superior sagittal sinus to the nose, passing through the foramen caecum. The first six of these

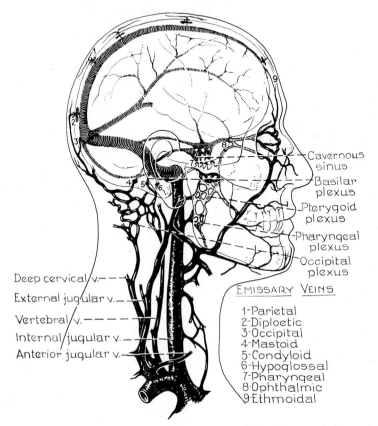

Deep cervical v.
External jugular v.
Vertebral v.
Internal jugular v.
Anterior jugular v.

Cavernous sinus
Basilar plexus
Pterygoid plexus
Pharyngeal plexus
Occipital plexus

EMISSARY VEINS

1-Parietal
2-Diploetic
3-Occipital
4-Mastoid
5-Condyloid
6-Hypoglossal
7-Pharyngeal
8-Ophthalmic
9-Ethmoidal

Fig. 20.—The emissary veins of the head and the extracranial venous drainage of the brain. (Courtesy of J. A. Gius and D. H. Grier.)

drain particularly to the vertebral system, the last three toward the external jugular veins.

Approximately 22 per cent of blood flowing in the external jugular veins under normal circumstances is derived from the brain (Shenkin *et al.*). In some animals, the entire intracranial drainage goes to the external jugular through the jugular foramen spurium. The potentialities of the vertebral venous system for collateral drainage of the brain is even greater, according to Batson, who estimated the cross-sectional area of this plexus to exceed that of the combined internal jugular veins. The vertebral veins extend from skull to coccyx, around the spinal cord and in the vertebrae, and connect with every internal venous channel. In the cadaver, injection of the dorsal vein of the penis will fill the intracranial sinuses.

The function of this posterior route may be increased by chronic lifting and straining with the glottis closed. The vertebral veins are best known for the role they play in the dissemination of malignancy and infection. Particularly since these vessels are valveless, sudden increases in pressure in body cavities can reverse the direction of flow in them. The value of the vertebral system in collateral drainage of the cerebral blood flow is well illustrated by the report of only temporary and mild increase in intracranial pressure after bilateral removal of both internal and external jugular veins (Gius and Grier). Vertebral venous connections are better developed in adults than in children.

MICROSCOPIC ANATOMY

Just as there are more veins than arteries, there are many more venules than arterioles. In distribution, a venule with its tributaries resembles a maple tree, being more stocky and angular than its arteriolar counterpart.

Microscopically, the cerebral and cerebellar veins have very thin walls in relation to their lumens, there is almost no muscle tissue in the media and the elastica is likewise poor. The collagenous nature of these venous channels is even more pronounced in the dural sinuses.

BIBLIOGRAPHY

Batson, O. V.: The function of the vertebral veins and their role in the spread of metastases, Ann. Surg. 112:138-149, 1940.

Gibbs, E. L., and Gibbs, F. A.: The cross-section areas of the vessels that form the torcular and the manner in which flow is distributed to the right and left lateral sinus, Anat. Rec. 59:419-426, 1934.

Gius, J. A., and Grier, D. H.: Venous adaptation following bilateral radical neck dissection with excision of the jugular veins, Surgery 28:305-321, 1950.

Padget, D. H.: Unpublished data.

Schlesinger, B.: The venous drainage of the brain, with special reference to the galenic system, Brain 62:274-291, 1938.

Shenkin, H. A.; Harmel, M. H., and Kety, S. S.: Dynamic anatomy of the cerebral circulation, Arch. Neurol. & Psychiat. 60:240-252, 1948.

Wolff, H. G.: Headache and Other Head Pain (New York: Oxford University Press, 1948).

Woodhall, B.: Variations of the cranial venous sinuses in the region of the torcular Herophilii, Arch. Surg. 33:297-314, 1936.

CHAPTER 4

Nerve Supply of the Intracranial Vessels

TWO TYPES OF nerves are seen on and in the walls of the cerebral vessels, particularly the arteries, in microscopic preparations especially stained by silver impregnation or with methylene blue. Nonmedullated fibers are considered to be largely but not exclusively autonomic in function. After sympathetic ganglionectomy a host of medullated fibers remain and are found in great number freely terminating on and in the adventitia of large arteries at the base of the brain and their proximal branches. McNaughton demonstrated the same type of nerve bundles on and in the walls of the major venous sinuses, the prominent entering veins in the choroid plexuses, in the dura at the base and vertex of the skull and around the meningeal arteries. These medullated fibers are principally peripheral branches of cranial sensory nerves and conduct pain sensation.

VASOSENSORY NERVES

Wolff summarized observations made during the course of craniotomies performed on conscious patients. All intracranial pain-sensitive structures on or above the tentorium cerebelli are innervated by the trigeminal nerve, and stimulation of them causes pain referred to various regions of the head or face anterior to a line drawn from the auditory meatus superiorly to the vertex. Painful sensations from the vessels and dura below the tentorium are referred to the scalp and head posterior to this line and to the neck and are conveyed by the sensory divisions of the glossopharyngeal, vagus and hypoglossal cranial nerves and the upper three cervical spinal nerves.

TRIGEMINAL NERVE.—The trigeminal nerve transmits sensation from most of the arteries of the circle of Willis, and sensory branches to the middle meningeal arteries are abundant. The trigeminal also supplies the superior sagittal, inferior sagittal and anteroinferior group of paired basal sinuses, the superior walls of the transverse and straight sinuses and torcular Herophili and the entering veins to all. Sensory fibers pass to meningeal arteries in the vicinity of each of the three divisions of the trigeminal nerve. The tentorial nerve of Arnold, a recurrent component of the ophthalmic trigeminal, runs through the sheath of the trochlear nerve to the superior leaf of the tentorium and posterior superior sagittal sinus. The nervus spinosus (v. Lushka) is the contribution of the mandibular nerve within the skull. Sensation (pain) from the large vessels within the domain of the trigeminal nerve is referred to external scalp areas corresponding to the trigeminal field involved.

Wolff and Ray found that traction applied to the large arteries at the base of the brain resulted immediately in headache. Pressure on or manipulation of the internal carotid and most major components of the circle of Willis was followed by pain in the region of the eyes, and displacement of the whole arterial system from right to left caused severe, generalized headache, chiefly on the right, extending from eye to neck. No primary sensation other than pain was experienced by the human subject.

LOWER CRANIAL, UPPER CERVICAL NERVES.—Of the glossopharyngeal, vagus, accessory and hypoglossal nerves, stimulation of the glossopharyngeal and vagus has been found to reproduce clinical types of posterior headache most exactly. These nerves conduct sensory impulses from the undersurface of the transverse sinus, the torcular confluence, the upper end of the occipital sinus, the dura in the region of the sigmoid and probably the termination of the basilar artery. Pain is felt behind the homolateral ear when these vessels and the pontile and internal auditory arteries are manipulated at operation.

The upper three cervical roots serve the lower part of the occipital sinus, the vertebral and posterior inferior cerebellar arteries, the posterior meningeal vessels and the dura of the floor of the posterior fossa near the foramen magnum. Stimulation of these structures and of the first cervical root causes pain in the vertex of the head. Pinching of the second and third cervical nerve roots results in pain and aching on the top and back of the head and in the neck. Injection of the second cervical root with hypertonic saline will also produce searing pain over the eye, a not uncommon referral of suboccipital headache.

HEADACHE OF INTRACRANIAL VASCULAR SOURCE.—The effective stimuli causing spontaneous painful sensations from the intracranial vessels are two: dilatation and displacement. Both types of change occur during withdrawal of cerebrospinal fluid by lumbar puncture performed in the sitting position. Arteries and especially veins enlarge as the surrounding cushion of fluid is removed, and the points of branching of large arteries and of the entrance of veins into sinuses are tugged on by the sagging brain. Expansile intracranial mass lesions displace both arteries and veins by the pressure which they exert on them.

Kuntz described a subcranial pathway which may be of importance in pain associated with dilatation of any part of the carotid system. Afferent (sensory) fibers pass down these vessels to the upper thoracic nerve roots in animals, and these may have their counterpart in man. If so, the "spreading" of headache into neck, shoulder and arm is validated anatomically.

VASOMOTOR NERVES

Sympathetic
(Vasoconstrictor) Innervation (Fig. 21)

The anatomic presence of a perivascular nerve supply to the intracranial vessels was first noted by Kolliker in 1863, and Brachet had earlier demonstrated (1830) cerebral congestion in the experimental animal following extirpation of the superior cervical ganglion. Despite repetitions and elaborations of these observations in modern times, the intracranial vasomotor influence of the sympathetic autonomic nerves remains a controversial subject. However, there is much experimental and clinical evidence that the intracranial sympathetic nerves are truly vasoconstrictor in action and help to regulate cerebral blood flow, although the upright head is endowed with a relative paucity of constrictive innervation compared to the dependent limbs.

Sympathetic centers in the brain.—The principal higher centers controlling the sympathetic supply to the cerebral vessels, in common with the entire thoracolumbar autonomic outflow, lie in the posterior hypothalamus and brain stem. Penfield and Stavraky found that electrical stimulation of the diencephalon between the third ventricle and the cerebral peduncle caused pial vasoconstriction. The vasomotor center in the medulla oblongata is equally or more important. It is probable that the prefrontal or infrafrontal cortex and cingulate gyrus exert autonomic influence from still more advanced levels.

Cervicothoracic spinal cord.—Pathways presumably stream downward through the lower brain stem and upper cervical cord to terminate in the intermediolateral cell column of the lowest cervical and upper three thoracic cord segments, from which preganglionic fibers destined for the head emerge in the anterior roots (Foerster). Passing outward in the white rami communicantes, these fibers then run upward

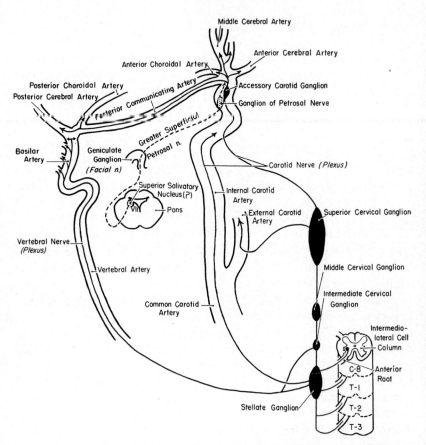

Fig. 21.—Autonomic innervation of cervical carotid, vertebral and intracranial arteries. *Solid,* sympathetic ganglions and nerves; *dotted,* parasympathetic ganglions and nerves. (Modified from McNaughton.)

through the thoracic paravertebral ganglions, directly outward to the stellate ganglion, where they synapse or continue still farther superiorly not ending until the middle and particularly the superior cervical sympathetic ganglions are reached.

Cervical sympathetic chain.—The cell bodies of the sympathetic neurons which supply postganglionic (gray, nonmedullated) nerves to the intracranial circulation lie in the cervical sympathetic chain. The chain is composed of four ganglions on each side: from above downward, the superior cervical, middle cervical, intermediate cervical and inferior cervical. The last named is usually fused with the first or the first and second thoracic sympathetic ganglions to form the stellate ganglion, so-called because of its resemblance to a star with projecting rays or fibers. The two largest cell masses, the superior and stellate ganglions, are also the most important. The cervical sympathetic chain runs from the base of the skull to the thoracic inlet between the transverse processes of the cervical vertebrae (behind) and the carotid arteries (in front).

STELLATE GANGLION.—The stellate ganglion is found just behind the subclavian artery at the site of origin of the vertebral artery. It extends downward to overlie the head of the first rib and in turn is overlain laterally by the dome of the pleura. The relation of the ganglion to the pleura in front requires that care be taken in performing stellate procaine block. The stellate is connected above to the small intermediate cervical ganglion by two branches which encircle the vertebral artery (valve of Vieussens) and by another loop around the subclavian artery. It sends gray rami to the nearby brachial plexus (sixth cervical to first dorsal), the somatic outflow to the arm, and gives off a prominent descending inferior cardiac nerve to the heart.

VERTEBRAL NERVE OR PLEXUS.—Fibers leave the stellate ganglion to pass upward superiorly and slightly laterally along the vertebral artery which they surround as the vertebral nerve or plexus. The vertebral nerve is the sympathetic supply to the intracranial vertebral arteries, the basilar artery and their branches. It runs upward with the cervical vertebral vessel, lying dorsal to it, and sends communications to the common carotid and internal carotid plexuses. There are many so-called anastomoses with the vagi, especially on the right. The vertebral nerve terminates sharply at the upper end of the basilar trunk and does not continue on to the posterior cerebral arteries (Williams). Removal of the inferior cervical or stellate ganglion in animals causes degeneration of most of the nonmedullated fibers on the posterior basal arteries supplied by the vertebral nerve (Christensen and Polley).

INTERMEDIATE AND MIDDLE CERVICAL GANGLIONS.—The intermediate cervical ganglion, next higher, contributes principally to the brachial plexus (fifth to seventh cervical nerves) but may send slender twigs to the vertebral and carotid plexuses. It is in turn connected above with the middle cervical ganglion (fourth to sixth cervical), subserving principally the heart (middle cardiac nerve) and thyroid gland. Fibers destined for the head pass upward through these two ganglions without synapse.

SUPERIOR CERVICAL GANGLION.—The long, fusiform or spindle-shaped superior cervical ganglion, the largest sympathetic cell cluster in the body, is situated at the base of the skull in front of the transverse processes of the second, third and fourth cervical vertebrae, and is intimately bound to the overlying internal carotid artery, the jugular vein being in front and lateral. The superior ganglion sends the usual connection to the cervical nerve roots (first to fourth), gives off the superior cardiac branch and also contributes gray rami to the glossopharyngeal, vagus, phrenic and superior laryngeal nerves.

INTERNAL CAROTID NERVE OR PLEXUS.—A well defined plexus leaves the upper pole of the superior cervical ganglion to course upward on and around the internal carotid artery. First, however, it acquires fibers from the stellate and intermediate ganglions, and the combination of superior ganglionic and stellate fibers is called the internal carotid nerve or plexus. The question of which cell mass sends the most axons into the plexus is undecided; some authorities maintain that the carotid nerve is composed entirely of postganglionic fibers from the superior cervical ganglion, and certainly removal of this structure has produced acute cerebral vasodilatation experimentally. On the other hand, stellate procaine block is capable of reversing human hemiplegia, and bilateral stellectomy has reduced cerebrovascular resistance in some patients.

The anatomic problem is further complicated by the finding of clusters of sympathetic ganglion cells in the adventitia of the intracranial carotid artery. It is of interest in this regard that the "sensitization phenomenon" of Cannon is not seen after removal of the superior cervical ganglion (Forbes and Cobb). Further, McNaughton has not found widespread degeneration of perivascular nonmedullated nerves after superior ganglionectomy, and he believes that cells of the small *intermediate intracranial carotid ganglions* continue to furnish intact axis cylinders.

The distribution of the sympathetic fibers continues peripherally to include vessels of at least 50 μ caliber and possibly farther. None crosses the midline, the vasomotor innervation of the brain remaining strictly ipsilateral.

COMMON CAROTID, EXTERNAL CAROTID PLEXUSES.—The common carotid plexus is formed by superomedial branches of the stellate ganglion. The external carotid plexus is derived entirely from filaments which leave the upper pole of the superior cervical ganglion in two bundles: one passes directly to the external carotid; the other descends inferiorly, then turns sharply upward again around the superior thyroid artery to join the first (Gardner). This plexus is not continuous with or derived from that of the common carotid below, and stripping of the common carotid artery will not denervate the vessels of the face and scalp.

PAIN CONDUCTION.—Conduction of pain-sensation is stated to be a property of the cervical chain by Leriche and Fontaine, who found that disagreeable sensations were experienced in back of the ear and in the lower jaw when the superior cervical ganglion was stimulated and that pain was referred to the arm and precordium when the stellate ganglion was pinched or electrified (operations under local anesthesia).

PARASYMPATHETIC (VASODILATOR) INNERVATION (FIG. 21)

Experimental stimulation of one vagus trunk in the neck results in bilateral cerebral pial vasodilatation (Cobb and Finesinger). When one facial nerve is cut, however, dilatation does not occur on that side. It is apparent that the function of the vagus is simply that of an afferent to the brain stem. Chorobski and Penfield have traced out and studied the pathways involved.

CEREBRAL CENTERS.—The higher control of parasympathetic activity affecting cerebral blood flow lies in the anterior hypothalamus, stimulation of the ventral portion of the tuber cinereum producing visible enlargement of pial vessels (Penfield and Stavraky). As in the sympathetic innervation, there is a possibility of still higher regulation by the inferior and medial frontal cortex.

FACIAL NERVE.—Presumably from the superior salivatory nucleus, since this is the parasympathetic cell station of the facial nerve, a bundle of fibers runs outward from the pons in the nervus intermedius to the geniculate ganglion. This special tract passes through the geniculate without interruption and leaves in the greater superficial petrosal nerve. The latter passes forward and medially from the hiatus of the fallopian canal, across the floor of the middle fossa beneath the trigeminal ganglion to the lateral aspect of the internal carotid artery, which is emerging from the petrous bone. One of the two divisions of the greater superficial petrosal nerve, containing vasodilator fibers, turns upward with the carotid plexus or nerve, and at this point there is a group of neurons. This collection undoubtedly represents the peripheral parasympathetic ganglion of the facial vasodilator nerve.

Unmyelinated fibers thought to be derived from the postganglionic tract have been traced within the brain as far as vessels of 20–30 μ diameter. Parasympathetic vasodilators are largely distributed to the parietal lobe, where pial vasodilatation is particularly prominent during stimulation of the central facial nerve.

GLOSSOPHARYNGEAL, VAGUS NERVES.—Branches of the glossopharyngeal nerve from the tympanic plexus by way of the caroticotympanic nerve and twigs from the nodose ganglion of the vagus nerve join with the internal carotid plexus. Since the parent nerve of each is as parasympathetic in function as is the facial nerve, these contributions may also be vasodilator. No branches from any of the three nerves (facial, glossopharyngeal and vagus) have been traced to the posterior vertebral-basilar circulation, where the question of active neural vascular dilatation remains unanswered.

BIBLIOGRAPHY

Chorobski, J., and Penfield, W.: Cerebral vasodilator nerves and their pathway from the medulla oblongata, Arch. Neurol. & Psychiat. 28:1257-1289, 1932.

Christensen, K., and Polley, E. H.: The nerves along the vertebral artery and the blood vessels in the hindbrain of the cat, Anat. Rec. 106:17-18, 1950.

Cobb, S., and Finesinger, J. E.: The vagal pathway of the vasodilator impulses, Arch. Neurol. & Psychiat. 28:1243-1256, 1932.

Forbes, H. S., and Cobb, S.: Vasomotor control of cerebral vessels, A. Nerv. & Ment. Dis., Proc. 18:201-217, 1938.

Gardner, E.: Surgical anatomy of the external carotid plexus, Arch. Surg. 46:238-244, 1943.

Huber, G. C.: Observations on the innervation of the intracranial vessels, J. Comp. Neurol. 9:1-25, 1899.

Kuntz, A.: The Autonomic Nervous System (Philadelphia: Lea & Febiger, 1934).

Leriche, R., and Fontaine, R.: Sur la sensibilité de la chaine sympathique cervicale et des rameux communicants chez l'homme, Rev. neurol. 1:483-487, 1925.

McNaughton, F. L.: The innervation of the intracranial blood vessels and dural sinuses, A. Res. Nerv. & Ment. Dis., Proc. 18:178-200, 1938.

Penfield, W.: Intracerebral vasomotor nerves, Arch. Neurol. & Psychiat. 27:30-44, 1932.

Williams, D. J.: The origin of the posterior cerebral artery, Brain 59:175-180, 1936.

Wolff, H. G.: Headache and Other Head Pain (New York: Oxford University Press, 1948).

CHAPTER 5

Physiology of the
Intracranial Circulation

THE HUMAN BRAIN weighs 1,400 Gm. on an average and represents only about 2 per cent of total body weight, yet it receives approximately one sixth of the cardiac output and consumes 20 per cent of the oxygen supply of the entire body. Man is a cerebral animal and his brain operates constantly at a high level and with the highest respiratory quotient, 1. Therefore, the circulation of the brain must be that of an organ in continuous maximal activity. The comparative peculiarity of cerebral circulatory activity is emphasized in the fact that a unit of cerebral tissue receives 25 times as much blood as an equivalent amount of resting skeletal muscle and takes about as much oxygen from the blood per unit that flows, yet capillary counts show a considerably richer vascular bed in muscle (2,000 mm. per cu. mm.) than even in cortical gray matter (1,000 mm. per cu. mm.) (Gerard).

It was the opinion of the earlier physiologists that the cerebrum was entirely at the mercy of the greater circulation and fully dependent on the body as a whole for its local blood supply. Although cerebral blood flow is essentially the product of the mean arterial blood pressure and the cerebrovascular resistance, in the metaphor of Lennox and the Gibbs, "the brain is an active and powerful monarch which, through its nervous emissaries, requisitions for itself from heart, lungs, endocrine glands and muscles a flow of blood not only adequate and relatively constant, but which contains the various food elements in proportions correct for its needs." The brain does not serve but is served.

CEREBRAL BLOOD FLOW

Accurate measurement of the cerebral blood flow under basal conditions in health, and as modified by physiologic and pathologic changes,

73

has been a signally important contribution. Two different technics have been used. One involves the determination of the degree of dilution of Evans blue dye injected into the internal carotid artery and recovered from the internal jugular vein as it passes through the brain (Gibbs *et al.*). The other measures the uptake of nitrous oxide by cerebral tissues per unit of time and weight of brain, with simultaneous recording of oxygen utilization and carbon dioxide formation (Kety). Samples of blood drawn from a peripheral artery, usually the femoral, and from the internal jugular vein are compared. So thoroughly is venous blood mixed by transcerebral anastomoses and at the torcular confluence that the arteriovenous oxygen and nitrous oxide differences are the same bilaterally. If the amount of gas diffusing out of each 100 cc. of blood and the amount diffusing per minute are known, the quotient of these will be the cubic centimeters per minute of cerebral blood flow. Most studies of cerebral blood flow in physiologic and pathologic states have been made by the nitrous oxide technic.

Normal values obtained in young men at rest average 54–65 cc. of blood per 100 Gm. of brain per minute, or approximately 750 cc. flow per minute through the entire brain. The normal range is from 500 cc. minimum to 1,000 cc. maximum (Kety; Himwich). Flows as low as 22 cc. per minute per 100 Gm. of brain have been recorded in polycythemia vera, and flows as high as 164 cc. per minute per 100 Gm. of brain have been found with cerebral arteriovenous anomalies.

The amount of blood actually present in the brain at a given moment is determined by the relative bulk of each of four components: cerebral tissue, arterial blood, venous blood and intracranial cerebrospinal fluid. Increase in amount of any one of the four noncompressible fluid substances causes a decrease in the other three. Inflow of arterial blood is the most important single factor in maintenance of intracranial pressure (Ryder *et al.*). The invariability of the total volume of intracranial contents, because of inexpansibility of the cranial boundaries, is known as the Monro-Kellie doctrine.

CIRCULATION TIME.—The velocity of flow of blood through the brain is dependent on pressure differences between the arterial and venous sides and the vascular volume. The systolic arterial tension in the carotids is equal to that of the systemic circulation, and pressure in the larger venous sinuses with the head upright is zero. Since the total mass of blood intracranially cannot be much greater at one time than at another, increase of supply of oxygen to the brain as a whole is effected by acceleration of the cerebral blood flow before enlargement of the capacity of the vascular bed. Blood flow is faster in the internal than in the external carotid because of its straight course and the absence of cervical branches. Local neuronal activity can increase the rate of local cerebral blood flow only.

The normal circulation time of the brain has been determined by angiography and by the radium-emanation method. Clinical roentgenographic studies of the brain during injection of radiopaque fluids into the carotid artery indicate that it takes three seconds for blood to pass from cerebral arteries to veins. This is confirmed by studies with radioactive substances. Four seconds must usually pass before good visualization of the major veins is attained. Six seconds after arterial injection, all visible dye has passed from the head.

DIRECTION OF ARTERIAL FLOW.—The direction of arterial flow of blood is fairly rigidly determined with all basal vessels open, although it is extremely difficult to estimate how much blood is carried by any particular artery. The circle of Willis is a potential but not actual anastomotic ring in the normal state, and blood entering the area of the circle via one artery leaves to go to the brain by the branches of the same artery and not another. With all arteries open, there is a perfect balance of tension, and it is as if the communicating vessels did not exist, stream of flow principles being maintained. Angiography normally demonstrates confinement of an injected substance to the derivatives of the artery injected. The presence of the two anterior cerebral arteries in an occasional unilateral carotid arteriogram usually means that blood flow to both vessels comes from one carotid trunk.

On the other hand, it is simple to demonstrate that the circle of Willis is a shunt capable of opening up and playing an important role when one of the main vessels is occluded. Compression of the opposite carotid artery during unilateral dye injection usually succeeds in filling both intracranial carotids and the middle and anterior cerebral arteries (Fig. 22). Indirect vertebral injection with the common carotid compressed above will sometimes show the supraclinoid carotid and middle cerebral arteries in a lateral film (Ecker). A more severe test of the anastomotic properties of the circle of Willis is the human tolerance for unilateral or even bilateral ligation of the cervical carotids, one artery supplying both cerebral hemispheres in the first instance and the vertebral circulation nourishing the entire brain in the second.

Intravital staining with methylene blue demonstrates that preferential terminal irrigation from the carotid system goes to the hemispheral cerebral cortex. Injection of the vertebral artery stains first the central gray masses, the cerebellum and the cortex at the inferior end of the sylvian fissure (cat) (Shimizu *et al.*).

VENOUS RETURN.—Circulatory return is predominantly but not exclusively homolateral. Dye put into one carotid artery comes through to the venous side with the block of blood into which it was injected, in concentrations much larger ipsi- than contralaterally. There is consider-

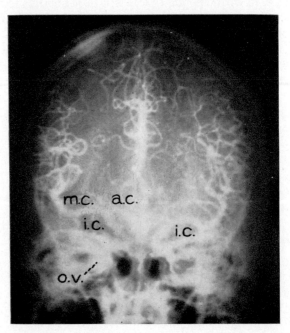

FIG. 22.—Bilateral filling of carotid, anterior and middle cerebral arteries on unilateral carotid angiogram with opposite carotid artery compressed. *o.v.*, carotid-cavernous fistula. (Courtesy of O. Sugar.)

able mixing of superficial and deep drainage through intracerebral anastomotic vessels and at the torcular confluence, so that each transverse sinus carries blood from both the cortex and the basal nuclei. Two thirds of the blood in one internal jugular vein is derived from the ipsilateral half of the brain.

However, not all blood coming from intracranial sources returns to the heart through the internal jugular veins; as mentioned previously, 22 per cent of the external jugular content is cerebral in origin. An extrajugular drainage pathway of particular importance during thrombosis in the neck or mediastinum is via the posterior emissary vessels to the vertebral venous plexus. Under special circumstances this back road can carry the entire venous return from the head.

Factors preventing a precipitate drop of blood from the brain to the heart, despite the absence of venous valves, include: rigidity and fibrosis of the walls of the intracranial sinuses; the large lumens of the sinuses compared with the small size of the veins; the entrance of venous blood against the flow of current in the collecting sinus; tortuosity of the course of the sinuses; splitting of the superior longitudinal sinus at right angles at the torcular; a lower level of the sigmoid sinus than of the jugular bulb, and constrictions at the entrance of the sigmoid sinus into the jugular bulb and where the jugular bulb exits from the skull (Loman and Damashek).

INTRAVASCULAR PRESSURES

PRESSURES IN THE CAROTID SYSTEM.—Much more blood is carried in man by the carotid than by the vertebral arteries. Pressures at various points in the carotid system have been determined by Sweet and by Woodhall and their collaborators relevant to the problem of therapeutic arterial ligation. Systolic and diastolic tensions in the supraclinoid segment of the carotid artery are exactly equal to those in the cervical region, which in turn are of the same values as the brachial blood pressure. Anterior cerebral pressure also is usually of the same value as that of the carotid in the neck. Frontal and parietal cortical branches have a tension 82 per cent of that found below.

When the common and external carotids are occluded, the systolic blood pressure in the internal carotid above falls to 50 per cent and the pulse pressure to 25 per cent of the initial values. Occlusion of the internal carotid itself reduces pressures recorded immediately above to levels no lower than those resulting from compression of the common carotid. These findings are objective tests of the anastomotic function of the circle of Willis. Simultaneous obstruction of the internal jugular vein does not elevate intra-arterial tension. Cervical vertebral artery occlusion does not lower intravascular pressures in distal intracranial derivatives (Bakay and Sweet).

Of particular importance in the problem of surgical treatment of intracranial aneurysm and arteriovenous anomaly is the observation of Bakay and Sweet that pressures in the distal small vascular branches of the anterior and middle cerebral arteries fall to within 1 per cent of values in the cervical internal carotid when the common carotid is ligated in the neck. Pressure in the anterior cerebral artery is reduced to 64 per cent of normal, a figure quite comparable to that obtained when the anterior cerebral itself is clamped just proximal to the point of measurement.

Carotid compression.—How much the blood flow may be increased in one carotid artery by compression of the other is of considerable importance in relation to anastomotic supply through the circle of Willis. Bilateral hemispheral filling after occlusion of one carotid or its branches may be due to dilatation of the circle from autonomic reflexes secondary to metabolic changes in the ischemic hemisphere. However, immediate visualization of both anterior and middle cerebral arteries during unilateral carotid angiography with the opposite cervical carotid compressed (Fig. 22) argues much more in favor of a simple physical explanation and is a function of the anterior communicating artery. Hydrostatic factors at the circle of Willis becoming preponderant on the open (injected) side, blood (or dye) flows into the field of decreased resistance.

On the other hand, it is evident in clinical experience that repeated compression of the carotid in the neck will often lengthen the time of tolerance for induced brain anemia, even if it is insupportable at first, and this maneuver is often used before final therapeutic ligation. This suggests metabolic (carbon dioxide) increase of collateral flow, although the opening of reluctant channels by repetitious force is possible.

The amount of increase in flow through one carotid during obstruction of the other in man is sufficient to maintain total cerebral blood flow at normal levels (Shenkin *et al.*). The Schneiders found in dogs that occlusion of one common carotid artery or its external branch proximal to the middle meningeal artery increased circulation through the opposite internal carotid by 70 per cent. Their assumption was that a reflex inherent in the middle meningeal artery controlled collateral flow from the other carotid. This has led to development of an operation involving ligation or resection of the meningeal artery for cerebral infarction.

Bouckaert and Heymans, repeating these experiments, demonstrated conclusively that, after ligation of the external carotid or meningeal artery, blood leaks from internal to external circulations ipsilaterally or from the other side through connections between the ophthalmic artery and the meningeal or external maxillary artery. Naturally, blood flow is increased in the opposite carotid artery, but not to the brain. In fact, ligation of the middle meningeal artery in man after thrombosis in the carotid tree eliminates a possible indirect source of cerebral supply.

EFFECTS OF GRAVITY.—The necessity of maintenance of a proper head of pressure in the large cervical-cranial arteries under conditions of gravitational stress is a current concern of aviation medicine. "Positive *g's*" of force, moving blood toward the feet during acceleration in a head-ward direction, as in coming out of a power dive, not only pool or hold blood on the lower venous side and thus sharply reduce cardiac output, but actually block flow upward by counteracting arterial propulsion. In tight turns and quick pullouts, the pilot of a modern aircraft is subject to a force as much as seven times the pull of gravity or more.

The average healthy man, unprotected, can take the force of 6 *g* for 15 seconds, 7.5 *g* for five seconds and 9 *g* for three seconds before "gray-out" proceeds to "blackout." But an increase from 1.5 *g* to only 3 *g* results in a measurable increase of instrument reading errors in pilots (Warrick and Lund). The mean arterial blood pressure may fall very low during gravitational stress; when it is reduced to 25 mm. of Hg consciousness is usually lost, but during high acceleration consciousness may still be re-tained. Simultaneous, exceptionally low venous pressures (20–60 mm. subatmospheric) found under such circumstances may preserve cerebral blood flow and consciousness by sucking blood through the brain despite the diminution of arterial thrust. Loss of vision before loss of conscious-ness is primarily due to the fall of tension in the ophthalmic artery. Air pressures on the eyeballs will duplicate blackout and suction on the eyes can prevent its appearance. The pilot of the modern jet aircraft is effec-tively guarded against these reactions by inflatable and compressive "*g*-suits."

The "redout" phenomenon, more rarely encountered, is the reverse of blackout. During the performance of an outside loop, the pilot experi-ences negative acceleration. "Negative *g's*" engorge the head and neck with blood, raising intracranial venous tension and arterial pressure, the latter by as much as 65 mm. Hg. Mental confusion may result, and retinal and even cerebral hemorrhages can occur. Two *g* is the usual limit of tolerance.

VENOUS PRESSURE.—The pressure in the intracranial sinuses and jugular and vertebral veins is purely passive and of values near or below zero in the upright position. When the body is recumbent, intravenous pressures rise to 6–8 mm. Hg. The valveless and toneless vessels readily accept backward thrust, such as that which takes place briefly during coughing, abdominal straining or in the head-down position. Chronic passive congestion of the brain is a side effect of cardiac failure or inade-quate pulmonary ventilation. Thrombosis or other occlusion of the intra-cranial sinuses or of the neck vessels also causes stagnation of blood on the venous side and raises intracranial pressure. Numerous intracerebral and intra-extracranial venous anastomoses as well as a compensatory rise in arterial tension may maintain cerebral blood flow and prevent cerebral symptoms.

EXTRACRANIAL FACTORS

CARDIAC OUTPUT.—Cardiac output is one of the interrelated factors determining systemic blood pressure, the other being general peripheral resistance. A familiar instance of acute reduction in cerebral blood flow associated with heart block is recognized in the syncope of the Stokes-Adams syndrome. Unconsciousness is quick in reflex-induced cardiac asystole during stimulation of a pathologic carotid sinus. The patient with mitral stenosis (small stroke volume) is plagued with fainting spells. In chronic low-output heart failure, cerebral blood flow may be reduced as much as 40 per cent and oxygen consumption cut by 13 per cent (Scheinberg and Jayne). The heart must drive out enough blood to supply the brain in order to maintain cerebral circulation. Severe personality changes may follow cardiac arrest.

BLOOD PRESSURE.—The sum total of all extracerebral factors playing on arterial supply to the brain results in a general increase in cerebral blood flow with a large rise of systemic blood pressure and a decrease in cerebral blood flow with a large fall. However, decrease during a slight elevation of blood pressure or increase during a slight drop may occur if active changes coincidentally take place in the intracranial vessels. A sharp rise in blood pressure after a previous rapid fall flushes the brain with arterial blood that comes through so fast that venules turn pink and only a small percentage of oxygen is removed. With severe and prolonged reduction of blood pressure to critical levels, there is a sudden extensive cerebrovascular dilatation; this is apparently an "agonal" or preterminal reflex designed to combat dangerous reduction of cerebral blood flow. With only 17 per cent reduction in mean arterial pressure, compensatory cerebral vasodilatation permits a normal cerebral blood flow (Hafkenschiel et al.). Observations by Morris and associates in operations performed during hexamethonium-induced hypotension indicate that there appears to be little danger of cerebral or renal anoxia in the supine patient if the mean arterial blood pressure falls no lower than 55 mm. Hg.

PERIPHERAL RESISTANCE.—Modification of the general peripheral resistance, principally in the arteriolar bed, readily and rapidly influences cerebral blood flow. Increasing general peripheral resistance increases cerebral blood flow, other factors being equal, and decrease in arteriolar tone throughout the body decreases circulation in the brain. Epinephrine increases cerebral blood flow even though it constricts intracranial arterioles, because the latter do not react to the same degree as the small vessels in the skin, muscles and splanchnic area. Cerebral vasodilatation is produced by inhalation of amyl nitrite; however, especially in the upright position, enlargement of the greater arteriolar bed causes mean blood pressure to drop and cerebral blood flow also falls. Carbon dioxide dilates intracranial vessels and constricts those elsewhere, making it an ideal substance to increase cerebral blood flow.

An acute increase in general peripheral resistance occurs when the bladder of the paraplegic patient is distended or otherwise irritated and after severe hemorrhage. Chronic increase in the tone of systemic arterioles distinguishes essential hypertension. An acute decrease in peripheral resistance causes emotional fainting, and chronic decrease in small vessel contraction accounts for postural hypotension after thoracolumbar sympathectomy. Orthostatic hypotension may be symptomatic of long-standing diabetes.

SYNCOPE.—Transient loss of consciousness associated with inadequacy of cerebral nutrition, when not epileptic or hysterical, is called syncope or fainting. Minor forms of true syncope are light-headedness and giddiness. A primary decrease in the head of arterial pressure is the commonest cause of syncope. Other factors are: (1) changes in cerebral metabolism due to a lack of nutrient materials such as oxygen or glucose or a failure to metabolize them (avitaminosis, diabetes, uremia); (2) a fall of effective arterial pressure secondary to a decreased venous return to the heart (pooling of blood in the splanchnic bed) or to loss of circulating blood volume (hemorrhage, shock), and (3) an increase in cerebrovascular resistance (hypertension, overventilation, arteriosclerosis, high blood viscosity, increased intracranial pressure, cerebral carotid sinus syndrome) (Shenkin). The critical level of systolic blood pressure at which syncope occurs appears to be 50–55 mm. Hg in normal persons and 75 mm. Hg in arteriosclerotic subjects (Bromage). Below these levels consciousness is lost; in the electroencephalogram, alpha activity disappears and is replaced by a delta (slow) rhythm.

Nonmetabolic mechanisms all operate to produce faintness by decreasing cerebral blood flow. The danger associated with syncope is that of cerebral infarction; lowering the head during a fainting spell is a protective mechanism of more importance than mere social convenience. Head-lowering seldom fails to raise the cerebral blood pressure or to halt its fall.

ANEMIA.—Evidences of cerebral malnutrition are common in acute or chronic anemia which is due either to a low erythrocyte concentration or to a reduced amount of blood actually in circulation. A considerable percentage of the total blood volume will remain in peripheral venules if muscular activity does not massage it back toward the heart. This explains fainting of the soldier standing at attention and of the invalid getting out of bed for the first time after a prolonged illness. Transfusion

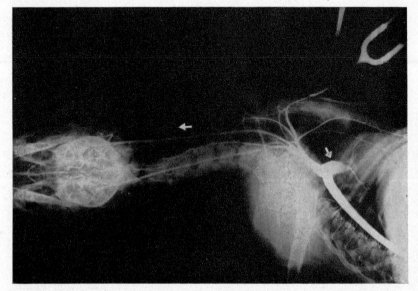

FIG. 23.—Intra-arterial angiogram (dog) demonstrating rapid injection of cerebral and coronary arteries in shock. (Courtesy of D. E. Hale.)

has benefited elderly patients with recent strokes and moderately low hematocrit values.

In shock due to hemorrhage or trauma, blood either is lost from the body or is retained in pools away from the heart, which speeds and sends smaller and smaller increments out the aorta. When reduced cerebral blood flow results in anoxic failure of the central nervous vasomotor centers, shock becomes irreversible. In such circumstances the giving of blood intra-arterially, particularly into the carotid artery, is much more effective in restoring the patient than is intravenous transfusion. The brain and coronary arteries may be reached directly and not through the cardiac cycle, owing to low resistance in the arterial tree (Fig. 23). The enlargement of pial vessels in experimental traumatic shock indicates that the brain is particularly well prepared to receive the arterial blood.

The induction of syncope by a change in position of the body is of value in recognizing significant hemorrhage. Consciousness is not lost in the intact person tilted abruptly upward from the supine position, since vasoconstrictor mechanisms possibly set off by the carotid sinus prevent fall of blood toward the feet. A significant reduction in cerebral blood flow is also attendant on the fall in mean arterial pressure induced by intravenous administration of hexamethonium (Finnerty et al.).

The merest trickle of blood is often sufficient to maintain vital centers under certain conditions. This explains the resuscitation without sequelae of patients presumably dead of cardiac asystole. In these patients impalpable cardiac impulses continue and send an imperceptible but effective aliquot of blood to the brain.

The symptoms of cerebral anemia are due to the alteration in brain metabolism and resemble those of the anoxic or hypoglycemic states.

CEREBROVASCULAR RESISTANCE

Local impedance of blood flow through the brain by friction of fluid against the internal walls of the vessels is called cerebrovascular resistance. It is calculated by dividing mean arterial blood pressure by the estimated cerebral blood flow and equals the force (in millimeters of mercury) required to drive 1 cc. of blood through 100 Gm. of brain in one minute. The normal value is 1.6 mm. Hg (Kety). Increase of cerebrovascular resistance equals decrease of cerebral blood flow, and decrease of cerebrovascular resistance, increase of cerebral blood flow if blood pressure remains constant.

Conditions Influencing Cerebrovascular Resistance

ARTERIAL, ARTERIOLAR DISEASE.—As might be anticipated, cerebrovascular resistance is increased as a result of diffuse or local arterial and arteriolar changes. In essential hypertension, the cerebrovascular resistance averages 88 per cent above normal (Kety). A significant increase of vascular impedance is likewise present in eclampsia. This high cerebrovascular resistance is assumed to be of humoral origin, because it is reversible and is reduced by bilateral thoracolumbar sympathectomy (Shenkin et al.). Heightened cerebrovascular resistance protects the brain against excessive arterial pressure.

Cerebrovascular resistance is increased in cerebral arteriosclerosis, especially if clinical signs of major neurologic involvement are present or hypertension coexists (Fazekas *et al.*). In many elderly subjects inhalation of a mixture of carbon dioxide and oxygen has been found to increase cerebral flow, indicating that the increased cerebrovascular resistance of age is not necessarily fixed (Scheinberg *et al.*).

Unilateral ligation of the common carotid artery raises resistance across the circle of Willis (Shenkin *et al.*). Frontal lobotomy in psychotic patients is followed by heightened cerebrovascular resistance either as a consequence of interference with reflex homeostasis (Shenkin *et al.*) or simply as a result of isolation of a part and contraction in size of the total intracranial bed. Inflammatory changes accompanying sclerosis build up cerebrovascular resistance in meningovascular neurosyphilis (Patterson *et al.*).

Arteriovenous shunts in cerebral vascular anomalies decrease cerebrovascular resistance measured as a function of the whole brain. Arterialized blood with a high oxygen content appears in the internal jugular vein, especially during hyperventilation (Logan *et al.*), allowing one method of diagnosis of these lesions. An increase in cardiac output and in size of the heart and a lowering of the diastolic pressure are secondary changes induced in the general cardiovascular system.

Practical considerations concerning intrinsic vascular disease and cerebrovascular resistance may be summarized thus: Arteriosclerosis in the absence of hypertension and hypertensive disease without arteriosclerosis may or may not reduce total cerebral blood flow. Cerebrovascular resistance is heightened by hypertension. Arteriosclerotic cerebral vessels are difficult to dilate by any means but can be constricted by hyperventilation. In hypertension unaccompanied by arteriosclerosis, the cerebral vasculature is much more pliable and may be modified readily in the direction of constriction or in that of dilatation by many means, chemical and other. In most persons, cerebral blood flow becomes reduced after age 50.

BLOOD VISCOSITY.—Viscosity of the blood regulates flow-friction to a major degree and is a secondary function of the erythrocyte concentration. The highest values ever recorded for cerebrovascular resistance were found by Kety in a patient with polycythemia vera. An increase in erythrocytes secondary to congenital cardiac lesions and chronic pulmonary fibrosis or arteriosclerosis (Ayerza's disease) must likewise mean a low rate of cerebral blood flow and high cerebrovascular resistance. Presumably, "sludging" of blood in the thromboembolic conditions should also imply increased cerebrovascular resistance. In patients with pernicious anemia, Scheinberg found a decreased cerebrovascular resistance when the hemoglobin value was less than 7 Gm. per 100 ml. and an increased cerebrovascular resistance above this level. Secondary anemia has been found to be accompanied by lowered cerebrovascular resistance.

VENOUS OBSTRUCTION.—Obstruction on the venous side, when anastomotic channels are not sufficient, decreases cerebral blood flow by resisting arterial thrust and therefore heightens total cerebrovascular resistance. Thus, thrombosis or other occlusion of major cerebral veins, dural sinuses, jugular veins or the superior vena cava will increase cerebrovascular resistance at least until compensation develops. Increased intracranial pressure, the result of an expansile mass or of obstructive hydrocephalus, likewise magnifies cerebrovascular resistance, primarily by preventing venous return.

METABOLIC REGULATION
OF CEREBROVASCULAR RESISTANCE

CARBON DIOXIDE.—Carbon dioxide is the chief physiologically operative local regulator of cerebral blood flow, acting to obtain oxygen. It is homeostatically ideal because it is always present as an end product of metabolism. Carbon dioxide tension exerts a considerable influence on the tone of intracranial vessels. When by hyperventilation carbon dioxide is reduced to the extent of 40 per cent, cerebrovascular resistance is increased by 70 per cent. Inhalation of carbon dioxide in low concentrations (5–7 per cent) sharply reduces cerebrovascular resistance and increases cerebral blood flow as much as 75 per cent.

Surprisingly, cerebrovascular resistance is lowered in diabetic coma, owing to the associated acidity. The slight increase in cerebral blood flow during natural sleep may be due to carbon dioxide accumulation but can occur in other ways. Cerebral blood flow is increased during carbon dioxide inhalation by direct enlargement of the cerebral vascular bed, and vasoconstriction induced elsewhere shifts blood to the brain. Intracranial pressure rises as arterial inflow to the brain is accelerated by an increase in carbon dioxide. Conversely, alkalosis, or loss of carbon dioxide, cuts down the available cross-sectional area of the intracranial circulatory bed. Cerebral vasoconstriction during hyperpnea may be looked on as a defense mechanism to conserve lowered stocks of carbon dioxide and to preserve an optimal pH (Lennox et al.).

When the cardiac reserve is poor or cardiac failure actually exists, inhalation of carbon dioxide may actually reduce cerebral blood flow by embarrassing the general circulation. Measurement of the peripheral venous (brachial) pressure will determine whether or not carbon dioxide should be administered to the stroke victim in questionable circumstances. When carbon dioxide is inhaled in a state of cardiac decompensation, peripheral venous pressure rises; if the heart is competent, there will be no change in the tension of the arm veins except a possible slight drop of pressure.

Alterations in carbon dioxide tension are immediately and frankly recognizable in the electroencephalogram. While the subject is breathing carbon dioxide in low concentrations, the electroencephalogram shows speeding, whereas during a period of hyperventilation and loss of carbon dioxide, marked slowing is seen. The effect of hyperventilation may be primarily on the brain cells, with loss of carbon dioxide increasing neuronal irritability, or the induced electroencephalographic slowing may be secondary to changes in cerebral blood flow. Experimental section of the vasodilator greater superficial petrosal nerve will eliminate slowing induced by hyperventilation in the ipsilateral hemisphere (Darrow et al.).

OXYGEN.—A decrease in oxygen increases cerebral blood flow by decreasing cerebrovascular resistance, whereas excessive oxygen intake causes cerebral vasoconstriction. These are also physiologic responses designed to preserve homeostasis; thus, although carbon dioxide, the product of oxygenation, is most effective in assuring the arrival of the parent substance in adequate amounts, oxygen itself helps regulate its own supply and distribution. Indeed, if the brain is already anoxic, still further decrements in oxygen tension will increase cerebral blood flow, carbon dioxide concentrations notwithstanding (Gibbs et al.).

Administration of 10 per cent oxygen reduces cerebrovascular resistance by 35 per cent, and cerebral blood flow is further increased due to simultaneous increase in heart rate and cardiac output (Kety and Schmidt). Electroencephalographic effects from hypoxia are minimal until the oxygen concentration of blood leaving the brain is less than 30 per cent of normal. Oxygen in complete saturation protects the brain against its own deleterious effects ("oxygen poisoning") by cutting down cerebral blood flow within the cerebrum.

OTHER METABOLIC INFLUENCES.—Barcroft declared, "In no organ excited by any form of stimulus can it be shown that positive work is done without the blood supply having to respond to a call for oxygen," and the brain is no exception. The increase of general metabolic activity during Metrazol seizures doubles the cerebral blood flow. But the converse is not necessarily true, cerebrovascular resistance being slightly lowered and cerebral blood flow slightly raised while the cerebral metabolic rate is depressed during thiopental anesthesia (Wechsler *et al.*). This response is in the direction of homeostasis.

Local metabolic processes are associated with a local increase in blood flow. Experimentally, shining a light on the retina increases cerebral blood flow in the visual system, and electrical stimulation of a certain cortical area leads to transient rise of flow in functionally related subcortical nuclei. Also, in animals killed while inhaling ammonia fumes, more capillaries are seen in the olfactory bulb than are found in controls. Fulton observed a patient with an arteriovenous anomaly of the occipital lobes who complained of an intolerable loudness of tinnitus while reading.

It is unlikely that vasodilator fibers are responsible for these changes, unless possibly through operation of the Lovén reflex. McCulloch and Roseman obtained direct evidence of an accumulation of carbon dioxide and a decrease of pH sufficient to cause vasodilatation when excessive cortical discharge is induced by Metrazol or electrically. An increase of cerebral blood flow in restricted areas is difficult to recognize in the usual procedure of total flow analysis unless the region is extremely vascular (arteriovenous fistula). Similarly, the fact that general cerebral blood flow is not magnified by stellate block does not preclude the possibility of an improvement of irrigation in a small region of cerebral infarction.

Neuroregulation of Cerebrovascular Resistance

"Blood supply controls brain controls blood supply." Five higher centers of vasomotor regulation are present in the cerebrum and brain stem: the frontal lobe and cingulate gyrus, the hypothalamus, midbrain, pons and medulla. The vasomotor center in the lower bulb is probably most active. A downward discharge activates neurons in the central gray matter of the medulla and spinal cord, and vasomotor impulses pass out the nerve roots to the arteries and veins. Peripheral loci of neurogenic reflex vasoregulation lie at various points along the walls of large vessels, acting as built-in governors of blood flow. The most important are in the carotid sinus, aortic arch and heart, but significant reflex zones include the pulmonary, caval and splanchnic areas as well. Were it not for these, fluctuations in blood pressure would always invade the cerebral circulation which is not equipped to handle them alone.

CAROTID SINUS.—The name carotid ("drowsy") was given to the artery by the ancient Greeks because of the recognized function of the carotid sinus. Rufus of Ephesus (second century) commented on the derivation of the name, saying: "Now, however, we realize that this is not an affection of the arteries, but of the sensory nerves which happen to be near." As Lennox and associates stated, it took 1,800 years to rediscover the importance of the carotid sinus.

The carotid sinus nerve of Hering arises in the glomus caroticus, a neurovascular structure responsive to changes in pressure and pH of the blood, and runs upward in the glossopharyngeal nerve to the brain stem circulatory and respiratory centers. An increase in intrasinal tension sets off a general vasodilatory response and a decrease of pressure causes vasoconstriction. Acidity of the blood results in hyperpnea to blow off carbon dioxide, and alkalinity results in apnea. In turn, induced chemical changes have a vasomotor effect.

Irritative stimulation of the pathologic carotid sinus may result in one or more of three clinical syndromes (Weiss): (1) cardiac or *vagal,* with slowing or arrest of the heart, an effect abolished by atropine; (2) *depressor,* featured by a fall in blood pressure due to paroxysmal enlargement of the vascular bed and controlled by epinephrine, and (3) an entirely *cerebral* reaction, independent of cardiovascular effects, which is characterized by temporary blindness, giddiness and weakness and accompanied by slowing in the electroencephalogram. The cerebral reaction is due to particular changes in cerebrovascular resistance or is the expression of an epileptiform discharge in the cerebral cortex.

The carotid sinus reflex may be increased by a local abnormality, such as arteriosclerosis or tumor of the carotid body, a lowering of the threshold of the central nervous system by drugs or anesthesia, or a change in the effector organ as in coronary sclerosis and myocardial infarction or cerebral arteriosclerosis. Excessive stimulation of an especially responsive carotid body may cause true convulsive seizures or thrombosis of intracranial arteries with cerebral infarction.

SYMPATHETIC AUTONOMIC NERVES.—Forbes and Wolff watched pial vessels through a window in the cat skull and saw these small arteries constrict during cervical sympathetic stimulation, although such narrowing after activation of vasomotor nerves was found to be 10 times as great in the skin as in the pia. Similar observations have been made in the monkey. Browne and associates demonstrated passive shift of blood to one side of the circle of Willis when sympathetic stimulation contracts cerebral vessels ipsilaterally. When one sympathetic nerve is cut, a striking increase in the number of capillaries is seen in the homolateral hemisphere compared with the control side. The sensitization phenomenon of Cannon—contractility of vessels to circulating adrenaline when postganglionic denervation is effected—does not take place in the cat brain after superior cervical ganglion removal (Forbes and Cobb).

Critical experiments have not been performed in man as yet, and the important problem is that of application to human physiology. Procaine infiltration of the stellate ganglions has been found clinically to increase cerebrospinal fluid pressure and to cause the exposed cerebral hemisphere to swell (Naffziger and Adams). Stellate block is being used all over the world in the treatment of hemiplegia due to cerebral embolism or infarction. Cervical sympathectomy has also been observed to increase the ipsilateral blood supply after thrombosis of the carotid (Pereira) and to decrease cerebrovascular resistance in patients with Parkinson's disease (Shenkin et al.). L-nor-epinephrine, a secretion possibly responsible for some features of high blood pressure in man, increases cerebrovascular resistance when injected systemically (King et al.). It is probable that the sympathetic innervation makes only a slight contribution to the maintenance of cerebrovascular tone in health, but it is also probable that this neural control may become quite significant in pathologic vascular states.

Participation of the sympathetics in the physiology of sensation has been proposed by Leriche and Fontaine. Stimulation of the superior cervical ganglion in man caused pain in back of the ear and in the lower jaw and stimulation of the stellate ganglion, pain in the chest and arm.

PARASYMPATHETIC AUTONOMIC NERVES.—The physiologic contribution of parasympathetic vasodilator nerves to the sum total of influences determining cerebrovascular resistance and cerebral blood flow in man has not been determined. Experimental stimulation of the central facial nerve produces homolateral cerebral vasodilatation (Chorobski and Penfield), and an indirect method of activating both right and left pathways reflexly is via the vagus. Agonal, paroxysmal increase in cerebral blood flow despite low systemic arterial pressure when the latter reaches critical levels may be explained as a vagus or glossopharyngeal-facial reflex of an emergency nature. Cutting of the greater superficial petrosal nerve has resulted in relief from pain in some patients subject to severe headache assumed to be vasodilatory in nature (Gardner et al.).

VASOCONSTRICTOR DRUGS.—Ergotamine has been proved to be a cerebral vasoconstrictor, which action may account for the delirium and hallucinations which feature ergot poisoning. The extracerebral beneficial effect of ergotamine derivatives on the headache of migraine is well known. Epinephrine weakly constricts pial arteries to which it is locally applied, and it raises cerebrovascular resistance when injected into the living carotid. When given systemically, however, epinephrine raises cerebral blood flow despite a contrary cerebral effect because of a preponderant elevation of systemic blood pressure. Therefore, cerebral blood flow is increased in the strong emotional stress of emergencies. Epinephrine will terminate convulsive seizures induced by Metrazol; if the blood pressure falls, convulsions begin again (Gellhorn *et al.*). The body may attempt to stop epileptic attacks by an increased production of epinephrine. L-nor-epinephrine, a more powerful pressor drug, does increase cerebrovascular resistance despite simultaneously elevating general blood pressure. However, this neurohormone (Arterenol) is valuable in treating severe shock. Both caffeine and aminophylline increase cerebrovascular resistance and decrease cerebral blood flow (Shenkin; Wechsler *et al.*), surprising findings in view of widespread use of both drugs as resuscitants in stroke. Probably the beneficial effects on the heart outweigh those in the brain. Slow injection of aminophylline has caused dramatic revival of more than a few patients in coma. Caffeine vasoconstriction may be secondary to hyperpnea and alkalosis. When ACTH therapy is continued for two weeks or more, cerebrovascular resistance is heightened (Schieve *et al.*).

VASODILATOR DRUGS.—Vasodilating substances are of great current interest therapeutically. Their ultimate effect on cerebral blood flow depends not only on a decrease in cerebrovascular resistance but also on a balance with usually simultaneously reduced systemic blood pressure. Therefore, to be benefited, the patient receiving a powerful cerebral vasodilating drug should be recumbent or even positioned with the heart higher than the head. With only a slight lowering of general blood pressure, cerebral blood flow may increase despite an upright position.

The *nitrates* enlarge the intracranial more than the peripheral vascular bed and increase cerebral blood flow and intracranial pressure. *Papaverine* is used extensively in the treatment of cerebrovascular disease or for acute arterial dilatation, as in arteriography or after ligation of the carotid artery. Objective studies have disclosed definite diminution of cerebrovascular resistance after its injection (Shenkin; Jayne *et al.*). *Nicotinic acid* is given with salutary effect to patients with minor cerebral accidents or signs of cerebral arteriosclerosis. Although Scheinberg found no increase in total cerebral blood flow after the administration of nicotinic acid, direct microscopy of the monkey cerebral cortex discloses multiplication of capillaries and enlargement of arterioles and venules in the brain after systemic injection of either papaverine or nicotinic acid (Huertas and Forster). There is thus afforded convincing proof that nicotinic acid, like papaverine, increases cerebral vascular irrigation (Fig. 24).

Histamine lowers cerebrovascular resistance rapidly. However, cerebral blood flow is increased only when mean arterial blood pressure is not decreased more than 12 per cent, and local flow is definitely reduced if the general arterial tension falls 50 per cent (Shenkin). Histamine is often injected intravenously in acute hemiplegia. *Anesthetics* such as ether or Pentothal decrease cerebrovascular resistance. *Alcohol* does not increase total cerebral blood flow (Battey *et al.*).

In evaluating the effect of vasodilating drugs and other substances in

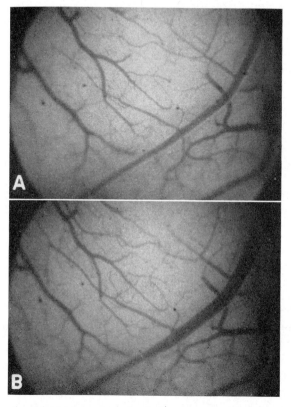

FIG. 24.—*A*, cerebral cortex of monkey before systemic administration of nicotinic acid. *B*, increase in visible cortical capillaries and dilatation of larger vessels seven minutes after injection. (Courtesy of J. Huertas.)

reversing the effects of local or general cerebral ischemia, it must be remembered that total cerebral blood flow studies are not necessarily more reliable than clinical observations. It is impossible to measure increase of blood flow in restricted cerebral areas by present methods. If capillary irrigation is doubled or tripled and arteriolar caliber simultaneously enlarged by chemical vasodilatation, the increased vascular capacitance is balanced by slowing of stream velocity. The ultimate arithmetic measurement of unit flow of blood per minute may therefore remain the same or may even be reduced although more nerve cells in more areas receive more blood.

Sympathicolytic drugs—tetraethyl ammonium nitrite, Priscoline, hexamethonium chloride (C6) and hydrazinophthalazine—exert powerful effects. They will reduce cerebrovascular resistance and increase cerebral blood flow, but so extensive is the lowering of blood pressure that special caution must be maintained to guard against cerebral anemia, especially in the aged. *Acetylcholine* enlarges pial arteries when applied locally or injected systemically, but it is of little practical clinical use because of its toxicity and the effect on the nervous system generally. *Procaine* intravenously does not alter cerebrovascular resistance.

INTRACRANIAL PRESSURE AND CEREBRAL BLOOD FLOW

Total intracranial pressure is a sum of partial tensions exerted by arteries, veins, brain mass and cerebrospinal fluid. The contribution of arterial pressure is the greatest, that of cerebrospinal fluid intermediate and venous pressure the least. Cerebral vasodilatation raises cerebrospinal fluid tension and vasoconstriction reduces it. The one variable with which intracranial pressure varies concomitantly is the volume flow of blood into the cranium from the arterial side. This is demonstrated dramatically in the immediate fall of experimentally increased intracranial pressure when the carotids are clamped or rapid hemorrhage is permitted (Ryder *et al.*). On the other hand, there is not a continuous linear relationship between arterial blood pressure and cerebrospinal fluid pressure. Patients with arterial hypertension do not exhibit a parallel increase in lumbar cerebrospinal fluid pressure unless hypertensive encephalopathy or other complication of cerebrovascular disease is present.

Venous stagnation or obstruction of any type may maintain or cause heightened intracranial pressure. Cerebrospinal fluid tension rises in uremia and congestive heart failure. Thrombosis of an intracranial sinus or of a jugular vein may simulate neoplasm or abscess. Withdrawal of cerebrospinal fluid causes immediate compensatory swelling of the brain due to enlargement of veins, but there is no observable dilatation of arteries. The physiologic pressure equilibrium between the brain veins and the cerebrospinal liquor is described as that of an elastic membrane separating two fluids which are normally under almost identical pressure but which can exist under very different tensions. Cerebrospinal fluid and venous pressures follow each other very closely when measured at the same level of the craniospinal system. In the standing or sitting position, both pressures are negative intracranially, positive in the lumbar region, with the zero point lying a little above the auricles of the heart and below the cisterna magna (Wolff).

Continuous intracranial manometry, devised to record intraventricular pressure and its variations, reveals large spontaneous fluctuations in intracranial pressure which may last as long as a minute. In disease, these pressure variations may range up to tens of centimeters of hydrostatic force. The oscillations are thought to be reflections of changes in vascular tonus (Guillaume and Janny). Intraventricular tension is increased during sleep, especially at the end of the night, and during vasomotor flushing of the face.

Heightened pressure within the skull means a coincident increase in the resistance offered to passage of blood through the intracranial vascular system. First venules and then small arteries are compressed and flattened if intracranial pressure is allowed to proceed unchecked. A level of 450 mm. of water (lumbar spinal puncture) must be reached before intracranial pressure begins to reduce cerebral blood flow significantly, and further increments cut down on cerebral blood flow more and more despite coincident elevation of systemic arterial tension (Kety et al.). As the brain shifts, especially with unequal pressure on one part of it, herniations occur and major veins and arteries are kinked or cut off against a rigid dural partition or bony shelf. Cerebrovascular resistance is thus increased still further.

The dictum that ischemia of the brain stem produced by increased intracranial pressure raises blood pressure by stimulation of the medullary vasomotor centers is known as Cushing's law. Cheyne-Stokes alternating type of breathing bespeaks complete dependence on carbon dioxide tensions for the maintenance of the respiratory cycle when the circulation of the medulla is compromised. A progressive elevation of the blood pressure accompanies slowing of the pulse and respiration, as compensatory factors force blood through a smaller and smaller vascular bed when increased intracranial pressure cannot be relieved.

Alterations of vital signs are particularly evident when intracranial pressure is increasing acutely. However, very rapid elevations to 1,000 and even 2,000 mm. of water do not immediately affect consciousness, pulse rate, blood pressure or respiration (Evans et al.). Some time must pass to fulfil requirements for the operation of Cushing's law. Brain shift with compression of the mesencephalon by downward herniation of the temporal lobe is probably the real cause of coma and death under these circumstances.

Injection of hypertonic solutions intravenously in the presence of high intracranial pressure shrinks the brain and also, if given in large quantities, decreases cerebrovascular resistance and increases cerebral blood flow without changing cerebral oxygen consumption. Ventricular drainage which reduces intracranial pressure to normal (brain tumor) may relieve headache but does not always change cerebrovascular resistance or cerebral blood flow (Shenkin *et al.*).

CEREBRAL METABOLISM

OXYGEN.—The brain is necessarily and constantly avid for oxygen, taking more of this vital gas from the blood than either the liver or kidney. The normal cerebral metabolic rate of young adults is 46–53 cc. of oxygen per minute, which represents about 20 per cent of the total oxygen consumption of the body. It is impossible to increase the normal basal cerebral respiratory quotient of 1, although increase in cerebral blood flow usually also means greater utilization of oxygen in a given period. Reduction of the cerebral metabolic rate and oxygen uptake occurs in the presence of a grossly deficient gaseous medium or when there is impairment of cerebral blood flow by a pathologic state of cerebral vessels or an interference with the enzymes of oxidation (insulin coma, senility, anesthesia).

About a five minutes' supply of oxygen remains available to the brain after total cessation of oxygen intake. Himwich emphasized the part played by anaerobic processes, more active in the newborn than in the adult, in keeping cerebral tissues alive and functioning in the circumstance of oxygen lack. Hypoxia also increases cerebral blood flow. The normal oxygen saturation of internal jugular venous blood is 60 per cent; changes in the electroencephalogram and unconsciousness do not appear until this value is reduced by more than one-half (Lennox *et al.*). Oxygenation of returning venous blood is increased during normal hyperventilation since parenchymal vasoconstriction reduces the amount of blood actually traversing the brain, and venous oxygen saturation is elevated during epileptic seizures. The normal arteriovenous (carotidjugular) oxygen difference in the adult is 6–6.7 volumes per cent.

ANOXIA.—As expressed by Haldane, "anoxia not only stops the machine but wrecks the machinery." Acute and complete arrest of the total arterial inflow to the brain in normal young men was found by

Rossen and co-workers to result in coma in six to seven seconds. Delta waves then suddenly appear in the electroencephalogram. When ischemia is allowed to persist for as long as 100 seconds, readmission of blood rapidly awakens the subject and there are no objective signs of injury thereafter. The brain can tolerate complete cessation of circulation for periods up to 3 minutes with perfect functional recovery (Stokes and Gibbon).

The most recently developed areas of the central nervous hierarchy are the most sensitive to oxygen deprivation. Of the laminae of the cere-

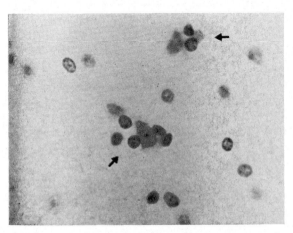

FIG. 25.—Satellitosis, necrobiosis and neuronophagia (arrows) in cerebral cortex after severe anoxia.

bral gray mantle, the third to fifth layers are particularly vulnerable. The occipital cortex and Purkinje cells of the cerebellum are the most susceptible of all superficial ganglion cells. Irreversible changes (death) are found in the ganglion cells of the cerebral cortex after five minutes of anoxia; in the midbrain, after 10–20 minutes, and in the medulla, which respires at one-quarter to one-third the rate of the cortex, only after 30 minutes (Gerard). On the other hand, gross experiments indicate that the total cerebral cortex can withstand complete anoxia for 15 minutes with subsequent restoration of electrical activity thereafter (ten Cate and Horsten). Histologic changes range from swelling, vacuolation, pyknosis, and hyperchromicity of nerve cells (Fig. 25) with early proliferative changes in the glia to gross, focal areas of necrosis which require 24 hours survival time to appear (Gildea and Cobb).

Much greater resistance to anoxia is shown by the brain of the newborn than by the adult cerebrum (Kabat). This is related by Himwich to greater proportionate activity of anaerobic metabolic systems in the infant. Were it not for this inborn mechanism, it is probable that no neonatal brain would be spared the damage of hypoxia. Follow-up studies on children apneic for three to 10 minutes at birth disclosed normal intelligence quotients at 13–14 years of age (Usdin and Weil). In cerebrovascular disease of the adult, increased oxygen extraction may compensate for decreased cerebral blood flow (Scheinberg and Jayne).

The clinical syndrome of *acute anoxia* is characterized by dimness of vision, drowsiness, exhilaration followed by mental depression, confusion, hallucinations and delusions, convulsions and coma. Anoxia acts like alcoholic liquor. In human experiments, deterioration in judgment is evidenced when arterial oxygen saturation, normally 100 per cent, falls to 75–85 per cent. Unconsciousness approaches at levels of 56–62 per cent, consciousness is lost at 51–65 per cent (King). Aviators who collapse from sudden and severe deprivation of oxygen either die, in minutes or hours, or recover completely (Titrud and Haymaker). Permanent residual injury to the nervous system after severe oxygen deprivation may be manifested in psychoneurosis, psychosis, choreoathetosis, decerebration, parkinsonism, blindness or other neurologic syndromes. In one-half of cases the myocardium is more sensitive to anoxia than is the cerebral cortex. Hypoxia accentuates the heart rate.

Individual variability and susceptibility modify the response to hypoxia. The coincident carbon dioxide tensions influence the tolerance of the brain for hypoxia to a considerable degree. Normal cerebral activity can be maintained for some time in an atmosphere of 2 per cent oxygen, compared with the 21 per cent oxygen content in ordinary air, if the carbon dioxide partial pressures in the body are unchanged. Carbon dioxide apparently protects by increasing pulmonary ventilation, causing cerebral vasodilatation and accelerating release of oxygen from hemoglobin (Gibbs *et al.*).

Chronic anoxia hampers the activities of persons from lowlands transplanted to great altitudes, causing lethargy and forgetfulness. Exceptionally high erythrocyte counts enable the residents of the mountainous regions to exist in a rarefied atmosphere. As in cerebral arteriosclerosis and chronic anemia, individuals subjected to chronic anoxia suffer from vertigo, irritability, depression, loss of memory retention and recall, sleeplessness and vertex headaches. *Asphyxia* combines anoxia with the anesthetic effects of carbon dioxide in high concentration. *Strangulation* adds to the results of asphyxia an acute passive congestion of the brain due to venous compression. *Oxygen poisoning,* a rare, largely experimental circumstance produced by inhalation of 80–100 per cent oxygen, results in weak cerebral vasoconstriction and is capable of producing nerve cell injury.

GLUCOSE.—Glucose is the chief fuel of the brain, which accounts for the cerebral respiratory quotient of 1. Seventy per cent of the total glucose output of the normal liver is utilized in cerebral metabolism. Oxidation of various carbohydrates, especially glucose, as well as of some noncarbohydrates such as lactic and pyruvic acids maintains the steady oxygen consumption of excised cerebral slices in a Warburg apparatus.

The general level of blood sugar is regulated by a neuroendocrine balance which involves the parasympatho-insulin system, the sympatho-adrenaline system, the anterior and posterior lobes of the pituitary, the adrenal cortex, ovary and thyroid. When the blood sugar level falls, the brain takes glucose first through its control of neuroendocrine relations. During hypoglycemia, three mechanisms function to prevent complete cessation of brain metabolism: (1) formation of glucose from cerebral glycogen, (2) release of hepatic glucose to the blood stream (hypothalamic activation due to cortical depression) and (3) a change in utilization from glucose to fat by non-nervous tissues, saving carbohydrate for the brain (Himwich).

Manifestations of *hypoglycemia* are similar to those of anoxia. As a low concentration of blood glucose is lowered further or is prolonged, signs appearing in order are those of: (1) depression of the cerebral and cerebellar cortex: motor excitement, staggering gait, clouded consciousness, coma; (2) subcortical and diencephalic release: spasms, dilated pupils, sham rage; (3) midbrain release: tachycardia, tonic spasms, torsion spasms; (4) upper medullary discharge: extension spasms, dilated pupils, tachycardia, and (5) lower medullary discharge: bradycardia, respiratory depression (Himwich). Induced hypoglycemia has been used widely in the treatment of schizophrenia. Spontaneous hypoglycemia results from the excess secretion of insulin by islet cell adenomas of the pancreas, from liver disease or from unknown causes. Clinical manifestations may suggest a disorder of the hypothalamus.

OTHER INFLUENCES.—Temperature, the presence of certain inorganic ions and particularly the ratio of potassium to calcium, the activity of respiratory enzymes, the level of general body metabolism and specific hormone controls all influence the cerebral metabolic rate. Fever exerts a profound acceleratory influence and, if prolonged, may actually destroy cerebral tissues. Scheinberg finds no accompanying increase of cerebral blood flow and believes that relative ischemia may account for febrile delirium. When chlorpromazine is administered to dogs and the body temperature is lowered to 80 F., the blood supply to the brain may be cut off completely for as long as 15 minutes without ill effects. Induced hypothermia down to 20 C. in monkeys has been reported to be without deleterious effect.

The giving of salts of potassium, when deprivation exists, has aroused the patient in otherwise irreversible coma. Poisoning of the enzymes of oxidation by carbon monoxide or cyanide destroys cerebral metabolic rate at its source and produces the same changes as profound anoxia. Catalytic substances cannot function properly in the absence of vitamins, particularly of the B complex. Anesthetic agents likewise depress cerebral metabolic rate at the enzymatic level. A chronically low level of cerebral enzyme activity probably accounts in part for the sluggish cerebral metabolic rate in the aged (Fazekas *et al.*).

Cerebral blood flow is retarded in myxedema; however, it is not speeded up, nor is cerebral metabolic rate above normal, in thyrotoxicosis (Scheinberg). Other hormonal effects include a decrease in cerebral metabolic rate and of cerebral blood flow during ACTH therapy (Scheinberg), a sluggish cerebral metabolic rate in pituitary deficiency, a high cerebral metabolic rate in preadolescent eunuchoidism (Bentinck *et al.*) and the inhibition of cerebral metabolic rate by testosterone. In the adrenalectomized rat there is a marked reduction in cephalic blood flow and slowing of the frequency of the electrocorticogram. These disturbances are rectified by the administration of 11-oxysteroids and pregnenolone but not by desoxycorticosterone (Hoaglund *et al.*).

DEPRESSION OF CEREBRAL METABOLISM.—Coma, even if not metabolic, may be considered the result of low cerebral metabolic rate as well as of other factors. Kety found the normal cerebral metabolic rate in healthy young men to be 3.3 cc. of oxygen per 100 Gm. of brain per minute. In states of stupor or confusion, this value falls to 2.5–3 cc., and in coma the rate is less than 2 cc. It is possible to differentiate between diabetic acidosis and diabetic coma by studies of cerebral oxygen utilization. The cerebral metabolic rate is higher in ketosis (2.4 cc. per 100 Gm. per minute) than in coma (2.1 cc. or less).

The cerebral metabolic rate is also reduced in eclampsia, general paresis, parkinsonism and cerebral arteriosclerosis. It is suspected of being low in psychosis with pernicious anemia, in heart failure, major pneumothorax, vitamin B deficiencies and heredocongenital brain disease. It is normal in schizophrenia, essential hypertension without complication, normal pregnancy and idiopathic epilepsy (Himwich).

ELECTROENCEPHALOGRAPHY

The electroencephalogram, recorded by electrodes placed on various areas of the scalp, is a summary of several electrical vectors playing on a particular point. It is composed of action potentials coming from the cerebral cortex as well as from interior nuclei projecting to and receiving impulses from the cortical ganglion cells ("reverberating circuits"). The ink-written strip obtained represents reception and amplification of electrical activity of the brain changed to mechanical force (Fig. 26, A).

Alpha waves originate in the parieto-occipital regions (areas 18 and 19, Brodmann) and are prominent deflections which have a frequency of 8 to 12 per second, most easily recognized in the occipital leads. They "scan" the brain at regular intervals. Alpha waves are of 50 microvolt potential average. They are slower and larger in infants and young children and disappear when the eyes are open, during intense mental concentration and in sleep. *Beta* waves ("background activity") range in frequency from 14 to 50 per second and are much lower in height. *Delta* waves, with a frequency of ½ to 5 per second, are very slow, very high, and usually pathologic in import. Amplitude and frequency are inversely related; that is, slow waves are large, fast waves are small.

The electroencephalogram in sleep is far different from that taken with the subject awake. It is featured by cessation of alpha waves and biparietal "humping" in the drowsy stage; sleep "spindles" (fast, high frequencies of 12–14 per second) and "K-complexes" (large, slow waves plus spindles, frontal and parietal in location) in moderately deep sleep; and large, very slow swings in the electroencephalogram of extremely deep sleep.

Carbon dioxide accumulation or acidosis of other type, diffuse increase in cerebrovascular resistance, sensory stimulation, light anesthesia and barbiturate derivatives all *speed* the frequency of the electroencephalogram. Carbon dioxide lack, or hyperventilation, oxygen deprivation, hypoglycemia and deep anesthesia all *slow* the electroencephalogram (Fig. 26, B). Increased intracranial pressure in itself has no effect until it is high enough to exceed arterial blood pressure (beyond the range of clinical experience), when the cortex becomes silent (Forster and Nims). Coma and syncope are both featured by widespread, high-voltage slow waves (Engel).

The cerebral reserve "cushion" is evident in the observations that the electroencephalogram is not altered until the oxygen saturation of jugular blood is less than 30 per cent (one-half normal) or the glucose level

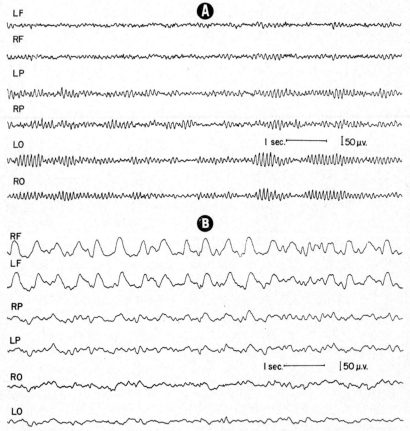

FIG. 26.—*A*, the normal human electroencephalogram. *B*, changes induced by chronic anoxia: general disorganization and slowing, with prominent delta waves in frontal leads. *F*, frontal; *P*, parietal, and *O*, occipital leads.

below 50 mg. per 100 ml. (Lennox *et al.*). Of the two physiologic gases, carbon dioxide has a greater direct influence on the electroencephalogram than does oxygen. If the oxygen tension of the brain is lowered and carbon dioxide concentration is maintained, consciousness is lost without a preceding confusion and without high-voltage, slow electrical discharge. But when cerebral carbon dioxide tension falls, even though the oxygen supply is kept constant, high-voltage, slow activity appears and is accompanied by mental confusion.

CEREBROSPINAL FLUID

It has long been taught that cerebrospinal fluid is formed largely by the choroid plexuses in the ventricles of the brain as a combination dialysate-secretion. The relative proportions of certain chemical constituents and comparative osmotic pressures in blood plasma and cerebrospinal fluid favor dialysis as the mode of formation, whereas inequities of other osmolytes and the autonomic innervation, cellularity and large surface area (over 1 sq. m.) of the choroid plexuses suggest a secretory elaboration. Cerebrospinal fluid, natural or stained, has been seen forming on tufts of the choroid plexuses.

Studies with the use of radioactive tracer substances indicate the significant, additional extrachoroidal formation of cerebrospinal fluid, as is evident clinically in infantile hydrocephalus which continues to progress despite total removal of choroid tissue. According to Sweet and Locksley, water and electrolytes are found to enter the cerebrospinal fluid rapidly, both in the ventricles and throughout the subarachnoid space, and at the same rate when diffusion is estimated by the tracing of radioactive ions and molecules. When the quantity of fluid and solutes elaborated from the vascular system of the entire neuraxis and subsequently reabsorbed within a 24 hour period is measured, it is found that the net amount of cerebrospinal fluid elaborated per day in the ventricles is of the order of 10–20 cc. per day in man.

The exact mode of reabsorption of cerebrospinal fluid on the venous side remains controversial. Key and Retzius believed that chief responsibility lay with the pacchionian granulations and other arachnoid villi which project principally into the superior sagittal sinus but also into other intracranial sinuses and into veins of the spinal cord. Weed demonstrated this pathway to be functional by recovering from the arachnoid villi large amounts of foreign substances injected into the subarachnoid space.

That other routes are available for passage of cerebrospinal fluid into the blood stream was suggested by Hassin and by Dandy, who did not find hydrocephalus in dogs after stripping the arachnoid membrane from the cerebral dura and sinuses. Tracing the passage of radioactive phosphorus confirms this suspicion (Adams). It is demonstrated in this manner that the main absorption bed is not in the granulations and villi at all but lies distal to this point, presumably in the capillaries and small veins of the pia-arachnoid. Prolongations of the subarachnoid space around the blood vessels and even to potential perineuronal spaces allows cerebrospinal fluid to bathe every vessel of the brain, microscopic as well as macroscopic.

Sweet and Locksley found that protein is absorbed by the arachnoid villi, in contrast to water and electrolytes which re-enter the vascular system on the venous side at any point. The villi thus seem to function in the cerebrospinal fluid system in a manner similar to that of the lymphatics of the body generally. The site and rate of protein reabsorption may be an important determinant of the rapidity of circular flow of the cerebrospinal fluid. It is of further interest to note that the protein content of the lumbar fluid is much greater than that of the fluid in the ventricles of the brain, suggesting transudation through the vessels of the pia as the source of protein in the cerebrospinal fluid.

BLOOD-BRAIN BARRIER.—The blood-brain barrier is the interface between the blood stream and the nervous parenchyma and is so called because it has selective properties not allowing the passage of all substances. It must function properly, otherwise the bringing of nutrients to cerebral tissues by the blood stream is all in vain. Colloidal particles suspended in plasma filter outward through pores in the intercellular cement of the capillary wall. They must then pass through a pia-glial membrane which surrounds precapillaries and through a glial membrane beyond. All materials entering the brain thus traverse an interface of epithelial-glial derivation which is therefore relatively impermeable to negatively charged ions. Cell membranes (capillary and neuronal) are even more resistive to the passing of cations, and since the membranes are fatty in composition lipid solubility is also important. Carbon dioxide, oxygen and water cross without difficulty. Some organic crystalloids, such as sucrose, are held back and therefore are effective osmolytes to use for dehydration of the brain. The capillary wall, the glial insertion on vessels and the capsule of the cell all contribute to the formation of the blood-brain barrier.

BIBLIOGRAPHY

Adams, J. E.: Tracer studies with radioactive phosphorus (P^{32}) on the absorption of cerebrospinal fluid and the problem of hydrocephalus, J. Neurosurg. 8:279-288, 1951.
Bakay, L., and Sweet, W. H.: Cervical and intracranial pressures with and without vascular occlusion: Their significance in treatment of aneurysms and neoplasms, Surg., Gynec. & Obst. 65:67-75, 1952.
Bakay, L., and Sweet, W. H.: Intra-arterial pressures in the neck and brain: Late changes after carotid closure, acute measurements after vertebral closure, J. Neurosurg. 10:353-359, 1953.

Battey, L. L.; Heyman, A., and Patterson, J. L., Jr.: Effects of ethyl alcohol on cerebral blood flow and metabolism, J.A.M.A. 152:6-10, 1953.

Bentinck, R. C., et al.: Steroidal control of cerebral metabolism in man, Proc. A. for Study of Internal Secretions, June 7, 1951.

Bouckaert, J. J., and Heymans, C.: On the reflex regulation of cerebral blood flow and cerebral vasomotor tone, J. Physiol. 84:367-380, 1935.

Bromage, P. R.: Some electroencephalographic changes associated with induced vascular hypotension, Proc. Roy. Soc. Med. 46:919-923, 1953.

Browne, K. M.; Stern, W. E., and Walker, A. E.: Cerebral arterial shunt, A.M.A. Arch. Neurol. & Psychiat. 68:58-65, 1952.

Chorobski, J., and Penfield, W.: Cerebral vasodilator nerves and their pathway from the medulla oblongata, Arch. Neurol. & Psychiat. 28:1257-1289, 1932.

Darrow, C. W., et al.: Parasympathetic regulation of high potential in the electro-encephalogram, J. Neurophysiol. 7:217-226, 1944.

Ecker, A. D.: The Normal Cerebral Angiogram (Springfield, Ill.: Charles C Thomas, Publisher, 1951).

Engel, G. H.: Fainting (Springfield, Ill.: Charles C Thomas, Publisher, 1950).

Evans, J. P., et al.: Experimental and clinical observations on rising intracranial pressure, A.M.A. Arch. Surg. 63:107-114, 1951.

Fazekas, J. F.; Alman, R. W., and Bessman, A. N.: Cerebral physiology of the aged, Am. J. M. Sc. 223:245-257, 1952.

Finnerty, F. A., Jr.; Witkin, L., and Fazekas, J. F.: Acute hypotension and cerebral hemodynamics, M. Ann. District of Columbia 22:115-116, 1953.

Forbes, H. S., and Cobb, S.: Vasomotor control of cerebral vessels, A. Res. Nerv. & Ment. Dis., Proc. 18:201-217, 1938.

Forbes, H. S., and Wolff, H. G.: The cerebral circulation: Vasomotor control of cerebral vessels, Arch. Neurol. & Psychiat. 19:1057-1086, 1928.

Forster, F. M., and Nims, L. F.: Electroencephalographic effects of acute increase of intracranial pressure, Arch. Neurol. & Psychiat. 47:449-453, 1942.

Fulton, J. F.: Observations upon the vascularity of the human occipital lobe during visual activity, Brain 51:310-320, 1928.

Gardner, W. J.; Stowell, A., and Dutlinger, R.: Resection of the greater superficial petrosal nerve in the treatment of unilateral headache, J. Neurosurg. 4:105-114, 1947.

Gellhorn, E.; Darrow, C. W., and Yesinick, L.: Effect of epinephrine on convulsions, Arch. Neurol. & Psychiat. 42:826-836, 1939.

Gerard, R. W.: Brain metabolism and circulation, A. Res. Nerv. & Ment. Dis., Proc. 18:316-345, 1938.

Gibbs, F. A., et al.: The value of carbon dioxide in counteracting the effects of low oxygen, C.A.M. Rep. No. 47, Apr. 5, 1942.

Gibbs, F. A.; Maxwell, H., and Gibbs, E. L.: Volume flow of blood through the human brain, Arch. Neurol. & Psychiat. 57:137-144, 1947.

Gildea, E. F., and Cobb, S.: The effects of anemia on the cerebral cortex of the cat, Arch. Neurol. & Psychiat. 23:876-903, 1930.

Guillaume, J., and Janny, P.: Continuous intracranial manometry, Presse méd. 59:953-955, 1951.

Hafkenschiel, J. H.; Crumpton, C. W., and Moyer, J. H.: The effect of intramuscular dihydroergocornine on the cerebral circulation in normotensive patients, J. Pharmacol. & Exper. Therap. 98:144-146, 1950.

Himwich, H. E.: Brain Metabolism and Cerebral Disorders (Baltimore: Williams & Wilkins Company, 1951).

Hoaglund, H., et al.: Studies of adrenocortical physiology in relation to the nervous system, A. Res. Nerv. & Mental Dis., Proc. 32:40-60, 1953.

Huertas, J., and Forster, F.: Pharmacodynamic responses of pial vessels, Fed. Proc. 13:72, 1954.

Jayne, H. W., *et al.*: Effect of intravenous papaverine hydrochloride on cerebral circulation, J. Clin. Invest. 31:111-114, 1952.

Kabat, H.: The greater resistance of very young animals to arrest of the brain circulation, Am. J. Physiol. 130:588-599, 1940.

Kety, S. S.: The physiology of the human cerebral circulation, Anesthesiology 10:610-614, 1949.

Kety, S. S., and Schmidt, C. F.: Effects of altered arterial tensions of carbon dioxide and oxygen on cerebral blood flow and cerebral oxygen consumption of normal young men, J. Clin. Invest. 27:484-492, 1948.

Kety, S. S.; Shenkin, H. A., and Schmidt, C. F.: Effect of increased intracranial pressure on cerebral circulatory functions in man, J. Clin. Invest. 27:493-499, 1948.

King, B. D.; Sokoloff, L., and Wechsler, R. L.: Effect of l-epinephrine and l-nor-epinephrine on cerebral circulation and metabolism in man, J. Clin. Invest. 31:273-279, 1952.

King, B. G.: Time available for protective measures in emergencies at high altitudes, Report of Air Transport Associations Conference, April, 1951.

Lennox, W. G.; Gibbs, F. A., and Gibbs, E. L.: The relationship in man of cerebral activity to blood flow and to blood constituents, A. Res. Nerv. & Ment. Dis., Proc. 18:277-297, 1938.

Leriche, R., and Fontaine, R.: Sur la sensibilité de la chaine sympathique cervicale et des rameaux communicants chez l'homme, Rev. neurol. 1:483-487, 1925.

Logan, M., *et al.*: Arterialization of internal jugular blood during hyperventilation as aid in diagnosis of intracranial vascular tumors, Ann. Int. Med. 27:220-224, 1947.

Loman, J., and Damashek, W.: Plethora of intracranial venous circulation in case of polycythemia: Pathologic physiology and diagnostic considerations, New England J. Med. 232:394-397, 1945.

McCulloch, W. S., and Roseman, E.: Cerebral blood flow and pH in excessive cortical discharge induced by metrazol and electrical stimulation, J. Neurophysiol. 5:333-347, 1941.

Morris, G. C., Jr.; Moyer, J. H., and Haynes, B. W., Jr.: Vascular dynamics in controlled hypotension, Ann. Surg. 138:706-711, 1953.

Naffziger, H. C., and Adams, J. E.: Role of stellate block in various intracranial states, Arch. Surg. 61:286-293, 1950.

Patterson, J. L., Jr.; Heyman, A., and Nichols, F. T., Jr.: Cerebral blood flow and oxygen consumption in neurosyphilis, J. Clin. Invest. 29:1327-1334, 1950.

Pereira, A. deS.: La chirurgie sympathique dans le traitement des embolies et thromboses cérébrales, Lyon chir. 44:271-280, 1949.

Rossen, R.; Kabat, H., and Anderson, J. P.: Acute arrest of cerebral circulation in man, Arch. Neurol. & Psychiat. 50:510-528, 1943.

Ryder, H. W., *et al.*: Influence of changes of cerebral blood flow on the cerebrospinal fluid pressure, A.M.A. Arch. Neurol. & Psychiat. 68:165-174, 1952.

Ryder, H. W., *et al.*: Observations on the interrelationships of intracranial pressure and cerebral blood flow, J. Neurosurg. 8:46-58, 1951.

Scheinberg, P., *et al.*: Effects of aging on cerebral circulation and metabolism, A.M.A. Arch. Neurol. & Psychiat. 70:77-85, 1953.

Scheinberg, P., and Jayne, H. W.: Factors influencing cerebral blood flow and metabolism, Circulation 5:225-236, 1952.

Schieve, J. F.; Scheinberg, P., and Wilson, W. P.: The effect of adrenocorticotropic hormone (ACTH) on cerebral blood flow and metabolism, J. Clin. Invest. 30:1527-1529, 1951.

Schneider, M., and Schneider, D.: Untersuchungen über die regulierung der Gehirndurchblutung: I. Mitteilung, Arch. exper. Path. u. Pharmakol. 175:606-639, 1934.

Shenkin, H. A.: Effects of various drugs on cerebral circulation and metabolism of man, J. Appl. Physiol. 3:465-471, 1951.

Shenkin, H. A.: Syncope, J. Philadelphia Gen. Hosp. 3:61-68, 1952.

Shenkin, H. A.; Cabieses, F., and van den Noordt, G.: Effect of bilateral stellectomy upon the cerebral circulation of man, J. Clin. Invest. 30:90-93, 1951.

Shenkin, H. A.; Harmel, M. H., and Kety, S. S.: Dynamic anatomy of the cerebral circulation, Arch. Neurol. & Psychiat. 60:240-252, 1948.

Shenkin, H. A., et al.: The acute effects on the cerebral circulation of the reduction of increased intracranial pressure by means of intravenous glucose or ventricular drainage, J. Neurosurg. 5:466-470, 1948.

Shenkin, H. A., et al.: Effects of frontal lobotomy on cerebral blood flow and metabolism, A. Res. Nerv. & Ment. Dis., Proc. 27:823-841, 1947.

Shenkin, H. A., et al.: Hemodynamic effect of unilateral carotid ligation on the cerebral circulation of man, J. Neurosurg. 8:38-45, 1951.

Shimizu, K.; Refsum, S., and Gibbs, F. A.: Effect on the electrical activity of the brain of intra-arterially and intracerebrally injected convulsant and sedative drugs, Electroencephalog. & Clin. Neurophysiol. 4:141-146, 1952.

Stokes, T. L., and Gibbon, J. H., Jr.: Experimental maintenance of life by mechanical heart and lung during occlusion of the vena cavae followed by survival, Surg., Gynec. & Obst. 91:138-156, 1950.

Sweet, W. H., and Locksley, H. B.: Formation, flow and reabsorption of cerebrospinal fluid in man, Proc. Soc. Exper. Biol. & Med. 84:397-409, 1953.

Sweet, W. H.; Sarnoff, S. J., and Bakay, L.: A clinical method for recording internal carotid pressure: Significance of change during carotid occlusion, Surg., Gynec. & Obst. 90:327-334, 1950.

ten Cate, J., and Horsten, G. P. M.: Influence of the cerebral circulation on the electroencephalogram, Folia psychiat., neurol. et neurochir. neerl. 56:447-450, 1953.

Titrud, L. A., and Haymaker, W.: Cerebral anoxia from high altitude asphyxiation, Arch. Neurol. & Psychiat. 57:397-416, 1947.

Usdin, G. L., and Weil, M. L.: Effect of apnea neonatorum on intellectual development, Pediatrics 9:387-393, 1952.

Warrick, M. J., and Lund, D. W.: Effect of moderate positive acceleration on ability to read aircraft-type instrument dials, Air Materiel Command Memo. Rep. TSEAA-694-10, 1946.

Wechsler, R. L.; Dripps, R. D., and Kety, S. S.: Blood flow and oxygen consumption of the human brain during anesthesia produced by thiopental, Anesthesiology 12:308-314, 1951.

Wechsler, R. L.; Kleiss, L. M., and Kety, S. S.: The effects of intravenously administered aminophylline on cerebral circulation and metabolism in man, J. Clin. Invest. 29:28-30, 1950.

Weiss, S.: The regulation and disturbance of the cerebral circulation through extracerebral mechanisms, A. Res. Nerv. & Ment. Dis., Proc. 18:571-604, 1938.

Wolff, H. G.: Headache and Other Head Pain (New York: Oxford University Press, 1948).

Woodhall, B., et al.: Direct measurement of intravascular pressure in components of the circle of Willis, Ann. Surg. 135:911-922, 1952.

The Acute Cerebrovascular Accident: Examination

THE PATIENT WITH an acute intracranial vascular accident presents a difficult and often troublesome problem of diagnosis and emergency care, which cannot be resolved by cursory inspection, casual management and complete reliance on watchful waiting. Improved knowledge of differentiation among the various types in a supposedly amorphous clinical group and the development of accurate diagnostic technics permit use of particularized programs of specific therapy, on which life and the degree of residual disability so often depend. All "strokes" are not alike, and the accurate evaluation of each patient will be amply repaid in terms of more effective treatment (Fig. 27).

GENERAL PHYSICAL EXAMINATION

VITAL SIGNS.—*Temperature.*—Elevation of the temperature may be incorrectly attributed to a primary infectious condition, such as meningitis, or a complication such as pneumonia. Intracranial hemorrhage, cerebral or subarachnoid, will in and of itself produce a high fever and leukocytosis. Most patients in coma are febrile. Hyperthermia is also associated with heat stroke, whereas possible causes of hypothermia are morphinism and freezing.

Pulse.—The pulse slows with increasing intracranial pressure, at which time it is often full and bounding. This may be reported as being a pulse of "extremely good quality" by nursing assistants but actually is a sign of ill omen. A very slow pulse in the absence of signs of tamponade of the brain suggests heart block or the previous use of morphine. Pulse rate usually parallels hyperpyrexia, as in any disease. When cerebral compensation breaks as the nutrition to the vital centers in the brain

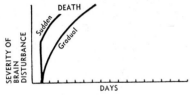

BRAIN HEMORRHAGE

Onset, sudden coma or gradually deepening stupor. Course, death in hours to days; recovery rare.

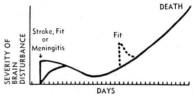

BRAIN ABSCESS

Onset, sudden with septic embolus, gradual with meningeal signs when related to ears or sinuses. Course, gradual progression over weeks with or without fits.

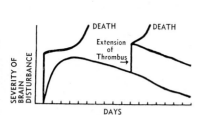

THROMBOSIS

Onset, sudden or over several hours. Course, death within days or gradual improvement; relapse with death or improvement may occur from extension of thrombus in same vessel.

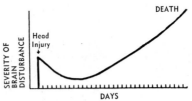

CHRONIC SUBDURAL HEMATOMA

Onset, head injury, may be slight. Course, gradual progression.

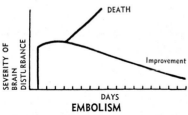

EMBOLISM

Onset, sudden. Course, death in days or gradual improvement; further emboli may occur.

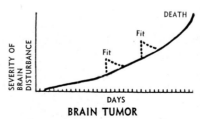

BRAIN TUMOR

Onset, gradual. Course, progressive, may be punctuated by convulsions.

FIG. 27.—Graphic contrast of various types of cerebrovascular accidents and other intracranial diseases. (Courtesy of R. D. Adams and M. E. Cohen.)

stem is reduced, the pulse speeds and may attain a fantastic rate. Irregularity should alert the physician to the presence of auricular fibrillation, a source of cerebral embolism, but is not uncommon with rapidly increasing intracranial pressure.

Respiration.—Respirations are often loud and stertorous with major cerebral accident, and the more phasic or alternately fast and slow they become, the more serious is the patient's condition. The use of accessory muscles of respiration is particularly ominous. Kussmaul breathing is characteristic of diabetic acidosis, whereas a Cheyne-Stokes cycle is associated with increased intracranial pressure of any cause. Rapid breathing occurs in febrile, infectious states and in the terminal stage of brain decompensation. Greatly depressed respirations are seen with early brain tension, morphine poisoning or freezing.

Blood pressure.—The blood pressure is almost invariably high in patients with cerebral hemorrhage and is elevated secondarily in the presence of high intracranial pressure. In the latter circumstance, the systolic pressure rises earlier and to a greater degree than the diastolic pressure. The blood pressure may fall after cerebral infarction, with or without accompanying coronary occlusion.

SKIN AND EXTREMITIES.—The skin, particularly of the head and neck, is suffused and red with cerebral hemorrhage but may be pale after cerebral thrombosis. Perspiration can be profuse in either condition. Plethora is especially striking in polycythemia. Chronic cyanosis suggests advanced cardiac or pulmonary disease. Acute cyanosis accompanies severe heart failure, methemoglobinemia and severely increased intracranial pressure (venous congestion). Carbon monoxide poisoning is evidenced in a cherry red skin. The face of the alcoholic is flushed, as is that of the patient in diabetic acidosis. Chronic pallor suggests nephritis. A cold, clammy, pale skin is associated with hyperinsulinism or with overdosage of morphine. Petechiae are signs of multiple embolism from endocarditis. Ecchymoses are common in the hemorrhagic blood dyscrasias. Chronic productive skin lesions may mark generalized disease of small blood vessels. Congenital vascular nevi (port-wine stains) are often surface concomitants of angiomatous malformations of the central nervous system.

Visible or palpable swelling of the lymph nodes accompanies leukemia, sometimes etiologic of intracranial bleeding in the acute stage, sarcoma, carcinoma or chronic inflammatory states.

The state of the blood vessels in the extremities should be evaluated. Cerebral arteriosclerosis is frequently but not necessarily associated with peripheral arterial degeneration. Thromboangiitis obliterans may be revealed as the cause of carotid or intracranial thrombosis. Edema of the ankles indicates cardiac incompetence or deep venous thrombosis, possible sources of cerebral embolism. Nodular enlargements may be sites of primary or metastatic malignancy.

HEAD AND NECK.—It is rare to have a head injury of significance without external signs of trauma, cuts, bruises or scalp depressions. Brain substance may be oozing through a deep laceration. A depressed skull fracture may be palpable, although x-ray confirmation is usually necessary because of confusion with pericranial hematoma. Orbital ecchymoses and blood and/or cerebrospinal fluid in the nose or ears are diagnostic of basal skull fracture.

The *nasal passages* should be examined for blood, watery fluid, purulent discharge from the paranasal sinuses and neoplasms which may invade the cranial cavity. Chronic obstruction may necessitate special care to secure an adequate airway. The *ears* must be inspected similarly. Otitis media of some chronicity can cause brain abscess. Hemorrhage behind the drum follows basal skull fracture.

Blowing out of one corner of the *mouth* often indicates contralateral stroke with consequent facial paralysis. A freshly bitten or scarred tongue is common in epileptics. Stomatitis may be caused by metallic poisons, and a blue line on the gums reveals lead toxicity. The odor of the breath is often helpful; the sweet smell of acetone discloses diabetic acidosis, and an ammoniacal odor distinguishes uremia. Alcohol is readily recognizable, but too often the patient with a cerebral accident or head injury is therefore dismissed as being simply intoxicated. Other poisons may be exhaled and detected on the breath.

The *eyes* should be examined with special care. Soft eyeballs are found in diabetic acidosis or with severe dehydration of other cause. An especially hard eyeball is associated with glaucoma or may be due to a glass prosthesis. Exophthalmos is often due to a retro-ocular mass which may be neoplastic or aneurysmal in type. Pulsation of the protruding eyeball indicates carotid fistula in the cavernous sinus. Fresh hemorrhages in the retina are of traumatic, nephritic, diabetic or hypertensive origin or result from increased intracranial pressure, cerebral hemorrhage, embolism or subarachnoid bleeding. In the last instance extravasations may be subhyaloid in location. Sclerosis of retinal vessels is the result of arteriosclerosis or of primary or secondary hypertension. Retinal scars from previous hemorrhages, emboli or nephritic or diabetic retinopathy may be evident.

Investigation of the *scalp* and *skull* is of importance in examination of the patient with cerebrovascular accident. Auscultation of the head should be a routine procedure. Bruits of intracranial arteriovenous malformation or carotid-cavernous aneurysm may be audible. Percussion of each half of the skull may reveal flatness over a subdural hematoma, especially in the very young patient. Palpation of soft masses in the scalp may distinguish them as being of neoplastic, inflammatory or congenital vascular origin. The open fontanel of infants is normally slightly depressed when the child is held upright and is quiet; if it is not, or if the soft spot is palpably tense, pressure inside the head is increased. Scalp veins are often distended with increased intracranial pressure of any cause, particularly sagittal sinus thrombosis.

Palpation of the *neck* may disclose primary or metastatic tumors or may reveal a shift of the larynx or trachea due to a mediastinal mass or thoracic disease. It is important to test pulsation of the carotid arteries. Cervical carotid thrombosis, sometimes responsible for cerebral infarction, will obliterate the thrust of the common or internal carotid. Aneurysms of the large neck vessels may be associated with intracranial fistula. Enlargement and palpable thrill of the arteries sometimes accompanies an intracranial arteriovenous malformation. Tenderness below the ear in the anterior triangle of the neck is found over thrombophlebitis of the jugular vein. All veins and venules of the head and neck are enlarged when the superior vena cava is occluded. Thrombosed and tender scalp arteries indicate temporal (cranial) arteritis.

HEART AND LUNGS.—Since cardiac disease so often causes or is associated with cerebrovascular accident, examination of the heart should be careful and supplemented with electrocardiography when indicated. Enlargement of the heart is common in hypertension or valvular disease. Murmurs may indicate endocarditis or stenosis of the valves and atrial enlargement, sources of embolism to the brain. Intracranial lesions are not infrequent in congenital heart disease. Electrocardiographic changes may be the only manifestations of myocardial infarction, often associated with simultaneous cerebral infarction or a later cause of embolism.

The lungs may be the primary origin of bland emboli, purulent or malignant metastases to the cerebrum and cerebellum. Pulmonary function must be assayed carefully for signs of deficient oxygenation, tracheobronchial obstruction and pneumonia. Concentration on the neurologic episode to the exclusion of pulmonary complications is a form of neglect responsible for many deaths.

ABDOMEN AND PELVIS.—Signs of thrombosis or thrombophlebitis in the abdominal and pelvic cavities should be looked for. Abdominal or pelvic malignancy may be the remote origin of an intracranial tumor. Pregnancy may correlate with thrombosis of intracranial veins or venous sinuses or with subarachnoid hemorrhage.

Urinary incontinence coincident with the onset of coma suggests an epileptic seizure. A full bladder may be one cause of restlessness in the unconscious patient. Rectal examination should not be omitted and may reveal neoplasm. Scars on the genitalia may be residuals from old syphilitic disease, newly evident in cerebral thrombosis.

NEUROLOGIC EXAMINATION

CONSCIOUSNESS.—The state of consciousness is of great importance prognostically. A person is spoken of as being *conscious* or alert if he is immediately and constantly aware of changes in his environment. When there is spontaneous drifting in and out of light sleep, the patient is said to be *drowsy.* A persistent state of quietude from which the sleeper may be aroused by vocal command or painful stimulation is called *stupor,* graded according to the intensity of excitation necessary for awakening. In *coma* no imminent arousal is possible by any means, and the condition is ominous.

MENINGEAL IRRITATION.—All irritants of the meninges, such as inflammation or hemorrhage, cause stiffness of the neck and back. Limitation of extension of the legs, due to resistance of the hamstring muscles, is evident in Kernig's sign in which passive straightening of the flexed knee is difficult or impossible. Brudzinski's sign is present when the lower extremities flex spontaneously in response to bending of the head toward the chest. Severe meningeal irritation may produce opisthotonos, an arching of the body backward, as in strychnine poisoning. The patient may prefer to lie on his side with head extended and knees bent fully in a position of greatest comfort.

CONVULSIVE SEIZURES.—Epileptic attacks are often symptomatic of cerebrovascular disease, particularly in the aged, but may be of other organic cause or idiopathic in etiology. There is no real differentiation between the terms epileptic attack and convulsive seizure. All convulsant phenomena are exaggerations of the function of brain systems normally in operation. The onset characteristics of a convulsive episode reveal the site of initiation of the electrical storm and may, though not necessarily reliably, point to the location of an intracranial process. Attacks may be generalized from the onset when there is an encapsulated hematoma over one hemisphere or a benign tumor in one frontal lobe, or they may be focal and even restricted to one extremity when the pathologic process is that of diffuse cerebral arteriosclerosis.

Types of attacks.—Generalized convulsions or grand mal originate with a cry, followed by arching of the back and neck, complete rigidity (tonus) and then repetitive jerkings of the entire body musculature (clonus). Biting of the tongue, incontinence, the Babinski sign, loss of the pupillary light reflex and coma are the most reliable stigmas of generalized grand mal epilepsy. The electrical discharge is assumed to be from both motor areas and later from the brain as a whole.

Focal convulsions, restricted to one part of the body, are usually purely motor in expression but may be sensory or mixed. Consciousness is frequently retained, although temporary loss of speech may be a part of the seizure. Clonic attacks which begin in the corner of the mouth, the thumb and index finger or the great toe and spread proximally; involving the whole face or extremity or the remainder of the side are called jacksonian seizures. Rhythmic jerkings are usually the peripheral phenomena, but the episode may be entirely paralytic. A spread of paresthesias constitutes a sensory jacksonian attack. Postconvulsive (Todd's) paralysis is a manifestation of cortical extinction if temporary, but may be due to thrombosis if persistent. The discharging electrical center in focal or jacksonian seizures is most often in one sensorimotor area of the cerebral cortex.

Petit mal attacks consist of rapid blinking and rolling upward of the eyes, loss of consciousness in staring or falling episodes and, occasionally, incontinence. They are featured by brief duration and are of a repetitive nature. Petit mal is most common in children and is rare above the age of 20. The origin of petit mal epilepsy is believed to be in the thalamo-diencephalic nuclear complex.

Psychomotor epilepsy is featured by dreamy states, confusion and periods of amnesia in which bizarre and often antisocial behavior occurs. These strange visitations may terminate in a true clonic convulsion. The areas of electrical discharge responsible are in the temporal lobe or associated internal nuclei.

Decerebrate or tonic postural seizures are a manifestation of uncontrolled release of the midbrain and lower brain stem, sometimes caused by increased intracranial pressure ("cerebellar fits"). The head is retracted, the back arched, jaws are clenched, pupils dilated and the entire body is in rigid opisthotonos.

Hysterical fits are sometimes difficult to distinguish from organic epilepsy. Theatrics, the presence of an audience, fluttering of the eyelids,

resistance to opening of the eyes and their rolling upward are characteristics. Incontinence usually does not occur in hysteria and Babinski's signs
are absent.

MENTAL STATUS.—Estimation of the mental status is of great value
in evaluating the patient and the relevance and validity of his responses
and as a guide to correct diagnosis and appropriate treatment. Certain
questions must be asked concerning orientation, memory and formal
disorders of mental content, since a superficial semblance of sanity may
conceal a profound organic mental defect. In all physical afflictions of
the brain which alter psychic function, recent remembrance, retention and
recall are lost first if memory is affected.

CRANIAL NERVES

Anosmia, due to loss of function of the *olfactory nerves,* is not uncommon after falls on the back of the head or with basal skull fracture
and, if chronic, may be diagnostic of an infrafrontal neoplasm.

Ophthalmoscopy; visual fields (Fig. 28).—The optic nerves are examined with respect to the reaction of the pupils to light, the appearance of
the nerve heads, visual acuity and a charting of the visual fields. Papilledema is indicative of increased intracranial pressure of at least four
hours' duration, usually much longer. Hemorrhages encircle the papilla
in acute choked disk, whereas the margins are fuzzy and gray with the
secondary atrophy of long-existing pressure. Primary atrophy produces a
chalky white and clearcut nerve head. Retinal hemorrhages often correlate with intracranial hemorrhage.

Visual acuity may be tested by comparing the patient's recognition of
objects at varying distances with one's own. Inability to name articles may
be due to agnosia or aphasia and not necessarily to perceptual blindness.
The visual fields should always be mapped roughly by gross confronta-
tion (wiggling fingers). In a stuporous or otherwise non-co–operative
patient the laterality of a hemispheral lesion can sometimes be determined by the absence of the blink reaction to threatening gestures on the
hemianoptic side. Conjugate deviation of the eyes toward the brain injury
may be due to a contralateral field defect, the patient being unaware of
events in the absent field of vision. Complete homonymous hemianopsia
means thorough interruption of the visual projection system. After hemispheral or capsular strokes, homonymous hemianopsia is usually total and
includes the macular field of vision. If the occipital lobe is involved, the
macular field is often spared on the side of blindness. Involvement of the

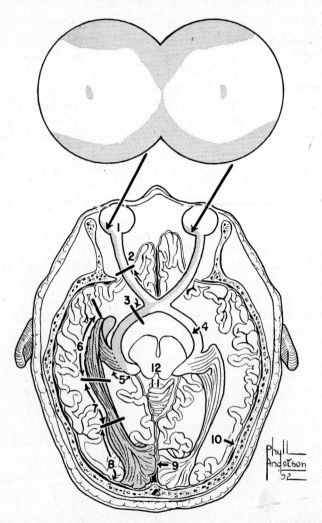

FIG. 28.—Arterial supply of the visual system. *1,* optic papilla and retina: central artery; *2,* optic nerve: ophthalmic artery; *3,* optic chiasm (arrows): internal carotid, anterior cerebral arteries; *4,* optic tract: anterior choroidal artery; *5,* geniculate body: anterior choroidal, posterior communicating arteries; *6,* anterior third optic radiation: anterior choroidal, middle cerebral arteries; *7,* middle third optic radiation: middle cerebral, posterior cerebral arteries; *8,* posterior third optic radiation: posterior cerebral artery; *9,* calcarine (primary visual) cortex: posterior cerebral, middle cerebral arteries; *10,* occipitoparietal (visual association) cortex: middle cerebral artery; *11,* superior colliculi, and *12,* oculomotor nuclei: posterior cerebral artery.

lower half of the geniculocalcarine tract results in heterolateral upper quadrantanopsia (temporal lobe lesion), whereas after upper fiber cut, lower homonymous quadrantanopsia is found contralaterally (parietal lobe lesion).

Extraocular innervation.—The oculomotor, trochlear and abducent nerves controlling motor pupillary reaction and the motion of the upper lid and eyeball are all examined together. Pure oculomotor lesions result in pupillary dilatation and loss of the light reflex, ptosis of the eyelid and external (temporal) rotation of the eye. Ocular palsies are common with a unilateral intrinsic or extrinsic cerebral expansile mass, since the third nerve is stretched by downward and medial herniation of the temporal lobe. The oculomotor syndrome is the commonest cranial nerve paralysis caused by congenital berry aneurysm of the circle of Willis. The Argyll Robertson pupil is often encountered in syphilitic taboparesis, and it is also seen with aneurysm or any process which similarly results in misdirection of regenerating oculomotor fibers. Primary or secondary brain stem hemorrhages produce tonically small pupils, as does morphinism. Wide pupillary dilatation accompanies barbiturate intoxication. Intrapontile lesions involving the abducens nerves and their supranuclear control paralyze conjugate gaze. Sixth nerve palsies, evidenced by inward rotation of one or both eyes, are also caused by a simple, nonspecific increase of intracranial pressure, a basal skull fracture or a neoplasm in the brain stem.

Conjugate deviation of the eyes and head toward the side of cerebral damage will occur after destructive lesions in the posterior frontal cortex, the knee of the internal capsule, the cerebral peduncle or the parieto-occipital area.

Other cranial nerves.—*Trigeminal* sensation is tested by pinprick on the face and by stimulation of the cornea. Absence of one corneal reflex and preservation of the other may be all that indicates cerebrovascular accident in a comatose patient. Pressure on the supraorbital nerve at the notch will elicit signs of hemiplegia, the nonparalyzed side moving in defense. In hemiplegia, paralysis of the *facial* nerve is incomplete and involves the lower half of the face, whereas in Bell's palsy it is total. *Acoustic* nerve function includes hearing, control of equilibration and balancing of eye movements. Violent nystagmus is characteristic of traumatic or inflammatory labyrinthitis or may indicate cerebellar or medullary stroke. Ménière's syndrome is often confused with minor pontile infarction, to which it may in fact be related.

The *glossopharyngeal* and *vagus nerves* supply sensation and motor power to the pharynx and larynx. Either nuclear or supranuclear (pseudo-bulbar palsy) lesions cause loss of the gag reflex, palatal palsy, a nasal voice or the squeaking hoarseness of flaccid vocal cords. The *carotid sinus reflex* is glossopharyngeal in its sensory arc. The sinus is tested by light massage, during which consciousness, pulse rate and blood pressure are checked. Weakness of the sternocleidomastoid or trapezius muscles indicates participation of the *accessory nerve* complex in hemiplegia. *Hypoglossal* paralysis is of interest in that the tongue points to the side of injury in unilateral nuclear (brain stem) damage and away from hemispheral hemorrhage or infarct in supranuclear lesions.

SPEECH

The functions of speech are manifold and complex. Failure at any level will alter communication: the delirious patient has hallucinations or illusory experiences, the confused individual speaks in irrelevancies, the comatose person is necessarily silent and the patient with bulbar poliomyelitis cannot articulate. Aphasia is the term restricted to any disturbance of language, motor or sensory, due to a lesion of the brain. It does not include disturbances due to faulty innervation of the necessary musculature or to involvement of the sense organs themselves, the general mental function being relatively intact. In this sense, aphasia also includes the agnosias, the apraxias, alexia and agraphia.

Ordinary conversation will usually suffice to determine the degree of auditory reception and interpretation and the extent of organization and expression of vocal speech. A newspaper and a magazine with brightly colored illustrations can be used to estimate the defects in visual recognition. Aphasic syndromes almost always result from pathologic processes in the left cerebral hemisphere, chiefly in the temporoparietal region. Most cases are of mixed expressive-receptive character.

MOTOR SYSTEM

The most common motor manifestation of cerebrovascular accident is *hemiplegia,* the paralysis of the lower face, arm, leg, neck and trunk muscles on one side of the body, or *hemiparesis,* a weakness of the members named. In an unconscious or semiconscious patient, strong sensory stimulation may be necessary to determine which side is paralyzed or weak. Blowing out of one cheek, an unchecked falling of an arm elevated and then released and outward rotation of the leg are all characteristic of hemiplegia. Flaccidity and a lack of resistance on passive manipulation of the musculature are present in the acute phase. Spasticity, a hypertonicity chiefly involving antigravity muscles, is a more chronic phenomenon. Flaccidity is worse prognostically than is spasticity; muscular atrophy indicates a severe or chronic paralytic lesion.

Reflexes.—In acute hemiplegia, the *deep* reflexes are often abolished, but hyperactivity of tendon jerks at the onset of stroke is better prognostically. Exaggeration of deep reflexes implies disease of the pyramidal tract or corticospinal system. *Cutaneous* reflexes are lost easily and their absence may be the only deficit indicative of pyramidal injury. These reactions are most sensitive, and loss of the abdominal reflexes may be of deceptive significance. Pathologic responses of great importance in hemiplegia are the *Babinski* (upgoing great toe, fanning of other digits) and *Hoffmann* (finger flexion) signs. Absence of the plantar reflex is sometimes equivalent to a Babinski sign. The Hoffmann sign in the hand is usually the equivalent of the Babinski in the foot, but false reflexes, often bilateral, are not unusual.

Gait.—Gait and station should be tested, if possible. The spastic fling of the hemiparetic patient is unmistakable. In-co–ordinate, staggering gait and swaying in the sitting position characterize the patient with disease of the cerebellum. The slapping walk of the tabetic may be recognized by its sound. The gait is shuffling and rigid in parkinsonism, and the patient with multiple small infarcts in the pons and basal nuclei advances with uncertain, small steps (*démarche à petit pas*).

Co-ordination.—Co-ordination implies control of force, range and direction of voluntary movement and involves intact proprioceptive sensation and motor power as well as proper regulation of motion. Cerebellar "tests" include the application of finger to nose, finger to finger, heel to shin, and the performance of rapidly alternating movements. The result of Romberg test (standing with the eyes closed) also aids in the evaluation of equilibration as well as of the integrity of proprioceptive systems.

SENSORY SYSTEM

Conduction from periphery.—In performing the sensory examination it is best to depend on objective evidences of sensory reception, such as wincing, whenever co-operation is absent or uncertain because of loss of consciousness, confusion, mental defect, aphasia or extreme youth. It is also wise to attach significance only to total loss or obviously severe reduction of the sensory modality under scrutiny, rather than to make important deductions from fine differences in discrimination. In all testing of sensation the two sides of the body should be compared. Touch is examined by stroking the skin with cotton wool. Pain appreciation is tested by light pin scratch in the conscious individual and by vigorous pricking when the patient is stuporous. Temperature conduction is readily evaluated with a piece of ice. Deep sensibility is examined with firm pressure and by the application of a tuning fork with vigorous vibrations to bony prominences.

Gnostic sensibilities.—The sensation of pain, temperature and, to some extent, light touch are conducted upward via the spinothalamic tracts; those of vibration, pressure and some of touch, are conducted through the posterior columns. All sensations reach the thalamus, from which epicritic and discriminatory sensibilities are relayed to the parietal cortex for interpretation and synthesis. The ability to recognize the texture and configuration of familiar objects by manipulation is called stereognosis. Appreciation of differences in weights is termed barognosis. The recognition of numerals or letters written on the palms and soles and identification of points on the hands or feet depend on topognosis. All these functions are properties of the parietal lobes.

In capsular hemiplegia all forms of sensation on the paralyzed side are often lost, with the occasional exception of deep pressure or vibration. Variations in the extent of denervation depend on the exact location and magnitude of the cerebrovascular accident. Brain stem lesions produce mixed and characteristic patterns. Parietal infarctions may result in loss of stereognostic and other cognitive functions alone. Anosognosia, the denial or failure of recognition of disease, is common in hemiplegia, especially when the right hemisphere is involved.

Autonomic Nervous System

Perspiration, temperature and the texture of the skin are manifestations of sympathetic autonomic activity. Pupillary responses, secretions of the lachrymal, salivary and bronchial glands and the skin color are controlled by the parasympathetic system. Heart rate, blood pressure and gastrointestinal activity are regulated in a balance between sympathetic and parasympathetic influences. Two autonomic syndromes commonly encountered in cerebrovascular disease are the Claude-Bernard-Horner complex (Horner's syndrome), in which there are unilateral ptosis, enophthalmos, miosis, flushing and dryness of the face, neck and arm, and the vasovagal attack recognizable in the sudden onset of faintness, pallor, weakness, slowing of the pulse and loss of consciousness.

LABORATORY EXAMINATIONS

HEMOGRAM.—Leukocytosis will be found in inflammatory processes, in the subacute stages of head injury and with spontaneous intracranial hemorrhage. The hematocrit reading will be low after severe blood loss and with chronic anemias but will be high in polycythemia and in shock of primary or secondary type. Sedimentation rates are accelerated in acute rheumatic and in inflammatory conditions. Cellular abnormalities in the blood smear may be diagnostic of blood dyscrasias, whereas hemorrhagic conditions will alter the bleeding, clotting or prothrombin times.

URINE, BLOOD CHEMISTRY.—Urinalysis will disclose sugar and acetone in diabetic decompensation; glycosuria is also occasionally the result of cerebral hemorrhage. Cells, casts and a low specific gravity indicate chronic nephritis or advanced nephrosclerosis.

Blood chemistry determinations may also reveal coma to be of metabolic origin. Sugar levels are high in diabetes and sometimes in intracranial hemorrhage, low in hyperinsulinism and Addison's disease. Creatinine, blood urea nitrogen and nonprotein nitrogen are elevated in uremia. Potassium levels are often depressed in all types of metabolic coma. Acidosis is indicated by reduced values for carbon dioxide and chlorides. Serologic test results prove the presence or absence of syphilis, and specific analyses of blood and urine disclose drug or metallic poisoning.

ROENTGENOGRAPHY.—X-rays of the *skull* show atrophy of the posterior sella turcica when increased intracranial pressure has been present for three months' time. Congenital aneurysms of the circle of Willis rarely erode the clinoid processes, superior orbital fissure or optic foramen. Whereas thickening of the cranial bones may be caused by meningioma, angiomas may thin the skull and increase its local vascularity. Pressure within or without one cerebral hemisphere will displace the pineal gland laterally from the lesion. Many arteriovenous malformations of the brain, some gliomas and a few aneurysms may be visualized as calcific masses in plain x-ray films of the cranium. Positive findings on x-ray are usually the only valid confirmation of skull fracture. Encephalography, ventriculography and arteriography are surgical procedures used in diagnosis (Chapter 20).

If roentgenograms of the *chest* reveal primary or secondary carcinoma in the lungs, the assumption may be made that a brain lesion is of malignant metastatic character.

CEREBROSPINAL FLUID.—*Spinal puncture* should be performed routinely, except when high-grade intracranial pressure is evident, and is of the greatest value in the differential diagnosis of cerebrovascular accidents.

Pressure above 150–180 in a relaxed patient correlates with congestion, edema or inflammation of the brain or an expanding lesion within or upon it. Bloody or red-yellow fluid indicates hemorrhage; faintly yellow fluid is seen with subdural hematoma, brain tumor and after cerebral infarction. Cloudy specimens are obtained in meningitis, and slightly hazy cerebrospinal fluid may result from mild subarachnoid extravasations.

The *cell content* of the cerebrospinal fluid is chiefly erythrocytic in intracranial hemorrhage, chiefly polymorphonuclear in acute inflammatory processes and predominantly mononuclear or lymphocytic in chronic infectious states or with the growth of neoplasms. Rarely, malignant cells are shed into the cerebrospinal fluid from primary or metastatic intracranial tumors. Increase of *protein* concentration above the top normal of 45 mg. per 100 ml. is often a result of the activity of many disease processes of the brain and may occur on occasion in all cerebral disorders.

Abnormal *colloidal gold* curves may also be found in patients with almost any type of intracranial pathologic change. "First zone" reactions are characteristic of syphilitic paresis but also occur in brain tumor; "mid-zone" determinations are typical of syphilitic tabes dorsalis but are likewise found in meningoencephalitis, glioma and many cerebrovascular disorders. Cerebrospinal fluid *serologic* reactions, when positive, are diagnostic of syphilis of the central nervous system unless serum-reagin from Wassermann-positive blood has leaked into the meningeal spaces.

ELECTROENCEPHALOGRAPHY.—Electroencephalography is a simple nontraumatic procedure of immediate diagnostic use. The electroencephalographic record consists of widespread, high-voltage slow waves (2–4 per second) in coma or syncope of any etiology. Reduction of amplitude of potential and infrequency of alpha waves on the side of the lesion are seen after cerebral thrombosis, vasospasm, embolism and subarachnoid hemorrhage and in the presence of subdural hematoma. Focal slow waves of intermittent appearance are common with glioma, abscess of the brain and intracerebral hematoma. Three per second spike-and-dome complexes are diagnostic of petit mal epilepsy. Grand mal is revealed in bursts of high-voltage diphasic spikes or in 3–4 per second medium or low-voltage activity during the interseizure phase. Local or random spiking is commonly present in focal or jacksonian attacks. Positive spike forms in the temporal or anterior temporal leads are characteristic of psychomotor seizures.

ELECTROCARDIOGRAPHY.—The electrocardiogram is of assistance in confirming the presence of auricular fibrillation (cerebral embolism) or heart block (Stokes-Adams syndrome) or in revealing coronary occlusion which may accompany cerebral infarction.

DIFFERENTIAL DIAGNOSIS

A summary of differential diagnostic features of the principal types of brain lesions resulting from cerebrovascular disease and of other syndromes with which they may be confused is given in Table 1. In general, the outlook for life and recovery after cerebrovascular accidents is determined by the age of the patient, the presence or absence of high blood pressure and heart disease, the rapidity of onset of symptoms and signs and the cause of the stroke.

CHAPTER 7

Cerebral Vasospasm

THE CONCEPT OF cerebral vasospasm as a cause of neurologic episodes in the course of cerebrovascular disease is a subject of clinical contention. The diagnosis of vasospasm is applied by some neurologists to explain all transient, evanescent and repetitive attacks of hemiplegia or other cerebral deficit; the probable or even possible existence of intracranial arterial spasm in any condition is denied by others. The truth undoubtedly lies somewhere between these extreme positions.

ETIOLOGY; PATHOGENESIS; PATHOLOGY

EXPERIMENTAL OBSERVATIONS.—Intracranial angiospasm has been observed experimentally many times. Villaret and Cachera produced widespread contraction of small pial vessels, locally and generally, after cerebral embolism with particulate matter. Prolonged, retrograde contraction of the internal carotid artery was seen by Harvey and Rasmussen when clips were applied to the middle cerebral artery of the monkey. Echlin also obtained intracranial arterial spasm in animals by mechanical and electrical stimulation and succeeded in causing true ischemic infarction in cortical zones supplied by the vessels involved.

Protracted angiospasm after exposure to simulated high altitude was found by Hoff *et al.* to result in parenchymatous changes if persistent for over two minutes. Gross and microscopic infarctions seen by Winternitz and associates in the brains of nephrectomized dogs after injection of tissue extracts were thought to be the result of vasoconstriction and alteration of the physical character of the circulating blood.

CLINICAL OBSERVATIONS.—Contraction of arteries of the human circle of Willis has been observed by Bassett during exploration of the chiasmal region and after the clipping of aneurysms. Arteriographic visualization of constricted intracranial vessels was made by Ecker and Riemenschneider in several patients; autopsy examination of some of these cases failed to reveal anatomic narrowing of vessels. The spiral muscular coat of arteries is felt by these authors to permit propagation of spasm. Many neurosurgeons have demonstrated the cervical carotid to be a narrow cord with hairlike lumen after and above ligation of the artery or following its direct injury (Ecker).

According to Ricker, several of the phenomena of cerebral vascular disease may be attributed to spasm of contractile elements which, if prolonged or especially severe, can lead to dilatation and stasis of the capillary network with diapedesis of plasma or of cellular elements and lengthy constriction of the arterioles. These phenomena are believed by Scheinker to account for brain edema in hypertensive crisis. Peripheral vasospastic manifestations familiarly observed in the extremities in Raynaud's disease, thromboangiitis obliterans and arteriosclerosis of the endarteritic obliterating type are considered by many clinicians to have their intracranial counterpart. It is quite possible that emotional crises may precipitate cerebral vasospasm in susceptible persons.

DISEASES ACCOMPANIED BY CEREBRAL VASOSPASM.—*Raynaud's disease.*—In 1862 Raynaud described retinal arteriospasm with loss of vision in the disease which bears his name. Osler later observed patients with Raynaud's disease who had epileptic attacks and hemiplegia with aphasia when exposed to the cold of winter.

Migraine.—Transient bouts of homonymous hemianopsia, loss of sensation of one side of the body or aphasia may precede headache or represent the entire attack. Frank occlusion of the central artery of the retina has occurred in migraine. Arteriographic and autopsy findings have been negative in patients with ophthalmoplegic migraine (Alpers and Yaskin), and cerebral infarction and hemorrhage of unverified origin have been described by Dunning in migrainous patients.

Simulated high altitudes, known to cause vasospasm, provoked the reappearance of the typical migraine syndrome including hemianopsia in susceptible subjects studied by Engel *et al.* Occipital changes in the electroencephalogram resembled those of spontaneous attacks. The fact that certain migraine patients respond favorably to psychotherapy, being relieved of organic neurologic attacks as well as headache, indicates a functional etiology for vascular occlusion in these individuals.

Hypertension.—When of the retinal angiospastic or the malignant type, the course of hypertension may be featured by recurrent, profound but temporary attacks of hemiplegia and aphasia or other brain deficit. Rosenberg found definite thrombotic lesions of microscopic character in all such cases, but such minute foci, even if multiple, cannot reasonably account for major hemiplegia. Kennedy and Riser and their associates have reported examples of multiple attacks of transient paralysis in severely hypertensive patients. At operation in one and at autopsy in another the middle cerebral trunks were found to be stenosed but patent. I have seen similar patients in whom serial attacks of hemiplegia, seconds in duration, occurred in not more than as many minutes. At autopsy in one such patient, a jellified cerebral hemisphere with open vessels was especially impressive.

Osler commented on the similarity of evanescent monoplegia and hemiplegia in hypertensive encephalopathic crises to cerebral episodes in Raynaud's disease. McAlpine attributes rapid onset of papilledema in young people with malignant hypertension to functionally contracted retinal vessels. Multiple areas of encephalomalacia in a patient with eclampsia examined by Holmberg were not associated with thrombosis.

Cerebral arteriosclerosis.—Spielmeyer believed that many of the multiple necrotic areas found in arteriosclerotic brains are of spastic etiology. Ricker felt that vessels with arteriosclerotic plaques are hypersensitive to localized vasomotor stimuli and therefore contract. Intramural hemorrhages from the rupture of vasa vasorum might also act as irritative foci. The unsolved question is whether or not they actually do.

Objection to the diagnosis of cerebral vasospasm is made largely in cases of cerebral arteriosclerosis. It is argued that existing stenosis of rigid vessels and defects in collateral circulation allow symptoms to be precipitated by a fall in blood pressure and that vasospasm is impossible because of the lack of sufficient muscularis in the vessel walls and because of arteriosclerotic thickening (Pickering). One cannot deny that such contentions are logical, but the same supposedly excluding factors operate in sclerosed vessels of the legs and arms, yet arteriospasm is easy to demonstrate when vasodilating drugs and sympathetic nerve block increase circulation here.

Cerebral embolism.—Spasm of branches of the parent vessel distal to the point of obstruction of an artery by an embolic plug is logical to assume as a clinical reproduction of the experiments of Villaret and Cachera. The type of stimulus (endovascular stretch) is ideal, and therapeutic response to stellate block is frequently most gratifying.

Epilepsy.—Although vasoconstriction preliminary to the discharge of an epileptic focus is denied by Penfield, he considers vasospasm in a brain scar to be a possible initiating cause of convulsions. Others have noted whitening of the exposed human motor cortex just before onset of an epileptic seizure. In 80 per cent of 126 epileptic brains Spielmeyer found microscopic areas of nerve cell atrophy and necrobiosis in the cerebral cortex, cornu Ammonis and cerebellum. Since there were no observable organic vascular abnormalities, the changes were attributed to vasospasm (Fig. 29).

Multiple sclerosis.—Brickner described retinal arteriolar spasm in

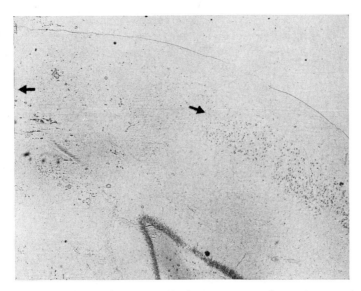

FIG. 29.—Necrobiosis of ganglion cells (between arrows), Sommer's sector of cornu Ammonis in epileptic brain.

patients with multiple sclerosis after exposure to a bright light or to a hot bath.

Vascular poisons.—When ergot derivatives are ingested in quantity, vasospasm is generalized. A most malignant and lethal form of hypertension is seen in severe lead poisoning, with pathologic changes in the brain similar to those of nephritic or essential hypertensive crisis.

SYMPTOMS AND SIGNS

Cerebral vasospastic episodes are often ushered in with feelings of apprehension, confusion, giddiness and headache. Fear is pronounced if attacks have occurred before and if consciousness is maintained, as it usually is. Physical manifestations depend on the part of the brain involved. Since the collateral circulation of the internal capsule and pons is extremely poor, symptoms and signs are frequently referred to the cortico-spinal system, and hemiparesis or hemiplegia results.

Ipsilateral sensory deficit may accompany or replace pyramidal tract deficit. A constriction of the temporal or parietal arteries of the left hemisphere results in aphasia. Parietal ischemia causes astereognosis, and temporal or occipital vasospasm is followed by loss of vision in the opposite homonymous fields. Cranial nuclear palsies and coma result from vascular contraction in the brain stem. Convulsive seizures may precede, accompany or represent an angiospastic episode.

LABORATORY STUDIES

The hemogram is not necessarily abnormal. The blood pressure is usually markedly elevated in hypertensive patients. If the blood pressure is chronically or paroxysmally low, relative anemia of the brain rather than spasm should be suspected. X-rays of the skull are not contributory. Cerebrospinal fluid findings are similar to those of cerebral arteriosclerosis or hypertensive disease. Pneumoencephalography may show atrophic changes in the brain compatible with vascular sclerosis, and angiograms reveal an open if narrowed arterial system. Electroencephalography may demonstrate flattening or infrequency of potentials in the occipital leads in migraine, or amplitude asymmetry and hemispheral slow wave activity with major vasospastic hemiplegia.

DIAGNOSIS

The chief diagnostic criteria of cerebral vasospasm are the temporary nature of neurologic manifestations and the completeness and rapidity of restoration of function. One cannot diagnose vasospasm logically except with reference to the time factor and in retrospect. Laboratory findings are essentially normal, and there should be a favorable response to antispasmodic therapy.

DIFFERENTIAL DIAGNOSIS.—The first condition to be differentiated is that of *thrombotic vascular disease,* particularly of the cervical carotid artery, in which state evanescent attacks often precede permanent hemiplegia. Others are transient hemiplegia associated with *hypotension* induced by posture, sleep or carotid sinus stimulation and *anemia* with or without reduced circulating blood volume. *Epileptic* attacks may be followed by temporary or long-lasting paralysis or may consist in paralytic phenomena only.

Cerebral embolism is accompanied by angiospastic phenomena but a source of emboli should be apparent. Cerebral hemorrhage, brain tumor and metabolic coma are mentioned simply for the sake of completeness; there should be no difficulty in distinction.

TREATMENT

GENERAL HYGIENIC MEASURES.—The patient subject to cerebral vasospasm should live a life of moderation. The problem of whether or not to forbid tobacco, coffee or tea is difficult. All increase cerebral vasomotor tone, but the relative value of eliminating mild vasoconstriction must be weighed against the upsetting consequences of attempts to break off social and sometimes lifelong addictions. Antihypertensive diets should be maintained if indicated. Alcohol, which Osler called the "milk of old age," may be beneficial if taken in moderation. The limitation of physical activity reduces metabolic needs and lightens the load of the brain.

DRUG THERAPY.—Carbon dioxide, 5–7 per cent, is a potent vasodilator, but coincidental excessive concentrations of oxygen (80–100 per cent) may defeat the purpose desired by causing weak cerebral vasoconstriction. Therefore, in administering carbon dioxide the accompanying oxygen pressure should be low but adequate (20–50 per cent).

Papaverine is ideal in an emergency; 0.065–0.13 Gm. may be given intravenously or by intramuscular injection every three to four hours. Papaverine given orally in large dosage has kept patients free from recurrent vasospastic episodes for many months (Russek and Zohman).

Nicotinic acid or nicotinic alcohol may be taken by mouth in doses of 100–300 mg. three times a day. Facial flushing is thought to be accompanied by intracranial vasodilatation. Histamine is given intravenously at a rate of 20–60 drops per minute of a dilute solution. The solution is prepared by adding 2.75 mg. of histamine diphosphate to 250 cc. of isotonic solution of sodium chloride, or 5.5 mg. histamine to 1,000 cc. of fluid (Horton; Furmanski et al.). Spontaneous (vasospastic?) stroke and postligation hemiplegia have been relieved in this manner. Benadryl and epinephrine should be at hand to counteract an anaphylactic or asthmatic reaction. Nitroglycerin sublingually or amyl nitrite as an inhalant may also be used for acute vasodilatation.

Sympatholytic drugs may be employed for their antihypertensive effect or as primary cerebral vascular relaxants. Tetraethyl ammonium bromide has reversed postarteriographic hemiplegia (Chusid et al.). Hexamethonium and hydrazinophthalazine may relieve cerebral vasospasm incident to high blood pressure, but caution in their use is urged in the presence of encephalopathy. Systemic arterial tension must not be reduced below a safe level, otherwise induced hypotension may produce exactly the wrong effect and a bad situation is worsened. Apresoline is particularly effective in lowering cerebrovascular resistance. Both hexamethonium and Priscoline have relieved hemiplegia when given intraarterially by carotid puncture.

SURGICAL THERAPY.—*Stellate block* was first advocated by Leriche

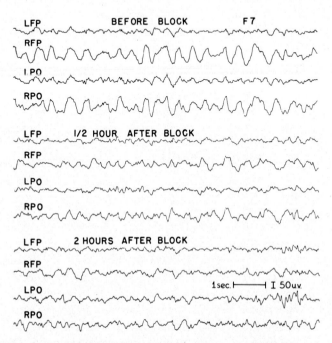

FIG. 30.—Reversal of electroencephalographic changes associated with cerebrovascular accident after stellate ganglion procaine block. (Courtesy of E. W. Amyes and S. M. Perry.)

and Fontaine in 1934 for treatment of hemiplegia associated with surgical shock and was extended by Mackey and Scott to the therapy of primary cerebrovascular episodes. Stellate block has been enthusiastically adopted for treatment of many nonhemorrhagic cerebrovascular accidents. In cerebral vasospasm the use of stellate infiltration would seem to be ideal and to have the greatest hope of success. Results are often startling and dramatic. Objective evidences of benefit may include revision of electroencephalographic abnormalities (Fig. 30).

Local anesthetization of the stellate ganglions should be undertaken as soon as possible in spastic episodes in order to try to prevent irreversible damage. Procaine may be injected into one or both stellate ganglions at four hour intervals, as indicated. Stellate block has the advantage of not producing general hypotension as do vasodilating drugs, but there may be complications. Therapeutic failure is not uncommon.

Cervical sympathectomy has been applied by Leriche to the problem of chronic cerebrovascular disease. The most logical use of sympathetic ganglion removal would seem to be to ward off recurrent episodes in patients subject to cerebral vasospasm. Shenkin and Gardner, who have extirpated cervical ganglions in such cases, believe benefit has been achieved. Pereira is most enthusiastic about results obtained in relief of neurologic disability assumed to be due to chronic cerebral vasoconstriction.

PROGNOSIS

The outlook in the cerebral vasospastic patient is dependent on the underlying pathologic state. Malignant nephrosclerosis and other decompensating hypertension are associated with a high mortality unless sympathicolytic drugs or thoracolumbar sympathectomy are effective. Arteriosclerotic spastic episodes often end in permanent thrombosis. Single attacks may be well controlled by the methods outlined; chemical sympathicolysis or cervical sympathectomy should be considered when vasospastic episodes are recurrent and inveterate.

BIBLIOGRAPHY

Alpers, B. J., and Yaskin, J. E.: Pathogenesis of ophthalmoplegic migraine, A.M.A. Arch. Ophth. 45:555-566, 1951.

Amyes, E. W., and Perry, S. M.: Stellate ganglion block in treatment of acute cerebral thrombosis and embolism: Report of 44 cases, J.A.M.A. 142:15-20, 1950.

Bassett, R. C.: Multiple cerebral aneurysms: Report of a case, J. Neurosurg. 8:132-133, 1951.

Brickner, R. M.: Management of acute episodes in multiple sclerosis, A.M.A. Arch. Neurol. & Psychiat. 68:180-198, 1952.

Chusid, J. G.; Robinson, F., and Margules-Lavergne, M. P.: Transient hemiplegia associated with cerebral angiography, J. Neurosurg. 6:466-474, 1949.

Dunning, H. S.: Intracranial and extracranial vascular accidents in migraine, Arch. Neurol. & Psychiat. 48:396-406, 1942.

Echlin, F. A.: Vasospasm and focal cerebral ischemia: An experimental study, Arch. Neurol. & Psychiat. 47:77-96, 1942.

Ecker, A. D.: Spasm of the internal carotid artery, J. Neurosurg. 2:479-484, 1945.

Ecker, A. D., and Riemenschneider, P. A.: Arteriographic demonstration of spasm of the intracranial arteries: With special reference to saccular arterial aneurysms, J. Neurosurg. 8:660-667, 1951.

Engel, G. L., et al.: Migraine-like syndrome complicating decompression sickness: Scintillating scotomas, focal neurologic signs and headache; clinical and electroencephalographic observations, War Med. 5:304-314, 1944.

Furmanski, A. R., et al.: Histamine therapy in acute ischemia of the brain, A.M.A. Arch. Neurol. & Psychiat. 69:104-117, 1953.

Gardner, W. J.: Personal communication.

Gilbert, N. C., and deTakats, G.: Emergency treatment of apoplexy, J.A.M.A. 136:659-665, 1948.

Harvey, J., and Rasmussen, T.: Occlusion of the middle cerebral artery: Experimental study, A.M.A. Arch. Neurol. & Psychiat. 66:20-29, 1951.

Hoff, E. C., Jr.; Grennell, R. G., and Fulton, J. F.: Histopathology of the central nervous system after exposure to high altitudes, hypoglycemia and other conditions associated with cerebral anoxia, Medicine 24:161-217, 1945.

Holmberg, G.: Extensive encephalomalacia after toxemia of pregnancy, Acta psychiat. et neurol. 24:175-198, 1949.

Horton, B. T.: Clinical use of histamine, Postgrad. Med. 9:1-23, 1951.

Kennedy, F.; Wortis, S. B., and Wortis, H.: The clinical evidence for cerebral vasomotor changes, A. Res. Nerv. & Ment. Dis., Proc. 18:670-695, 1938.

Leriche, R., and Fontaine, R.: L'anesthésie isolée du ganglion étoilé: Sa technique, ses indications, ses résultats, Presse méd. 42:849-850, 1934.

Mackey, W. A., and Scott, L. D. W.: Treatment of apoplexy by infiltration of the stellate ganglion with novocaine, Brit. M. J. 2:1-4, 1938.

McAlpine, D.: Hypertensive cerebral attack, Quart. J. Med. 2:463-481, 1933.

Penfield, W.: The circulation of the epileptic brain, A. Res. Nerv. & Ment. Dis., Proc. 18:605-637, 1938.

Pereira, A. deS.: Chirurgie du sympathique et affections vasculaires du cerveau, J. internat. chir. 11:301-304, 1951.

Pickering, G. W.: Transient cerebral paralysis in hypertension and in cerebral embolism, J.A.M.A. 137:423-430, 1948.

Ricker, G.: Sclerose und Hypertonie der Innervierten Arterien (Berlin: Julius Springer, 1927).

Riser, M.; Mériel, P., and Planques: Les spasmes vasculaires en neurologie: Etude clinique et expérimentale, L'Encéphale 26:501-528, 1931.

Risteen, W. A., and Volpitto, P. P.: Role of stellate ganglion block in certain neurologic disorders, South. M. J. 39:431-435, 1946.

Rosenberg, E. F.: The brain in malignant hypertension, Arch. Int. Med. 65:545-576, 1940.

Russek, H. I., and Zohman, D. L.: Papaverine in cerebral angiospasm (vascular encephalopathy), J.A.M.A. 136:930-932, 1948.

Scheinker, I. M.: Hypertensive cerebral swelling: Characteristic clinicopathologic syndrome, Ann. Int. Med. 28:630-641, 1948.

Shenkin, H. A.: Personal communication.

Spielmeyer, W.: Vasomotorisch trophische Veränderungen bei zerebraler Arteriosklerose, Monatsschr. Psychiat. u. Neurol. 68:605-620, 1928.

Spielmeyer, W.: Die Pathogenese der epileptischen Krampfes, Ztschr. ges. Neurol. u. Psychiat. 109:501-520, 1927.

Villaret, M., and Cachera, R.: Les répercussions vasculaires tardives de l'embolie cérébrale en pathologie expérimentale, Presse méd. 47:267-271, 1939.

Winternitz, M. C., et al.: The brain in experimental vascular disease, Yale J. Biol. & Med. 13:579-594, 1941.

CHAPTER 8

Cerebral Thrombosis; Infarction

CEREBRAL INFARCTION, or softening, is the type of cerebrovascular accident most frequently encountered in clinical practice. Infarctions, thrombotic and nonthrombotic, comprise approximately two thirds of all strokes. Distinction must be made between true thrombosis of intracranial arteries and infarction of areas of the brain without discoverable thrombosis. Surprisingly, in 60 per cent of instances of cerebral softening no occlusion of the vessel supplying the region can be found (Hicks and Warren). More complete autopsy investigation might reveal unsuspected thrombosis of the cervical carotid artery in such cases. However, most encephalomalacia without evident vascular obstruction would probably still prove to be due to relative ischemia, the result of disproportion among metabolic needs of the brain, the availability of open arterial channels and the level of efficiency of the heart and other factors modifying systemic blood pressure and circulation.

ARTERIAL THROMBOSIS

ETIOLOGY; PATHOGENESIS

ARTERIOSCLEROSIS.—Since the average age of patients with cerebral infarction is 64 years (Merritt and Aring), it is apparent that the principal etiologic factor in most cases of intracranial arterial thrombosis, representing 40 per cent of all brain infarcts, is arteriosclerosis. Cerebral vessels participate in the common pathologic changes characteristic of atherosclerosis. These are: fibrosis, hyalinization and calcification of the media, notably poor in muscular tissue; splitting and degeneration of the elastica; subintimal cholesterol deposition and new growth of fibroblastic tissue, narrowing the vascular lumen; and ulceration of the endothelium. Proliferated vasa vasorum are numerous in all coats. The arterial wall may be weakened by faulty nutrition, the lumen may be narrowed by

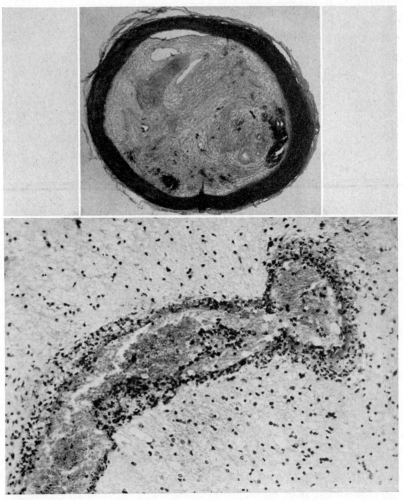

FIG. 31 *(above)*.—Thromboangiitis obliterans of cervical carotid artery. (Courtesy of H. Krayenbühl.)

FIG. 32 *(below)*.—Vasoparalysis and vasothrombosis in cerebral infarct. (Courtesy of I. M. Scheinker.)

intramural hemorrhage, or clotting can be initiated by intimal exudation (Winternitz *et al.*).

True thrombosis develops on damaged intima, on the site of internal rupture of an atheromatous plaque, or results when the plugging of tiny channels in a recanalized section of vessel almost entirely obstructed by fibroblastic growth completes the process of occlusion. Contrary to popular belief, propagation of thrombosis in cerebral arteries is uncommon, except in unusual circumstances. The course of events interpreted clinically as propagation is usually either final closure of a previously narrowed vessel or multiplicity of thrombotic episodes.

INFLAMMATORY VASCULAR DISEASE.—*Thromboangiitis obliterans* (Buerger-Winiwarter disease) not only attacks the cervical carotid artery (Fig. 31) but also involves intracranial vessels, major or cortical, particularly the middle cerebral artery (Lippmann). *Syphilis* is a well known cause of cerebral thrombosis, especially in relatively young persons. *Rheumatic fever* may inflame large and small intracranial arteries and veins as well. A proliferative panvasculitis resembles the construction of rheumatic lesions elsewhere. The syndrome of *febrile thrombosis* resulting in hemiplegia, usually with convulsive seizures, is associated with infectious illnesses in infants and children and is due to venous or arterial vascular occlusion. Various etiologies include endothelial inflammation, transient bacteremia and embolism. Scheinker discovered widespread *vasoparalysis* and vasothrombosis in the brains of children thought to have died of encephalitis (Fig. 32). *Insect stings* also have caused cerebral thrombosis.

TRAUMA.—Direct or indirect physical injury has caused thrombosis of the cervical carotid and intracranial arteries. Missile or other wounds or injuries of the neck are not uncommonly complicated by occlusion of the common carotid or of its primary divisions. Dissecting aneurysm of the circle of Willis, laceration of cerebral arterial walls and simple cerebral thrombosis have all occurred after severe head injury. Occlusions of the basilar, vertebral and cerebellar arteries with hemorrhagic infarction of the hindbrain have followed chiropractic manipulations of the head and neck (Pratt-Thomas and Berger), sprains or dislocations of the cervical spine.

OTHER CAUSES.—*Dissecting aneurysm of the aorta* extending into the innominate or carotid vessels can effect complete closure of these arteries without actual thrombosis, an intramural hematoma occluding the lumen from without (Fig. 33). Of 26 patients with this unusual condition examined by Moersch and Sayre, eight had cerebral involvement and five were hemiplegic. Thrombosis may begin in a *congenital berry aneurysm* of the circle of Willis and extend peripherally into the brain, a rare instance of true propagation of arterial occlusion intracerebrally. *Blood dyscrasias,* particularly polycythemia vera and sickle cell anemia, may cause arterial thromboses as well as many other types of cerebrovascular disease. *Congenital cardiac* disorders predispose to intracranial clotting, arterial as well as venous, in children who have polycythemia secondary to chronic cyanosis and who are subject to syncopal attacks (Ford). *Diabetes* is usually associated with arteriosclerosis and

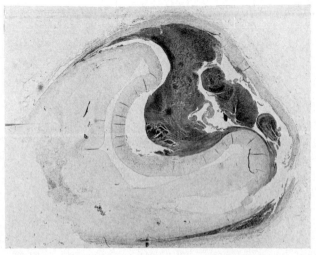

FIG. 33.—Dissecting aortic aneurysm with extension into and occlusion of carotid artery.

therefore with cerebral occlusions, and chronic *nephritis* also is accompanied by intracranial arterial degeneration. *Emotional crisis* may be a precipitant of cerebral infarction.

"Pulseless disease" (Takayasu's syndrome) is a rare cause of hemiplegia in young or middle-aged women. Progressive stenosis of the great vessels arising from the aortic arch obliterates the peripheral radial pulses long before cerebral infarction eventuates. The etiology is unknown. In one of my patients the entire carotid system was found to be thrombosed at operation.

PREDISPOSITION TO THROMBOSIS.—The middle cerebral artery is

involved in 75 per cent of intracranial arterial thrombotic occlusions, the posterior cerebral artery and basilar artery each in 10 per cent and the anterior cerebral artery in 5 per cent. Any cerebral or cerebellar arterial channel may become thrombosed.

Vulnerability of the *middle cerebral* circulation, particularly of its important ganglionic branches which run to the internal capsule and striate bodies, has long intrigued pathologic anatomists. Cohnheim declared that the ganglionic vessels are end-arteries, without any collateral source; hence, occlusions of these vessels are more likely to result in tissue destruction than is true elsewhere in the brain. This analysis was affirmed by Young and Karnosh, who found no precapillary anastomoses among the arterioles of the internal capsule and basal ganglions, final blood supply to this especially influential region being via a common capillary pool. Kristenson made the further significant observation that basal ganglionic derivatives from the terminal carotid and middle cerebral arteries run to their destination in retrograde fashion, the direction of stream being turned backward at an angle of 45 degrees or less. This investigator believes that the formation of valvelike bands at points of bifurcation or departure of vessels, the oblique passage of branches through the wall of the parent trunk and constriction of the lumen of the ganglionic artery at its origin also predispose to thrombosis (Figs. 9 and 16).

In 200 brains examined by Fetterman and Moran infarctions of thrombotic or nonthrombotic origin were found in 32 per cent of specimens in which *anomalies of the circle of Willis* coexisted; the incidence of cerebral softening was lower when such congenital abnormalities were not present. The posterior communicating arteries, the principal connection between basilar and carotid circulations, were often absent or were threadlike on one or both sides. Developmentally hypoplastic vessels at or distal to the circle are also prone to occlusion.

SUPERFICIAL ANASTOMOSES.—The importance of surface anastomoses between and among major arterial trunks of the cerebrum and cerebellum has been emphasized by Vander Eecken *et al.* Previously described by Duret, Heubner, Testut and Beevor, these communications are end-to-end and side-to-side from one arterial field of irrigation to the next, even across the midline. These anastomotic connections may serve to limit the extent of infarction, and the possibility of increasing collateral flow is a conceivable explanation for the therapeutic success of stellate block after stroke has occurred.

PATHOLOGY

When an artery of the cerebrum or cerebellum has been occluded, parenchymal infarction may be either of the "white," bloodless or the "red," hemorrhagic variety. The former type of infarct occurs principally in the white matter and is due to complete ischemia; the latter involves the cortex or central gray matter and results from partial ischemia.

WHITE INFARCTION.—The parenchyma in white infarction (encephalomalacia or cerebral softening) is mushy, opaque and yellow-white in color with occasional petechiae (Fig. 34). Discrimination between

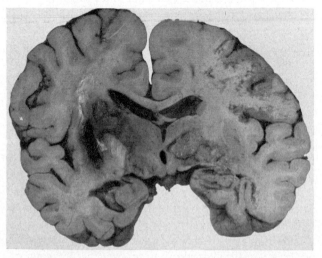

FIG. 34.—Ischemic (white) infarction of cerebral hemisphere *(right)* with capsular hemorrhage *(left)*. (AFIP #BR 6218-2.)

fiber tracts and supporting tissues is lost. Brain swelling may be extreme, especially in the acute stage. Hypertrophy of capillary endothelial cells, congestion and stasis of small vessels with perivascular edema and liquefactive necrosis of small veins and capillaries as well as nervous elements are visible microscopically. Ganglion cells are pale, ghostlike and contain pyknotic nuclei.

Neuronophagia and microglial activity are evident within 48 hours. Necrotic tissue liquefies and absorbs, and old softenings consist of cysts of yellow fluid, in which a spider-web framework of vessels and connective tissue floats (Fig. 35). Fat and iron-containing phagocytes are numerous. The perivascular adventitia is increased. The chronic process takes at least five weeks for completion.

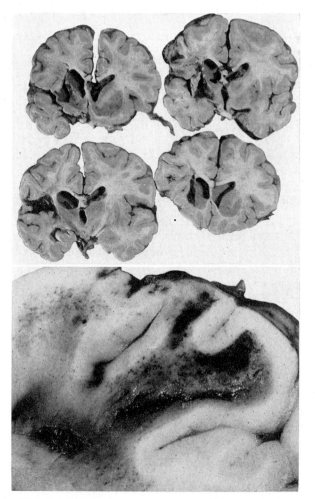

FIG. 35 *(above)*.—Ancient cystic infarct of insula *(left)*. (AFIP #L 4955-2.)
FIG. 36 *(below)*.—Hemorrhagic (red) cerebral infarction. (George Washington University Laboratory of Neurology.)

RED INFARCTION.—Red infarction is featured by grossly visible hemorrhages and congestion of all small vessels in the cortical mantle and basal nuclei, particularly the caudate nucleus and putamen (Fig. 36). Subarachnoid blood staining is seen on the exterior of the brain. Affected gyri are swollen and purple-brown in color. Extravasations extend into the immediate subcortex, but the central area of infarction is pale. All varieties of small vessel damage are found microscopically. Neurons are better preserved in hemorrhagic areas than in adjacent zones of total ischemia.

COLLATERAL CIRCULATION.—Collateral circulation modifies the appearance of infarction; if 5 per cent of the normal blood supply of an area continues to reach it after arterial occlusion, the rupture of venules will make the infarct hemorrhagic (Cobb). Experimental study of the problem of red and white softening by Hain *et al.* led to the conclusion that the activity of collateral flow determines the degree of the hemorrhagic component. Hence, the superficial location of red infarction where cortical collaterals are numerous. Evans and McEachern determined that red infarcts develop with slowing of circulation and that white necrosis with eventual cyst formation results when the arrest of supply is sudden.

Harvey and Rasmussen observed hemorrhagic change in the brains of monkeys when clips were applied to the middle cerebral artery and later removed. No gross cortical changes were visible after 30 minutes of ischemia or less. Fifty minutes of temporary occlusion produced the same degree of permanent brain damage as did section of the vessel. Coincident vasospasm is believed to render the whole hemisphere relatively anemic, increasing the vulnerability of tissue deprived absolutely of its blood supply.

INFARCTION WITHOUT THROMBOSIS

ETIOLOGY; PATHOGENESIS

In the larger group of cases in which cerebral infarction is not found to be due to intracranial arterial thrombosis, explanations are diverse and largely unsubstantiated. Arteriosclerosis is usually the basic fault. Explanations of what then occurs are of two persuasions: one school of thought contends that vasospasm produces brain lesions, the other that stenosis of major or minor vascular trunks in the presence of temporary or long-lasting circulatory insufficiency results in encephalomalacia. Both analyses are probably correct under appropriate circumstances.

VASOSPASM.—The concept of vasospastic thrombosis supported by Ricker was that irritative constrictor impulses fatigue and eventually paralyze peripheral arterioles and capillaries which leak blood, proximal main arteries remaining constricted. Hicks and Warren subscribe to the vasoconstrictive explanation of both hemorrhagic and infarctive apoplexy. They were unable to implicate systemic circulatory failure or significant arterial stenosis in 60 cases of brain softening without physical occlusion. Aring likewise considers that angiospasm fulfils the clinical and pathologic requirements in such instances. Goodman called attention to the frequency of recurrent infarctive episodes without final occlusion in hypertensive brain disease. The argument that "sclerosed vessels cannot contract" does not jibe with observations made elsewhere in the body, particularly in the heart and extremities. Arteriographic evidences of cerebral vasospasm are found much more frequently in patients with recent strokes than those with other types of intracranial pathology (Ecker and Riemenschneider).

STENOSIS OF VESSELS.—Nonthrombotic infarction has been attributed to stenosis of sclerosed arteries by Foix and his followers. Denny-Brown denies the possibility of vasospasm as a cause of recurrent cerebrovascular attacks and believes all such episodes result when hypotension occurs in the presence of vascular narrowing and defects in collateral circulation. Impaired constriction of brain vessels allowing cerebral edema and not angiospasm causes hypertensive brain disease, in the opinion of Pickering.

INTERMITTENT CLAUDICATION.—It is not beyond the realm of possibility that regional vascular inadequacy may cause local ischemia when functional exaltation in one brain system or area calls for more blood than can be supplied at the time. Complete and immediate dependence of brain tissue on a constant provision of oxygen or glucose can account for a reversible cerebral deficit when the circulatory deficiency is partial or is complete although temporary.

SYSTEMIC CIRCULATORY FACTORS.—The frequent association of *heart disease* with ischemic brain infarction is becoming evident. Dozzi found that in a series of 107 cases of cerebrovascular accident, 12 patients had had unsuspected coronary occlusions. Fifteen of 100 patients with acute stroke examined by Race and Lisa had lesions in both heart and brain. Cerebral anoxia from shock was implicated. Cardiocirculatory insufficiency was revealed at autopsy in 83 per cent of all types of intracranial accident studied by Wilson et al., and massive cerebral infarction precipitated by coronary thrombosis was reported by Cole and Sugarman.

Acute or chronic systemic circulatory inadequacy caused by myocardial infarct, valvular stenosis or left ventricular failure can produce small, disseminated or large, diffuse encephalomalacic lesions in the cerebrum or cerebellum, with neurologic or psychiatric consequences. The delirium of cardiac failure (anoxia) and the convulsive seizures of the Stokes-Adams syndrome (heart block) may terminate in hemiplegia or death. Cardiac symptoms may be concealed by cerebral signs. Alvarez suggests that the hand-shoulder reflex dystrophy which sometimes follows a myocardial attack is really a form of thalamic hyperpathia due to a complicating cerebral ischemic focus.

Neurologic sequelae of brief syncopal episodes in the elderly have been described by Alvarez as *little strokes* or "strokelets." Most of these seizures are due to minute pontile or capsular infarcts, on the basis of severe atheromatous change and tortuosity in the basilar, carotid or middle cerebral arteries (Fig. 104). Minor ischemic lesions in the internal capsule, basal ganglions and elsewhere may coalesce into the clinical picture of parkinsonism or pseudobulbar palsy. Syncope resulting from a hypertensive carotid sinus reflex has caused hemiplegia and even death after external massage of the carotid artery or during a tonsillectomy.

Systemic *hypotension* of other etiology may also have its neurologic aftermath. Episodes of transient paresis are common in patients with greatly thickened cerebral vessels and chronically low blood pressure. Lima observed a patient with a verified thrombosis of one of the arteries of the sylvian group in whom intracranial hypertension and focal neurologic signs appeared whenever the blood pressure fell. All abnormalities cleared when the arterial tension rose again. Corday *et al.* found that experimental hypotensive cerebral changes were related to low blood pressure as such and not necessarily to anemia.

Tabes dorsalis, syringomyelia, thoracolumbar sympathectomy and the use of powerful ganglion blocking agents, such as hexamethonium, predispose to hypotensive infarction. Extensive and fatal anoxic brain lesions have followed prolonged and shock-producing surgical operations, particularly those performed in the sitting position. Symmetrical softenings occur in the parietal lobes when acutely lowered cerebral blood pressure is intolerable (Foix *et al.*).

Current reports indicate that planned surgical hypotension may be responsible for infarcts in the brain and heart. Reduction of blood pressure by caudal anesthesia in patients with arteriosclerotic and hypertensive brain disease not only does not improve their neurologic status but makes it worse (Russek and Zohman). Acute, brief drops of arterial tension induced in hypertensive patients aged 50 or over usually decrease cerebrovascular resistance while cerebral blood flow and metabolic rate remain the same, indicating compensatory intracranial vasodilatation (Bessman *et al.*). When such reduction of vascular tone does not occur, there exists a susceptibility to hypotensive stroke. The frequency with which ischemic cerebral infarct develops during sleep is probably related to the physiologic reduction of blood pressure.

Sudden, severe *blood loss* will accomplish the same deprivation of cerebral nutrition and may also produce cortical necrosis, chiefly parietal in location. This has occurred after venesection in the elderly and arteriosclerotic, and after attempted suicide by severance of the jugular vein. If cerebrovascular disease, hypertension or general debility pre-exist, only a moderate hemorrhage is necessary to bring on cerebral infarction. How-

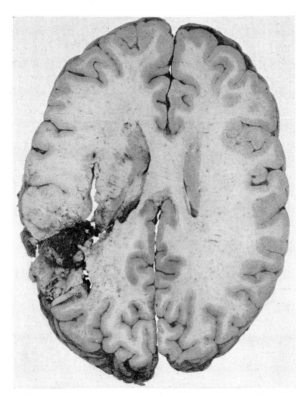

FIG. 37.—Hemorrhagic infarction. Catatonic schizophrenia.

ever, in the previously healthy patient, the total blood volume must be reduced severely to cause neurologic complications. Chronic *anemia* may be causally related to nonhemorrhagic stroke in older patients. Thompson and Mosberg have demonstrated that clipping of the anterior cerebral artery in the monkey is likely to be followed by paraplegia when the circulating blood volume is coincidentally acutely reduced but not if hypotension is produced instead by sympathetic blockade.

Miscellaneous conditions or circumstances in which cerebral infarction of either thrombotic or nonthrombotic type has occurred include migraine headache, exposure to heat, injection of a mercurial diuretic, postoperative or idiopathic thrombocytosis, the development of cold agglutinins after virus pneumonia, hemorrhage into the pituitary gland with compression of the anterior and middle cerebral arteries (Schnitker and Lehnert), and the acutely excited form of catatonic schizophrenia (Fig. 37).

Pathology

Most infarctions of nonocclusive etiology are of the white, ischemic, interior variety since collaterals are most lacking in perforating fields. Superficial, vasoparalytic softenings may be of the hemorrhagic kind.

SYMPTOMS AND SIGNS

The age group afflicted by cerebral thrombosis or nonthrombotic infarction of the brain is that from 50 to 80 years (average, 64 years), although occasionally younger persons are affected in special circumstances. The incidence is two to three times greater in men. About one third of patients have had previous cerebrovascular accidents. Many infarctive strokes tend to develop at rest. There is no seasonal incidence.

Prodromal symptoms, such as headache, vertigo, paresthesias and the like, occur in 10 per cent of patients with major infarctions but may constitute clinical manifestations of a "little stroke" in entirety. In general, the whole attack is less florid and devastating than is that of cerebral hemorrhage. Onset is often slow, sometimes over a period of hours and, rarely, days. Many patients remain entirely conscious throughout the episode, but coma develops in one-third. Convulsive seizures appear in about 10 per cent, particularly when syphilis is the cause or the lesion is near the motor cortex. Severe headache is rarely present but "spot pain" on the exterior of the head may be troublesome chronically. Vomiting is uncommon. The blood pressure is likely to be normal or exceptionally low, although hypertension does not rule out infarction by any means. Papilledema is extremely unusual and retinal hemorrhages are hardly ever seen, but sclerosed vessels are often visible in the eyegrounds.

Specific Arterial Syndromes

Neurologic symptoms and signs and other clinical phenomena characteristic of specific arterial syndromes depend on the location of parenchymal damage of the brain. Even when a particular artery is occluded there is lack of absolute consistency in the neurologic syndrome from case to case. This is due to anomalies of the cerebral circulation, comparative richness of basal and cortical anastomoses, dominance of certain brain areas, anatomic variations in fields of irrigation and the tendency of lesions in cerebral arteriosclerosis to be multiple. The overlap of functional representation in the cortex (Murphy and Gellhorn) likewise modifies the end result of local ischemia.

Carotid artery thrombosis

Arteriosclerosis is the commonest etiologic agent of carotid artery thrombosis although thromboangiitis obliterans and trauma may also be responsible. Carotid thrombosis is more common than present statistics would indicate, and there is little doubt that a number of cases of cerebral infarction without local arterial thrombosis are due to cervical occlusion. The proximal carotid artery is one of the places where the changes of atherosclerosis appear early in life, particularly in the interior of the carotid sinus. Thrombosis begins on ulcerated intima of the bifurcation and usually extends superiorly in the internal carotid for variable heights approaching the circle of Willis, sometimes into the ophthalmic artery. The common carotid may be occluded instead. In cases reported by Frøvig and by Takahashi the lumens of both common or internal carotids were completely obliterated, the patients existing with relatively few symptoms because of the basilar arterial supply alone.

Pathology.—The cervical carotid becomes a firm, pulseless cord. Fragments of clot may break off from the interior of the carotid sinus and cause cerebral embolism. The thrombus may be solid or may be recanalized, particularly with Buerger's disease. When brain infarction occurs, it follows the course of the middle cerebral artery and usually that of the anterior cerebral as well: sometimes the territory of the anterior choroidal vessel is included (Fisher). The frontal and temporal lobes are especially affected, or the whole hemisphere exclusive of the posterior cerebral distribution may become necrotic (Fig. 38).

Anastomoses.—The extent of cerebral damage is determined by the anastomotic properties of the circle of Willis and by the patency of the intracranial arteries themselves. Not only does blood reach the affected hemisphere from the opposite open carotid through the anterior communicating artery, owing to a reduction of pressure-head on the affected side, or from the vertebral-basilar system through the posterior communicating artery, but it can come through collateral connections between the external and internal carotids (Fig. 4). Such collaterals may sometimes be demonstrated by arteriography (Marx). The function of all these anastomotic connections may be so effective, particularly with slow obstruction of the internal carotid, that, as in surgical ligation of the vessel, no true infarction of the brain ever occurs. Indeed, Hultquist found gross changes in the cerebrum in only one third of carotid thrombosis patients.

Clinical syndromes.—Three different clinical patterns may be presented, each of which mimics occlusion of the anterior cerebral, middle

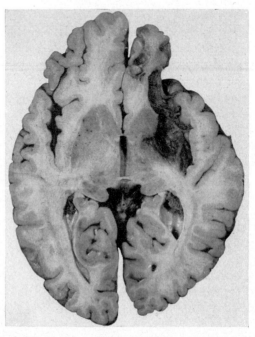

FIG. 38.—Fibrogliotic atrophy of cerebrum, right frontotemporal. Cervical carotid thrombosis. (Courtesy of M. Fisher.)

cerebral or anterior choroidal arteries (Johnson and Walker). (1) *Transient* attacks of headache, hemiparesis, paresthesias and aphasia often terminated by hemiplegia occur in 40 per cent of patients. The initial episode may precede final conclusion by months or even years. (2) *Sudden,* catastrophic onset of apoplectiform infarction with coma, hemiplegia and aphasia is the rule in 35 per cent of patients. (3) A *slowly progressive* course, featured by headaches which are severe and recur over a long period, contralateral sensory phenomena, convulsive seizures, mental regression and speech impairment, forms the syndrome in the other 25 per cent of patients presenting signs of cerebral ischemia.

The chief age group involved is that from 30 to 60 years, although King and Langworthy have reported carotid thrombosis in a 7 year old boy. The incidence in males outnumbers that in females, and the left carotid is involved more often than the right.

Pulsation of the internal or common carotid is often absent. Dunning suggests interior palpation of the posterolateral pharynx where the normal internal carotid throb is easily felt; if this is absent, the diagnosis is confirmed. Headache may be excruciating and migraine-like, is maximal above the eye on the affected side and is associated with tearing. Most often headache precedes or accompanies a hemiplegic attack. Periods of temporary blindness have been found to be associated with intraocular vasospasm (snow-white retina), and permanent amaurosis with optic atrophy may develop in the eye contralateral to the side of paralysis because of thrombotic occlusion of the ophthalmic artery (Walsh). The retinal blood pressure is low. Temporary digital occlusion of the uninvolved carotid will cause immediate syncope. This diagnostic maneuver is not recommended for fear of precipitating intracranial infarction.

Mental depression, insomnia, loss of memory, irritability and carelessness are common organic psychiatric symptoms. Fisher has suggested carotid thrombosis as an etiologic factor in senile dementia, having found narrowing or occlusion of one or both arteries in elderly psychotic patients. True epileptic seizures may alternate with episodes of exertional syncope. Persistent hemiplegia is usually profound, involves the arm much more than the leg and includes the face. Fractional additive paralysis, temporary or permanent, may precede total hemiplegia. Aphasia results from left-sided infarction and is expressive-receptive in mixture. There are usually evidences of arteriosclerosis or of thromboangiitis obliterans elsewhere in the body.

Anterior cerebral artery thrombosis

Complete occlusion of the anterior cerebral artery is rare, but obstruction of one or several of its branches is not uncommon. Closure of the vessel below the anterior communicating artery will not result in brain ischemia if the anterior communicating artery is patent, since one anterior cerebral artery will then supply the field of distribution of both. Just above the anastomosis, thrombosis of the main vessel will produce infarction of the anterosuperior frontal lobe, the anterior corpus callosum, the forward limb of the internal capsule and the medial surface of the cerebral hemisphere, including the paracentral lobule.

The neurologic syndrome (Critchley) includes mental disturbances, transient expressive aphasia (left side), apraxia of the arm, forced grasping and groping, paralysis and loss of sensation of the contralateral leg, arm or face and lack of control of the urinary bladder (Fig. 39). Beyond the ganglionic branches, obstruction of the artery causes only weakness of the lower extremity. Should one anterior cerebral artery supply the medial surface of both hemispheres, thrombosis will cause paraplegia because of infarction of the two paracentral lobules.

Medial striate artery thrombosis

Heubner's artery is an inconstant, recurrent branch of the anterior cerebral artery, which may replace the lenticulostriate artery of Charcot, running to the basal ganglions and the anterior limb of the internal capsule (Fig. 8). Occlusion of the medial striate artery results in paralysis of the face and arm, more severe proximally than distally in the extremity (Nielsen).

Anterior choroidal artery thrombosis

This vessel supplies a portion of the posterior limb of the capsule and the mesencephalon (Fig. 8). Infarction in its distribution results in contralateral hemiplegia and hemianesthesia, without aphasia or coma; contralateral hemianopsia which may be complete or only involve the upper quadrants; vasomotor changes, including edema, and partial thalamic sensory disturbances, especially in the arm (Steegman and Roberts). The syndrome resembles that of obstruction of the middle cerebral artery but is less severe and the prognosis for recovery is much better. Therapeutic ligation of the anterior choroidal artery, performed in Parkinson's disease, is said to leave no permanent hemiplegia, hemianesthesia or visual field defect (Cooper).

Middle cerebral artery thrombosis

Infarctions in the distribution of the middle cerebral artery represent 65–75 per cent of the total number of such lesions in the brain. Softenings are superficial in location in 50 per cent of cases, deep in 30 per cent and of mixed locale in 20 per cent. True thrombosis is notable in its absence.

Main artery thrombosis.—Occlusion of the primary trunk of the middle cerebral artery results in encephalomalacia of the bulk of one cerebral hemisphere, only the fields of irrigation of the anterior and

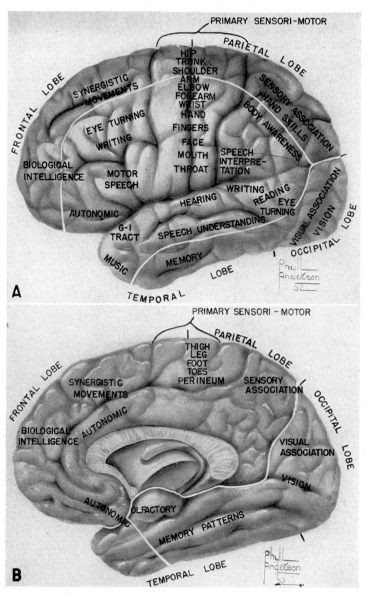

FIG. 39.—Cortical localization maps. *A,* lateral surface of cerebral hemisphere, showing areas supplied by anterior cerebral *(upper rim),* middle cerebral *(center)* and posterior cerebral *(lower rim)* arteries. *B,* medial surface of cerebral hemisphere, with distribution of anterior cerebral *(upper left),* posterior cerebral *(lower right)* and middle cerebral *(lower left tip)* arteries.

147

posterior cerebral arteries being preserved (Fig. 40). Changes are maximal on the surface along the sylvian fissure and interiorly in the basal
ganglions and internal capsule. Actual closure is more common in branch
vessels; lesions are not infrequently multiple and even symmetrical in the
two hemispheres.

The clinical syndrome of complete occlusion or softening is made up
of mental confusion and somnolence; hemiplegia with voluntary paralysis of the lower face and arm contralaterally but usually with only
severe paresis of the leg; an increase of deep reflexes after the state of

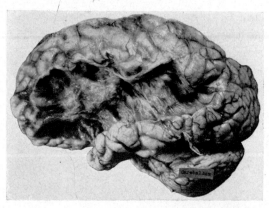

FIG. 40.—Atrophy of cerebral hemisphere after occlusion of middle cerebral artery.
(AFIP #L 4955-2.)

shock has passed away and a loss of superficial reflexes; the appearance
of pathologic reflex signs (Babinski and Hoffmann); loss or decrease of
all forms of sensation on the hemiplegic side; vasomotor changes in the
paralyzed limbs; complete contralateral hemianopsia with macular splitting, and global aphasia (Fig. 39). Sparing of the leg in hemiplegia is
probably due to continued nutrition of the medial hemisphere through
the anterior cerebral artery, blood coming from the ipsilateral or contralateral carotid artery. Anosgnosia, a term applied to denial of disease or
lack of recognition of paralyzed extremities, may be present if infarction
of the parietal lobe, especially in the right hemisphere, is severe.

Ganglionic thrombosis.—Encephalomalacia in the domain of the ganglionic derivatives of the middle cerebral artery, particularly the lenticulostriate arteries, will include the lenticular nuclei, internal capsule and
the white matter of the pre- and postcentral convolutions to some extent
(Fig. 8). The syndrome is comprised of initially severe hemiplegia which

may recover remarkably, hemisensory loss and hemianopsia of varying degrees and aphasia of a transient character. Multiple ganglionic occlusions produce the pathologic change described by Pierre Marie as *état lacunaire,* in which tiny necrotic cysts form around small vessels in the basal ganglions, the capsule and thalamus (Fig. 104). Serial thromboses in this region represent one type of "little stroke." Shuffling gait, parkinsonism and emotional overactivity are the clinical consequences.

Cortical thrombosis.—Infarctions in the territory of small cortical branches of the middle cerebral artery are often responsible for isolated cerebral functional disorders, such as alexia, agraphia, agnosia, apraxia and word deafness, or account for the appearance of epileptogenic foci of inveterate nature.

Communicating artery thrombosis

Thromboses restricted to the anterior or posterior communicating arteries of the circle of Willis are apparently without neurologic consequence, although medial ganglionic arterioles originating from these arteries are distributed to basal forebrain nuclei, to adjacent tracts and to the midbrain (Fig. 8).

Posterior cerebral artery thrombosis

This vessel and its area of distribution are involved in 10–15 per cent of all cases of cerebral infarction. A rapid fall of blood pressure sometimes causes symmetrical necrosis of the occipital poles in the elderly. Transtentorial herniation of the temporal lobe, a result of sudden hemispheral expansion or compression, will pinch off the posterior cerebral artery against the tentorium as it winds around the mesencephalon. Both the posterior and the middle cerebral arteries may be occluded simultaneously. However, strong anastomoses with the two other main arterial trunks often restrict infarction in the posterior cerebral field to a minimum.

Complete occlusion.—Obstruction of the main posterior cerebral artery renders ischemic the medial and inferior occipital lobe, the undersurface of the temporal lobe and a large part of the thalamus and the pes pedunculi (Figs. 39 and 52). The typical syndrome includes contralateral homonymous hemianopsia, usually with macular sparing, cortical blindness or visual agnosia, alexia, sensory aphasia, loss of feeling in and clumsiness of the opposite side of the body and a contralateral weakness and hypertonia (Foix and Masson).

Calcarine thrombosis.—Thrombosis of the calcarine branch of the posterior cerebral artery will effect isolated hemianopsia. If the terminal twig above the calcarine fissure is occluded, inferior quadrantanopsia results, whereas if the twig below the fissure is obstructed superior quadrantanopsia is found. Macular sparing in all instances is ascribed to collateral supply of the fissure from the middle cerebral artery or to bilateral representation of macular fibers.

Thalamic syndrome.—Occlusion of the thalamogeniculate arterial derivative of the posterior cerebral artery (Fig. 8) results in the thalamic syndrome of Déjerine-Roussy. This syndrome is featured by temporary flaccid hemiparesis, immediate complete hemianesthesia involving all mo-

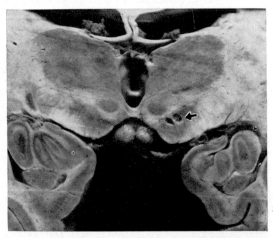

FIG. 41.—Cystic infarct in subthalamic body of Luys. Clinical hemiballismus. (Courtesy of F. P. Moersch and J. W. Kernohan.)

dalities of sensation and partial or complete return of superficial sensibility while vibratory and position sense remain absent. Aggravating sequelae are "thalamic hyperpathia," a constant, burning pain in the insensible or partially anesthetic areas of the body, and reflex dystrophy of the shoulder girdle and arm.

Hemiballismus.—Infarction in the territory of the thalamoperforating artery (from the posterior cerebral or posterior communicating arteries) injures the anterolateral thalamus, the cerebellorubrothalamic and pallidothalamic fibers and the subthalamic body of Luys (Fig. 41). The rare syndrome of hemiballismus results. This is a particularly violent type of unilateral chorea, which exhausts and may kill the patient when functions of the face, speech, swallowing and respiration are included (Moersch and Kernohan).

Posterior choroidal artery.—Occlusion of the posterior choroidal artery results in loss of the contralateral lower homonymous half-fields of vision.

Thrombosis in the midbrain

Mesencephalic infarctions may be severely disabling and can present a host of neurologic signs when occlusion of a small perforating vessel

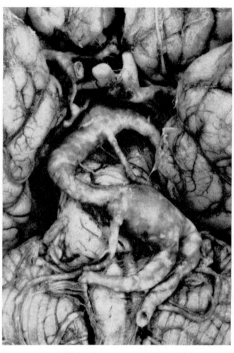

FIG. 42.—Basilar artery thrombosis. Note tortuosity of vessel and stretching of branches. (Courtesy of J. C. Richardson and H. H. Hyland.)

causes destruction of even a few cubic millimeters of tissue. Not only are many functionally important nuclei, afferent sensory and efferent motor tracts packed tightly together in the midbrain, but there is little anastomotic circulation among the mesencephalic arterioles and none across the midline. The blood supply is obtained from all regional arteries via an interpenduncular plexus (Fig. 12).

Weber's syndrome consists of ipsilateral oculomotor paralysis and contralateral hemiplegia due to involvement of the third nerve nucleus and adjacent pyramidal tract. In *Benedikt's syndrome* there are homolateral oculomotor paralysis, gross spontaneous tremor and contralateral paresis. The lesion affects the red nucleus, the neighboring fibers of the third nerve and the cerebral peduncle. The *syndrome of Claude,* consisting of oculomotor palsy and hemiataxia of the opposite extremities, is due to injury of the third nerve complex and the cerebellorubrothalamic system.

Basilar artery thrombosis

Thrombosis of the basilar artery accounts for 10 per cent of nonhemorrhagic strokes. Occlusion may be primary in the main trunk or may begin in the posterior inferior cerebellar or vertebral arteries and then extend superiorly. Syphilis or atherosclerosis are usually causative (Fig. 42). Although infarction destroys much of the pons, caudal mesencephalon and cerebellar vermis, the pontile tegmentum may be spared because of collateral circulation from the carotid via the posterior communicating, posterior cerebral and thence the superior cerebellar arteries.

The typical syndrome is characterized by drowsiness or coma, fleeting blindness or hemianopsia, miosis and extraocular palsies, bilateral complete paralysis (tetraplegia), dysarthria and dysphagia, sensory changes on the face and body, and decerebrate rigidity or tonic extensor spasms. Most patients with complete basilar occlusion die quickly. Syncopal, bradycardiac or vertiginous attacks often precede final thrombosis. Occasionally a patient may survive.

Pontile syndromes.—When the blood supply of the pontile tegmentum (Fig. 13) is interrupted, the medial longitudinal fasciculus is destroyed. The result is the *syndrome of Foville,* in which conjugate gaze to the side of the lesion is lost and convergence is preserved (Fig. 43). Infarction of the nucleus of the seventh nerve and of the pyramidal tract results in crossed paralysis of face and extremities, with or without lateral rectus weakness, comprising the *syndrome of Millard-Gubler.* The *Claude-Bernard-Horner syndrome* may appear with infarctions anywhere from the superior brain stem to the upper thoracic spinal cord. In this symptom complex the homolateral cervical sympathetic outflow is severed, with consequent constriction of the pupil, enophthalmos, drooping of the eyelid, congestion and a lack of sweating in one-half the head and arm on the same side.

Other specific manifestations of injury in the pontile tegmentum include ipsilateral facial sensory loss, deafness, cerebellar signs, contralateral hemisensory deficit and palatal myoclonus (Freeman *et al.*).

"Little strokes".—Cystic lesions in the pons are among the commonest neuropathologic findings in the brains of persons with sclerosing vascular

disease. Clinical features of occlusive episodes are fainting spells with neurologic residuals, Ménière-like attacks of atypical presentation or minor weaknesses and paresthesias. Abdominal complaints, personality change and even irrational behavior may also be significant manifestations. The succession of small infarctions is a slow, inexorable mecha-

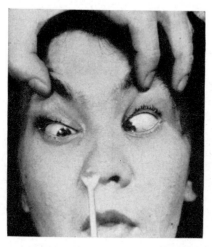

FIG. 43.—Foville's syndrome. (Courtesy of W. Freeman.)

nism of eventual fatality; a patient of Alvarez said to him, "Death keeps taking little bites of me."

Anterior inferior cerebellar artery thrombosis

The anterior inferior cerebellar artery has so many anastomoses that occlusion of this vessel is usually asymptomatic. When collateral connections are not present, thrombosis results in infarction of the lateral tegmental area of the pons and of the middle and inferior cerebellar peduncles, the flocculus and the undersurface of the hemisphere of the cerebellum (Fig. 13). Clinical syndromes include ipsilateral cerebellar asynergy, Horner's syndrome, deafness, loss of pain and temperature sensation and diminution of light touch on the face; and contralateral, incomplete reduction of pain and temperature appreciation on the body.

Superior cerebellar artery thrombosis

The superior cerebellar artery supplies the superior and middle cerebellar peduncles, the superior surface as well as all interior nuclei of the cerebellum and the lateral pontile tegmentum (Fig. 13). After occlusion, signs include homolateral ataxia, choreiform movements, Horner's syndrome, loss of hearing and nystagmus; and contralateral loss of pain and temperature sensibility over face and body, partial deafness and facial weakness.

Posterior inferior cerebellar artery thrombosis

Thrombosis of the posterior inferior cerebellar artery is much commoner than involvement of either of the other two principal arteries to

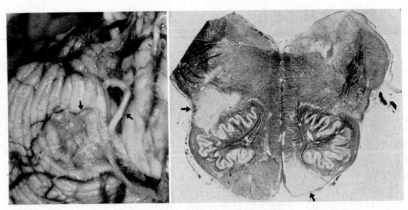

FIG. 44 *(left)*.—Arteriosclerotic thrombosis of posterior inferior cerebellar artery (arrow, right) with cerebellar infarction (arrow, left). (George Washington University Laboratory of Neurology.)

FIG. 45 *(right)*.—Infarction of descending root of trigeminal nerve (arrow, left), Wallenberg syndrome. Atrophy of medullary pyramid (arrow, right), old capsular hemiplegia.

the hindbrain. This important vessel irrigates the inferior cerebellar peduncle (restiform body), the lateral tegmentum of the medulla, especially the retro-olivary space, and the inferior surface of the vermis and adjacent cerebellar cortex (Fig. 14).

With obstruction of the posterior inferior cerebellar artery (Figs. 44 and 45) there result ipsilateral cerebellar ataxia, Horner's syndrome, loss of pain and temperature but preservation of light touch on the face, dysphagia and dysphonia. Contralaterally, pain and temperature sensibilities are absent on the body below the face and pyramidal signs may also be present. This symptom complex is called the *Wallenberg syndrome*. Foix and associates objected to attributing the syndrome to occlusion of the posterior inferior cerebellar artery and offered cogent evidence that thrombosis of the "artery of the lateral fissure of the bulb" or anterior inferior cerebellar vessel is often responsible instead.

Vertebral artery thrombosis

Not far different from the Wallenberg syndrome is the *syndrome of Babinski-Nageotte* which is ascribed to occlusion of the vertebral artery at the point of emptying into the basilar trunk. There occur ipsilateral hemiasynergia, lateropulsion, miosis and palatal paresis and contralateral hemiplegia and hemianesthesia.

The sequelae of occlusion of one or more of the paramedian branches of the vertebral arteries depend on the extent of infarction of the lower cranial nerve nuclei, the cerebellar connections and the sensory and motor tracts in the brain stem (Fig. 15). Paralysis and atrophy of the homolateral tongue and hemiplegia and sensory loss on the opposite side of the body commonly appear, with clinical signs added or subtracted according to the exact location of the lesions.

Specific paramedian syndromes include that of *Avellis,* which comprises ipsilateral paresis of soft palate and vocal cord and contralateral loss of pain and temperature sensation in the trunk and extremities. The *syndrome of Cestan-Chenais,* with paralysis of the homolateral palate, vocal cord and cervical sympathetics and of the opposite arm and leg may appear, as may *Schmidt's syndrome,* also expressive of a medullary infarction, which is restricted to pareses of the palate, the vocal cord and the sternocleidomastoid and trapezius muscles all on the same side. (*Vernet's complex,* an impairment of function of the ninth, tenth and eleventh cranial nerves, is usually found with lesions of the jugular foramen, and *Villaret's syndrome,* a paralysis of the ninth through the twelfth nerves and of the cervical sympathetics, is most often due to involvement of the retroparotid space.)

Anterior spinal artery thrombosis

Occlusion of the anterior spinal artery near its origin results in partial destruction of the ipsilateral pyramid, the medial lemniscus, the ventral portion of the inferior olivary body and fibers of the hypoglossal nerve. There occur, contralaterally, pyramidal signs in arm and leg and loss of discriminative ability. Where the two anterior spinal arteries join on the undersurface of the medulla oblongata, thrombosis usually obstructs both vessels. Bilateral involvement of pyramidal tracts and posterior columns results. Impairment of stereognostic sensibility in the presence of posterior fossa tumors is often due to interference with arterial supply as the cerebellar tonsils herniate downward.

LABORATORY STUDIES

The white blood cell count in cerebral thrombosis is ordinarily much lower than that in cerebral hemorrhage, although it may reach 12,000 per cu. mm. or slightly higher and can exceed 20,000 if infarction is

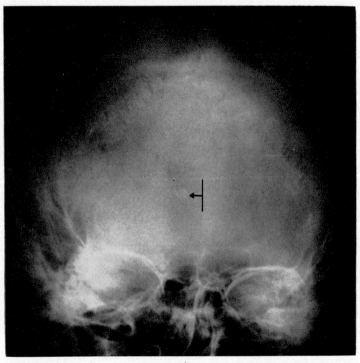

FIG. 46.—Lateral displacement of pineal gland to the right after thrombosis of left internal carotid artery.

massive. Anemia of acute or chronic type may be associated with non-hemorrhagic stroke.

Abnormalities of urinalysis may correspond to diabetic or nephritic disease, as may changes in blood chemistry. The blood pressure can be at any level but is normal or low more often than elevated.

CEREBROSPINAL FLUID.—Cerebrospinal fluid pressures were below 200 in 78 per cent of 500 patients examined by Merritt and Aring. In 90 per cent the specimens were clear and in 10 per cent xanthochromic.

With brain swelling and displacement the lumbar pressure rises, and when an infarct is largely hemorrhagic the fluid may be pink or darker red but it is never as bloody as that in cerebral or subarachnoid hemorrhage. The protein content may rise, though seldom above 100 mg. per 100 ml. Cells in the cerebrospinal fluid are increased in number in 10 per cent of patients. Very rarely, ventricular infarction may augment the cerebrospinal fluid cellular concentration to as much as 10,000–30,000 per cu. mm. (cloudy fluid). Colloidal gold curves are often midzonal in type.

ROENTGENOLOGY.—X-rays of the skull sometimes show calcification of the intracranial carotid (Fig. 105). The pineal gland, if visible, may

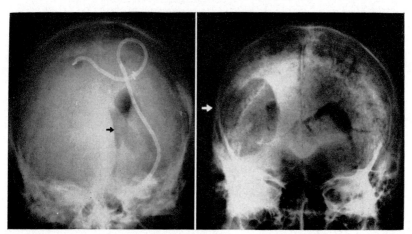

FIG. 47 *(left)*.—Ventricular shift due to massive cerebral infarction. (Courtesy of A. B. King.)

FIG. 48 *(right)*.—Porencephalic cyst, the probable result of fetal thrombosis.

be displaced laterally with a hemispheric infarct of large size (Fig. 46). Cervical roentgenograms may reveal calcification of the carotid sinus. Thickening of the skull vault, overdevelopment of the paranasal sinuses and comparative smallness of hemicranial volume are late bony evidences of infantile cerebral hemiplegia.

Encephalograms and *ventriculograms* disclose lateral ventricular enlargement and cortical atrophy, particularly in carotid or middle cerebral occlusion. In other chronic vascular syndromes, hydrocephalus ex vacuo and widening of the subarachnoid spaces parallel general ischemic brain atrophy (Fig. 106). Local deformations or dilatations correspond to specific parenchymal damage. In acute major infarction, air studies may simulate those of brain tumor (Fig. 47). Porencephaly or a grossly enlarged ventricle may be a late aftermath of infantile or juvenile febrile thrombosis (Fig. 48). With hemispheral atrophy, there is a shift of the septum pellucidum and third ventricle toward the side of the lesion.

Arteriography can establish the diagnosis with certainty, but risks from this procedure in a patient with degenerative vascular disease must be calculated. Good cervical films must be taken, because only in this way may thrombosis of the common or internal carotid artery be visualized. In the latter instance, the internal carotid is usually seen as a short stump

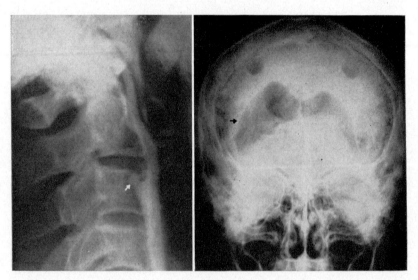

FIG. 49.—Thrombosis of cervical internal carotid artery. *Left,* arteriogram showing stump of vessel in the neck; *right,* ipsilateral ventricular dilatation. (Courtesy of H. C. Johnson and A. E. Walker.)

arising from the bifurcation, the external vessels filling alone (Fig. 49). Obstruction of the internal carotid may also be found in the siphon (Fig. 50). Intracranial branches may fill late through communicating channels, particularly the ophthalmic artery (Marx). Contralateral carotid injection will visualize both sets of anterior and middle cerebral arteries, but this procedure has caused death in patients with cervical thrombosis.

The consistent absence of the middle cerebral artery in lateral films may be interpreted as a true confirmation of thrombosis (Fig. 54); scanty branching indicates stenosis, advanced sclerosis or fractional occlusion (Fig. 107). Failure to visualize the anterior cerebral artery does not have the same significance, however, for on repeated arteriograms this vessel is often revealed. The posterior cerebral artery is seen in only 25 per cent of standard carotid angiograms; however, it is almost always visualized when a rapid, multiple exposure technic is used.

Injection of the cervical vertebral artery is necessary to reveal the vertebral-basilar circulation and to confirm or deny the diagnosis of major infratentorial thrombosis. This is seldom undertaken, since the risks to life and function are great and clinical confusion between vascular and neoplastic conditions of the posterior fossa is uncommon.

RADIOACTIVE STUDIES.—Injection of radioactive diiodofluorescein and subsequent Geiger recording of emanations from the head has been

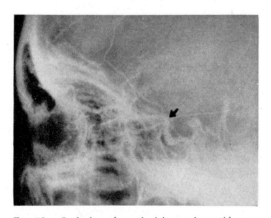

FIG. 50.—Occlusion of terminal internal carotid artery.

found by Ashkenazy and collaborators to aid in differentiating cerebral infarct from tumor. In 95 per cent of non-neoplastic cases, cerebral thrombosis included, the dye is not concentrated in the lesion as it is in intracranial growths. The procedure is said to offer no particular hazard in the presence of cerebrovascular disease.

ELECTROENCEPHALOGRAPHY

A cerebral infarct must involve the cortex to produce more than a minor, rapidly disappearing electroencephalographic abnormality. Small and purely capsular lesions may be entirely negative electroencephalographically. With extensive cerebral thrombosis there are focal, hemispheral or generalized delta (slow wave) activity and reduction of amplitude or disappearance of alpha waves on the side of the lesion (Fig. 51). Frontal slow waves may appear acutely, to be replaced in a few days by a more appropriate focus (Cohn *et al.*). When the middle cerebral artery was occluded in dogs by Epstein and co-workers, prominent slow wave production was picked up at the boundaries of large lesions, whereas electrical activity was decreased in the midzone. The site of injury determines the effect on the amplitude of alpha waves; the closer infarction lies to the place of alpha origin in the posterior parietal or parieto-occipital region, the greater the suppression of 8–12 per second waves and the reduction of their height. Porencephalic lesions presumably due to fetal thrombosis show flattening of potential ipsilaterally.

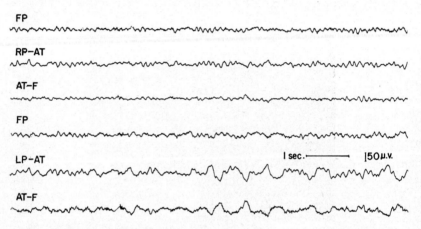

FP

RP–AT

AT–F

FP

LP–AT   I sec.————— |50 µ.v.

AT–F

FIG. 51.—Fresh cerebral infarction, left, with continuous irregular delta activity from left anterior temporal lead in channels 5 and 6.

In 55 per cent of 95 patients with strokes studied by Strauss and Greenstein the electroencephalogram was normal. In 29.5 per cent there were various types of delta activity, and in 15.5 per cent abnormal asymmetry of alpha waves. In all persons with clouding of consciousness there is a slowing of the electroencephalogram, and in most patients with focal delta in their records there is accurate correspondence to the anatomic location of the lesion. In sleep tracings, Cress and Gibbs noted absence of 14 per second spindles (normal during somnolence) on the affected side in all cases, a finding also true in experimental infarction.

In serial studies, Cohn and collaborators found that slow waves tend to disappear as the clinical course stabilizes after cerebral infarction. This restitution is most likely to occur in patients age 40 or younger. Although there is often little correlation of the electroencephalographic abnormality with the degree of neurologic involvement at the onset of illness, the more severe and persistent electrical changes are prognostic of a long hospital stay and severe residual disability (Van Buskirk and Zarling).

Rapid resolution of delta activity has been noted two to five days after episodes of cerebral vasospasm (Roseman *et al.*). Focal slow waves may increase at first with thrombotic lesions, owing to cerebral edema, but they begin to recede at the end of two weeks and are usually completely resolved by the third month after the cerebrovascular accident. Amplitude asymmetry also changes with the passage of time; voltage increases after slow activity has disappeared. Six months must pass before permanent stability of amplitude can be said to be achieved.

Thrombosis vs. tumor.—A particularly helpful role of electroencephalography is in the distinction of cerebral thrombosis from brain tumor. Patients in the middle and older age groups are subject to both non-hemorrhagic stroke and infiltrative glioma, and the differential diagnosis is often difficult. Strauss and Greenstein found that focal delta favors neoplasm over thrombosis in a ratio of 8:1, although they do not believe that there is any type of pattern specific for either. When infiltrative glioma and cerebral infarction records were compared, we found *inconstant,* irregular slow discharges, regional with the lesion, in 86 per cent of tumor patients, whereas irregular slow waves of *constant* appearance were present in 70 per cent of those with thromboses (Murphy and Duggins). Further, baseline sway was seen in 36 per cent of glioma records; fast, spiky activity was evident in 36 per cent of vascular cases.

The taking of repeated tracings can be a simple, innocuous and informative method of following a patient in whom differential diagnosis is difficult. Clearing or stabilizing of electrical abnormality indicates a vascular cause of hemiplegia or other neurologic sign, whereas repeated records obtained during the course of growth of an infiltrative glioma will almost always show progression in and focalizing of abnormality, often in a surprisingly short time.

Specific EEG syndromes.—Electroencephalographic changes vary in frequency with thrombotic lesions above the tentorium; infarctions in the brain stem and cerebellum are electrically silent. Specific cerebral artery occlusions will produce corresponding alterations in the electroencephalogram. After thrombosis of the *internal carotid,* when neurologic disability is evident, high-voltage slow waves appear in the frontotemporal leads (Elvidge and Werner), or there is a marked hemispherical dysrhythmia. Uncomplicated occlusion of the cervical carotid artery, as in successful ligation for congenital aneurysm, is not followed by electroencephalographic changes. Generally, the effects of *middle cerebral* infarction are manifested in temporal, frontal and parietal tracings in that order. *Anterior cerebral* thrombosis is revealed, if at all, frontally, infrafrontally and in the central (parietal) lead, and *posterior cerebral* occlusion causes slowing in occipital and parietal recordings.

DIAGNOSIS

The patient with a nonhemorrhagic stroke is usually 50–70 years of age or older and is most often male. Arteriosclerosis, diabetes and syphilis are common predisposing conditions. Three of every 10 patients have had a previous cerebrovascular accident. The episode is likely to occur at rest or at night, almost always without warning. Onset is frequently slow and fractional. Consciousness is retained in two thirds of the patients. Headache is rarely severe. Convulsions develop in 8 per cent. Vomiting is uncommon. The blood pressure is not necessarily elevated; in fact, it is normal or low twice as often as it is high. Retinal vascular sclerosis is the only abnormality to be anticipated in the eyegrounds. Neurologic findings correspond to the size of infarction.

X-rays of the skull may be normal, may reveal calcification of the basal carotid or, rarely, may demonstrate shift of the (calcified) pineal gland. The cerebrospinal fluid is clear, the cell count is increased only slightly if at all, the protein content is above 100 mg. per 100 ml. only exceptionally and the gold curve is flat or of the midzone type. Air studies may disclose brain swelling in the acute phase, local or general atrophy in the chronic state or may be normal. Arteriograms may reveal the site and degree of obstruction, may show narrowed vessels or with small lesions may appear unmodified.

Electroencephalographic abnormalities, when present, consist of focal or hemispherical slow activity, regional with brain injury, and a reduction of amplitude of alpha waves on the affected side. This is most apt to be true of cerebral infarctions extending to the cortex and is less characteristic of subcortical lesions; infarcts below the tentorium are negative electrically.

DIFFERENTIAL DIAGNOSIS.—Cerebral *hemorrhage* is distinguishable from thrombosis chiefly by the almost invariable presence of hypertension, a dramatic onset of stroke, the frequency of severe headache and coma, the profundity of neurologic disability and the common finding of bloody cerebrospinal fluid under increased pressure. Cerebral *embolism* occurs in the presence of a source of embolic material (cardiac disorders) in younger people, with previous or associated bouts of embolism in the brain or elsewhere in the body. Episodes are of fulminating onset and are neurologically severe; the accompanying headache is extreme. Cerebrospinal fluid is xanthochromic, bloody or cloudy (septic embolus). Cerebral *vasospasm* accounts for brief, evanescent attacks of neurologic deficit in the absence of most objective laboratory confirmations of organic brain disease, and it sometimes occurs as a part of a general disorder known to be spasmogenic. *Subarachnoid hemorrhage* lives up to its name, and oculomotor signs of congenital aneurysm are often present.

Cerebral *arteriosclerosis* without major complication is a pervasive syndrome of deterioration, with multiple chronic neurologic signs which are often the compendium of diffusely scattered "little strokes." In *primary brain tumor* there is slow development with interspersed episodes. Evidences of increased intracranial pressure are manifest, the cerebrospinal fluid protein concentration is elevated and gold curves are often abnormal. Electroencephalographic changes are progressive. *Metastatic neoplasm* comes from another source and is frequently but not always productive of intracranial hypertension. Tumor cells may be shed into the cerebrospinal fluid, and x-rays of the chest often reveal a primary bronchogenic origin or pulmonary metastases.

Hypertensive encephalopathy is a crisis in the course of malignant nephrosclerosis, and clinical stigmas are principally those of acute cerebral edema. *Traumatic* brain disease, such as epidural or subdural hematoma and cerebral laceration, results from head injury. *Epileptic* attacks are usually self-limited episodes on a lengthy clinical background. *Metabolic coma* is demonstrated in characteristic alterations of the blood chemistry and urine. *Drug poisoning* comes to light in the analyses of gastric contents, blood and urine.

TREATMENT

MEDICAL THERAPY.—General medical and nursing care, so important in the management of the confused, crippled and sometimes unconscious patient who has sustained a cerebral infarct, are discussed in Chapter 19.

The heart must be supported if there is any question of cardiac failure. Chronically low blood pressure, a potential cause of stroke, may be elevated by administration of Paredrine, ephedrine or amphetamine or, if postural in appearance, may be prevented by an abdominal support. Hyperactive carotid sinuses should be denervated or treated by roentgen irradiation. If the patient is at all anemic, blood transfusion may have a prompt and salutary effect. Specific antianemic treatment should follow.

Vasodilators, other drugs.—The use of vasodilators and other substances is predicated on an assumption that intracranial angiospasm is at least contributory to ischemic brain deficit. Administration of 5–7 per cent carbon dioxide in a mixture of oxygen not above 75 per cent partial concentration is physiologically ideal but usually needs to be supplemented.

Papaverine, given intravenously or intramuscularly in 0.065–0.13 Gm. amounts has been proved to lower cerebrovascular resistance and to increase cerebral blood flow. Histamine intravenously may relieve vasospasm and open up collaterals. Repeated treatments will give a favorable clinical response. A dilute solution, prepared by adding 2.75 mg. to 250 cc. of normal saline solution, is administered at a rate of 32 drops per minute. Care must be taken not to lower systemic blood pressure drastically (patient supine), and Benadryl and Adrenalin must be available to counteract an anaphylactic reaction. Oral nicotinic acid, 100–300 mg. three times daily, may be beneficial. Nitrites in the form of amyl nitrite as an inhalant or nitroglycerin sublingually will relieve angiocontraction temporarily.

Use of sympathicolytic ganglion blocking agents should be reserved for cases of fairly definite vasospastic origin. Infarction can be increased by the powerful general hypotensive action of these drugs. Although aminophylline has been proved to increase cerebrovascular resistance and slow cerebral blood flow, its use in stroke with cardiac failure or Cheyne-Stokes respiration is still justified, since it stimulates the respiratory center directly. Iodides by mouth or vein are an old and valuable remedy, and intravenous administration of trypsin may prove helpful (Innerfield et al.).

Anticoagulant therapy.—Propagation of intracranial arterial thrombosis is uncommon, but it does occur in at least three particular sets of circumstances. The first is cervical carotid thrombosis, the second is extension of thrombotic occlusion into the brain from an aneurysm of the circle of Willis and the third is progressive occlusion of the basilar artery. The use of anticoagulant drugs is permitted in these peculiar situations. Enthusiastic reports concerning the success of anticoagulants in *all* patients with cerebral infarction are exaggerated and unjustified. Furthermore, there is a definite danger of converting an anemic infarct into a hemorrhagic one or of causing further bleeding if brain damage is already complicated by extravasation.

SURGICAL THERAPY.—*Stellate block.*—The value of stellate procaine nerve block in the treatment of thrombotic infarction remains a matter of debate, although statistics argue in favor of the procedure, good results having been obtained in over one-half the reported cases. There is the supportable contention that some patients who improve after stellate block were going to do so anyway (Millikan *et al.*). Although no increase of total blood flow has been found after bilateral stellate block (Scheinberg), the possibility of local increase in circulation in any small area of the brain is not eliminated thereby.

The only hope of relief from symptoms and signs of cerebral ischemia by the use of sympathetic nerve block is through the revival of ganglion cells lying in the border zone of angiospasm which are not yet necrotic. It is evident that such restitution of function is more possible than had been supposed (Fig. 30). There is no infallible method of determining the exact extent of salvageable reserve in any area of the brain. The theoretic possibility of worsening brain injury by draining blood from areas already ischemic when normal channels are opened further is not evidenced clinically. Aside from technical complications, stellate block has not made any patient worse neurologically. There is therefore little to lose and a great deal of possible potential gain in using stellate block in patients with cerebral infarction.

Risteen and Volpitto who performed 3,000 stellate injections in 275 patients, observed that most patients with cerebral thrombosis were able to walk thereafter. In two instances of posterior inferior cerebellar artery occlusion, symptoms disappeared immediately after blockade. Amyes and Perry observed clearing of electroencephalographic abnormalities after stellate block in five of seven patients. In Naffziger and Adams' series 59 per cent of 155 patients with vasospasm, embolism and thrombosis had complete recovery and an additional 24 per cent were partially improved.

Cervical sympathectomy.—A further development of stellate anesthesia, cervical sympathectomy, is also being applied to the problems of cerebral thrombosis. A definite decrease of cerebrovascular resistance after bilateral stellectomy has been confirmed by Shenkin and collaborators. Pereira suggests that sympathectomy may be in order when improvement occurs repeatedly after stellate blocks but is not maintained.

Corréa de Barros found that the diastolic blood pressure in the central retinal artery, reduced ipsilaterally following cerebral thrombosis, is elevated to normal after bilateral cervical ganglionectomy. Gardner's opinion is that sympathetic removal is not superior to local anesthetic block in immediate effects but probably wards off future attacks of infarction.

Arterial resection.—Operating on the theory expressed by Babinski that an "obliterated artery is a sympathetic nerve," Leriche resected throm-bosed portions of the common, internal and external carotid arteries when cervical occlusion was responsible for cerebral ischemia. Favorable re-sponses have also been reported by others (Krayenbühl). Reichert advo-cates extirpation of diseased vessels from brain scars and encephalomalacic foci. Learmonth advises preliminary sympathectomy and end-to-end su-ture of external to internal carotid when the region of the carotid bifur-cation is removed for thrombosis or tumor. Replacement of a resected artery by an autogenous femoral or saphenous vein graft may be at-tempted to restore carotid circulation (Conley).

Endarteriectomy (dos Santos), in which thrombus and surrounding intima are removed, has also been undertaken with benefit in some cases of carotid occlusion. Since recanalization of thrombus in the carotid is fairly certain to occur, there may be little point in resection. It is so difficult to evaluate late results in strokes, treated and untreated, that judgment as to the efficacy of arteriectomy must be reserved at present.

Myopexy.—Experimental studies by German and Taffel demonstrated that new collateral channels to the ischemic cortex can be induced by the attachment of pedicled muscle grafts (temporal, suboccipital). This tech-nic of "myopexy" has been applied by Kredel to patients with cerebral infarction in the chronic state. Of 35 patients so treated, one-half seemed to have benefited, as manifested by increased neurologic function and cessation of convulsive seizures. This form of surgical therapy is obviously *sub judice.*

Physiotherapy.—The value of modern physiotherapy in the re-habilitation of the patient with subacute or chronic cerebral infarction is inestimable. It is not an exaggeration to state that almost any patient with post-thrombotic hemiplegia can be taught at least to walk again. Assist-ance from psychotherapy in refractory psychic or psychosomatic situations may be necessary. Discussion of these therapeutic methods as applied to cerebrovascular accidents is given in Chapter 19.

Life management.—It goes without saying that a general hygienic program must be set up for the person who has had a stroke. This neces-sarily implies curtailment of activities obviously associated with emo-tional tension or physical strain, an evaluation of the new status and responsibility of the individual as related to his environment and regula-tion of factors of diet and of habit, such as smoking, that would seem deleterious to the blood vessels. Alvarez has made a plea for the preserva-tion of the patient's enjoyment of life, and he sees little reason for the physician to make the final days or declining years of the stroke victim miserable by denying him such small pleasures as can only make his life worth living. Everyone's end is inevitable, and the most abstemious, Spartan-like regime cannot be guaranteed to prolong existence even 24 hours.

PROGNOSIS

Infarctive cerebrovascular accidents recur with a predictable frequency of 30 per cent of cases. Concerning the immediate prognosis of cerebral thrombosis, the outlook is much better than that of cerebral hemorrhage. However, so frequently is the clinical diagnosis of cerebral thrombosis inaccurate and so rapid has been improvement in therapy, that it is impossible to give an accurate estimation of percentages of survival and disability among these patients. It is obvious that the future of the stroke victim is becoming brighter. Of historical interest is the famous case of Pasteur, who sustained a severe hemiplegia 27 years before his death, in which interval he performed a great deal of useful work.

Considering autopsied cases, Newbill found the average survival period after thrombosis to be 15 times as long as that after hemorrhage or embolism. White persons live longer than Negroes, and women outlast men. The location and extent of lesions are important factors determining the length of life after infarct. Prognosis is best with hemispherical or capsular lesions, worst with major occlusions in the brain stem.

Prediction of survival and degree of residual disability after cerebral infarction must be predicated on the signs and symptoms which indicate the degree of involvement of the brain in the individual case, the presence or absence of such acute or chronic complicating conditions as pneumonia, cardiac failure, uremia, diabetes mellitus and pulmonary infarct, and the intelligence and vigor with which the patient is supervised and treated.

BIBLIOGRAPHY

Alvarez, W. C.: Cerebral arteriosclerosis with small, commonly unrecognized apoplexies, Geriatrics 1:189-216, 1946.

Amyes, E. W., and Perry, S. M.: Stellate ganglion block in treatment of acute cerebral thrombosis and embolism: Report of 44 cases, J.A.M.A. 142:15-20, 1950.

Aring, C. D.: Vascular diseases of the nervous system, Brain 68:28-55, 1945.

Ashkenazy, M.; Davis, L., and Martin, J.: An evaluation of the technic and results of the radioactive diiodo-fluorescein test for localization of intracranial lesions, J. Neurosurg. 8:300-314, 1951.

Bessman, A. N.; Alman, R. W., and Fazekas, J. F.: Effect of acute hypotension on cerebral hemodynamics and metabolism of elderly patients, A.M.A. Arch. Int. Med. 89:893-898, 1952.

Cobb, S.: Cerebral circulation: A critical discussion of the symposium, A. Res. Nerv. & Ment. Dis., Proc. 18:719-750, 1938.

Cohn, R.; Raines, G. N.; Mulder, D. W., and Neumann, M. S.: Cerebral vascular lesions: Electroencephalographic and neuropathologic correlations, Arch. Neurol. & Psychiat. 60:165-181, 1948.

Cole, S. L., and Sugarman, J. N.: Cerebral manifestations of acute myocardial infarction, Am. J. M. Sc. 223:35-40, 1952.

Conley, J. J.: Free autogenous vein graft to internal and common carotid arteries in treatment of tumors of the neck, Ann. Surg. 137:205-219, 1953.

Cooper, I. S.: Ligation of the anterior choroidal artery for involuntary movements: Parkinsonism, Psychiatric Quart. 27:317-319, 1953.

Corday, E.; Rothenberg, S. F., and Putnam, T. J.: Cerebral vascular insufficiency, A.M.A. Arch. Neurol. & Psychiat. 69:551-570, 1953.

Corréa de Barros, E.: Retinal tonoscopy and arterial occlusions of the brain, Ophthalmologica 121:211-216, 1951.

Cress, C. H., and Gibbs, E. L.: Electroencephalographic asymmetry during sleep, Dis. Nerv. System 9:2-4, 1948.

Critchley, M.: The anterior cerebral artery and its syndromes, Brain 53:120-165, 1930.

Curtis, J. B.: Rapid serial angiography: Preliminary report, J. Neurol., Neurosurg. & Psychiat. 12:167-182, 1949.

Denny-Brown, D.: The treatment of recurrent cerebrovascular symptoms and the question of "vasospasm," M. Clin. North America 35:1457-1474, 1951.

dos Santos, J. C.: Note sur la désobstruction des anciennes thromboses artérielles, Presse méd. 57:544-545, 1949.

Dozzi, D. L.: Unsuspected coronary thrombosis in patients with hemiplegia: Clinical study, Ann. Int. Med. 12:1991-1995, 1939.

Dunning, H. S.: Detection of occlusion of the internal carotid artery by pharyngeal palpation, J.A.M.A. 152:321, 1953.

Ecker, A., and Riemenschneider, P. A.: Arteriographic evidence of spasm in cerebral vascular disorders, Neurology 3:495-502, 1953.

Elvidge, A. R., and Werner, A.: Hemiplegia and thrombosis of the internal carotid system, A.M.A. Arch. Neurol. & Psychiat. 66:752-782, 1951.

Epstein, J. A.; Lennox, M. A., and Noto, O.: Electroencephalographic study of experimental cerebrovascular occlusion, Electroencephalog. & Clin. Neurophysiol. 1:491-502, 1949.

Evans, J. P., and McEachern, D.: The circulatory changes in cerebral vascular occlusion and in cerebral cicatrization, A. Res. Nerv. & Ment. Dis., Proc. 18:379-393, 1938.

Fetterman, G. H., and Moran, T. J.: Anomalies of the circle of Willis in relation to cerebral softening, Arch. Path. 32:251-257, 1941.

Fisher, M.: Occlusion of the internal carotid artery, A.M.A. Arch. Neurol. & Psychiat. 65:346-377, 1951.

Fisher, M.: Senile dementia: New explanation of causation, Canad. M. A. J. 65:1-7, 1951.

Foix, Ch.; Chavanny, and Bascourret: Foyers de ramollisement simultanés dans les deux hemispheres, Rev. neurol. 2:77, 1925.

Foix, Ch.; Hillemand, P., and Schalit, I.: Sur le syndrome latéral du bulbe et l'irrigation du bulbe superieur, Rev. neurol. 1:160-179, 1925.

Foix, Ch., and Masson: Le syndrome de l'artére cérébrale postérieure, Presse méd. 31:361, 1923.

Ford, F. R.: *Diseases of the Nervous System in Infancy, Childhood and Adolescence* (Springfield, Ill.: Charles C Thomas, Publisher, 1937).

Freeman, W.; Ammerman, H. H., and Stanley, M.: Syndrome of the pontile tegmentum, Arch. Neurol. & Psychiat. 50:462-471, 1943.

Frøvig, A. G.: Bilateral obliteration of the common carotid artery; thromboangiitis obliterans? Contribution to clinical study of obliteration of the carotids and to elucidation of cerebral vascular circulation, Acta psychiat., et neurol., supp. 39, pp. 3-79, 1946.

Gardner, W. J.: Personal communication.

German, W. J., and Taffel, M.: Surgical production of collateral intracranial circulation, Yale J. Biol. & Med. 13:451-459, 1941.

Goodman, L.: Recurrent hypertensive cerebral thrombosis: Clinicopathologic analysis of six cases with discussion of pathogenesis, Arch. Neurol. & Psychiat. 62:445-478, 1949.

Hain, R. F.; Westhaysen, P. V., and Swank, R. L.: Hemorrhagic cerebral infarction by arterial occlusion, J. Neuropath. and Exper. Neurol. 11:34-43, 1952.

Harvey, J., and Rasmussen, T.: Occlusion of the middle cerebral artery: An experimental study, A.M.A. Arch. Neurol. & Psychiat. 66:20-29, 1951.

Hicks, S. P., and Warren, S.: Infarction of brain without thrombosis: Analysis of 100 cases with autopsy, A.M.A. Arch. Path. 52:403-412, 1951.

Horton, B. T.: The clinical use of histamine, Postgrad. Med. 9:1-23, 1951.

Hultquist, G. T.: Über Thrombose und Embolie der Arteria carotis und hierbei vorkommende Gehirn veranderungen (Jena: Gustav Fischer, 1942).

Innerfield, I.; Angrist, A., and Schwarz, A.: Parenteral administration of trypsin, J.A.M.A. 152:597-605, 1953.

Johnson, H. C., and Walker, A. E.: Angiographic diagnosis of spontaneous thrombosis of the internal and common carotid arteries, J. Neurosurg. 8:631-659, 1951.

King, A. B., and Langworthy, O. P.: Neurologic symptoms following extensive occlusion of the common or internal carotid artery, Arch. Neurol. & Psychiat. 46:835-842, 1941.

Krayenbühl, H.: Zur Diagnostik und chirurgischen Therapie der zerebralen Erscheinungen bei der Endarteriitis obliterans v. Winiwarter-Buerger, Schweiz. med. Wchnschr. 75:1025-1029, 1945.

Kredel, F. E.: Collateral cerebral circulation by muscle graft, South. Surgeon 11:235-244, 1942; and personal communication.

Kristenson, A.: The question of pathogenesis of cerebral insultus, Acta med. scandinav. (supp. 196) 128:200-211, 1947.

Learmonth, J.: Collateral circulation, natural and artificial, Surg., Gynec. & Obst. 90:385-392, 1950.

Lima, P. A.: Cerebral Angiography (London: Oxford University Press, 1950).

Lippmann, H. I.: Cerebrovascular thrombosis in patients with Buerger's disease, Circulation 5:680-692, 1952.

Marx, F.: Arteriographic demonstration of collaterals between internal and external carotid arteries, Acta radiol. 31:155-160, 1949.

Merritt, H. H., and Aring, C. D.: Differential diagnosis of cerebral vascular lesions, A. Res. Nerv. & Ment. Dis., Proc. 18:682-695, 1938.

Millikan, C. H.; Lundy, J. S., and Smith, L. A.: Evaluation of stellate ganglion block for acute focal cerebral infarcts, J.A.M.A. 151:438-440, 1953.

Moersch, F. P., and Kernohan, J. W.: Hemiballismus: Clincopathologic study, Arch. Neurol. & Psychiat. 41:365-372, 1939.

Moersch, F. P., and Sayre, G. P.: Neurological manifestations associated with dissecting aortic aneurysm, J.A.M.A. 144:1141-1148, 1950.

Murphy, J. P.: Neuropsychiatric sequelae of partial exsanguination, Arch. Neurol. & Psychiat. 49:594-598, 1943.

Murphy, J. P., and Duggins, V.: EEG differentiation between cerebral thrombosis and infiltrative glioma, Paper presented to Harvey Cushing Society, 19th Annual Meeting, April, 1951.

Murphy, J. P., and Gellhorn, E.: Multiplicity of representation versus punctate localization in motor cortex, Arch. Neurol. & Psychiat. 54:256-273, 1945.

Murphy, J. P., and Neumann, M. S.: Fatal cerebrovascular accident associated with catatonic schizophrenia, Arch. Neurol. & Psychiat. 49:724-731, 1943.

Naffziger, H. C., and Adams, J. E.: Role of stellate block in various intracranial pathologic states, Arch. Surg. 61:286-293, 1950.

Newbill, H. P.: The duration of life after cerebrovascular accidents, J.A.M.A. 114:236-237, 1940.

Nielsen, J. M.: *A Textbook of Clinical Neurology* (New York: Paul B. Hoeber, Inc., 1946).

Pereira, A. deS.: La chirurgie sympathetique dans le traitement des embolies et thromboses cérébrales, Lyon chir. 44:271-280, 1949.

Pickering, G. W.: Transient cerebral paralysis in hypertension and in cerebral embolism, J.A.M.A. 137:423-430, 1948.

Pratt-Thomas, H. R., and Berger, K. E.: Cerebellar and spinal injuries after chiropractic manipulation, J.A.M.A. 133:600-603, 1947.

Race, G. A., and Lisa, J. R.: Combined acute vascular lesions of brain and heart: Clinicopathologic study of 15 cases, Am. J. M. Sc. 210:732-737, 1945.

Reichert, T.: Influence of vessel resection on neuropsychiatric syndromes, Zentralbl. Chir. 5:462-469, 1948.

Ricker, G.: *Pathologie als Naturwissenschaft. Relations pathologie* (Berlin: J. Springer, 1924).

Risteen, W. A., and Volpitto, P. P.: Role of stellate ganglion block in certain neurologic disorders, South. M. J. 39:431-435, 1946.

Roseman, E.; Schmidt, R. P., and Foltz, E. L.: Serial electroencephalography in vascular lesions of the brain, Neurology 2:311-331, 1952.

Russek, H. I., and Zohman, B. L.: Hypertensive encephalopathy and cerebral arteriosclerosis, New York J. Med. 49:1411-1414, 1949.

Scheinberg, P.: Cerebral blood flow in vascular disease of the brain: Observations on effects of stellate block, Am. J. Med. 8:139-147, 1950.

Scheinker, I. M.: Vasoparalysis and vasothrombosis of brain in infancy and early childhood, Arch. Neurol. & Psychiat. 55:216-231, 1946.

Shenkin, H. A.; Cabieses, F., and van der Noordt: Effect of bilateral stellectomy upon cerebral circulation of man, J. Clin. Invest. 30:90-93, 1951.

Schnitker, M. T., and Lehnert, H. B.: Apoplexy in a pituitary chromophobe adenoma producing the syndrome of middle cerebral artery thrombosis, J. Neurosurg. 9:210-213, 1952.

Steegman, A. T., and Roberts, D. J.: Syndrome of anterior choroidal artery, J.A.M.A. 104:1695-1697, 1935.

Strauss, H., and Greenstein, L.: The electroencephalogram in cerebrovascular disease, Arch. Neurol. & Psychiat. 59:395-403, 1948.

Takahashi, K.: Die percutane Arteriographie der arteria Vertebralis und ihrer Versorgungsgebiete, Arch. Psychiat. 111:373-379, 1940.

Thompson, R. K., and Mosberg, W. H.: Unpublished data.

Van Buskirk, C., and Zarling, R. V.: EEG prognosis in vascular hemiplegia rehabilitation, A.M.A. Arch. Neurol. & Psychiat. 65:732-739, 1951.

Vander Eecken, H. M.; Fisher, M., and Adanis, R. D.: Arterial anastomoses of the human brain and their importance in delimitation of human brain infarction, J. Neuropath. & Exper. Neurol. 11:91-94, 1952.

Walsh, F. B.: *Clinical Neuro-ophthalmology* (Baltimore: Williams & Wilkins Company, 1947).

Wilson, G., *et al.*: Factors influencing the development of cerebral vascular accidents: I. Role of cardiocirculatory insufficiency, J.A.M.A. 145:1227-1229, 1951.

Winternitz, M. C.; Thomas, R. M., and Lecompte, P. M.: *The Biology of Arteriosclerosis,* (Springfield, Ill.: Charles C Thomas, Publisher, 1938).

Young, A. F., and Karnosh, L. J.: The anterior perforating arterioles and their relation to the internal capsule, Dis. Nerv. System 10:99-103, 1949.

CHAPTER 9

Cerebral Embolism

CEREBRAL EMBOLISM, in which blood vessels of the brain are occluded by solid, fluid or gaseous bodies brought to the intracranial circulation by the blood stream, is usually seen in clinical practice as a complication of heart disease. The incidence of cerebral embolism is 5 per cent or less of all major cerebrovascular accidents, and this is decreasing as methods of treatment of endocarditis and intracardiac thrombosis improve. Although statistically the frequency of embolic episodes is highest in middle age (Merritt and Aring), cerebral embolism is a not uncommon cause of hemiplegia in young adult life because of rheumatic fever and its sequelae. In 1,000 autopsies of infants and children dying of cerebrovascular lesions, Irish found 133 cases of embolism of the brain.

ETIOLOGY; PATHOGENESIS

In experimental studies Villaret and Cachera observed widespread and persistent pial angiospasm after cerebral embolization with glass particles 80–150 μ in diameter. Hemorrhages and infarctions were the permanent results. Vasoparalysis and perivascular extravasations were seen by Chase following air embolism in animals, and severe depression of the electroencephalogram was produced by experimental embolization of the cerebral circulation (Loeb and Sacchi).

HEART DISEASE.—Embolic lesions of the brain are almost invariable in patients dying with active *rheumatic endocarditis* (Kernohan *et al.*). Of 194 patients with *rheumatic heart disease* complicated by embolic phenomena studied by Daley and associates, 97 per cent had mitral valvulitis and 90 per cent auricular fibrillation. In 50 per cent of the patients, emboli reached the intracranial circulation. *Bacterial endocarditis,* acute or subacute, always produces cerebral embolization, minute though the lesions may be. In *hypertensive or coronary occlusive* heart disease, fragments of clot may break off from the interior of a fibrillating auricle or damaged ventricle and pass upward to the brain. Cerebral or other embolism can be the first sign of an otherwise silent cardiac infarct. Intracranial vascular episodes are common in *congenital* heart disease; emboli may be either bland or infected, and brain abscess occurs on an embolic basis.

Emboli from the heart valves or cardiac chambers are distributed preferentially to the right cerebral hemisphere and particularly to the territory of irrigation of the middle cerebral artery. However, any intracranial arterial channel may be the recipient. Of the cerebellar arteries, the superior cerebellar is usually selected.

CAROTID THROMBOSIS.—Fragmentation of thrombi deposited on atheromatous ulcerations of the interior of the carotid sinus may result in attacks of cerebral embolism, as first noted by Chiari in 1905. Such episodes may be responsible for evanescent paralysis which often precedes the complete and lasting hemiplegia resulting from thrombosis of the cervical carotid artery. Embolism may also occur from a thrombus at the site of recent carotid ligation.

OTHER CAUSES.—*Air* or other gas *embolism* blocks the intracranial vessels with frothy bubbles, although an "air lock" in the heart is the most serious or lethal consequence. Air embolism has been reported to occur after or during chest operations, injury to the jugular or vertebral epidural veins, pneumothorax, pneumoencephalography, perirenal insufflation, inflation of the maxillary antrums and eustachian tubes, catheterization of the right heart, assumption of the knee-chest position post partum and violent coughing. In diver's bends, free nitrogen is the offender. Aeroembolism may affect the unprotected aviator, but such an event is extremely rare.

Fat embolism affects the small vessels (capillaries) of the brain. The condition is usually traumatic in origin and is seen most often after skeletal fractures and extensive contusions of adipose tissue. It can also result from various surgical operations, anesthesia, electric shock therapy, poisoning and the diagnostic or therapeutic injection of oily substances.

Rarely, *venous emboli* pass from systemic veins in the extremities, pelvis, abdomen or thorax to the cerebral veins via the "back road" of the vertebral venous plexus, by-passing the heart. It is unnecessary to assume a patent foramen ovale to account for such paradoxical embolism. Sudden changes of intravenous pressure, such as those occurring during coughing, facilitate venous embolization, hence the frequency of suppurative and malignant metastases from lung to brain. Experimentally, glass beads of 500 μ diameter have been found to pass through the pulmonary circulation and reach the brain.

Clumps of *tumor cells* may also act as intracranial emboli. Secondary growth of malignant tissue can then commence in a new locus, or the tumor emboli may remain in the vessels of the brain with resultant cerebral softening or hemorrhage (Madow and Alpers). Venous metastases are likely to be superficial in location, whereas arterial tumor emboli are found in the white matter.

Parasites free in the blood stream may lodge in the brain. Malarial organisms and trypanosomes fill cerebral capillaries, and toxoplasmic protozoa proliferate in minute intracranial vessels. The immature forms of the pork tapeworm (cysticercosis), dog tapeworm (hydatid disease), Japanese river fluke (schistosomiasis), and trichina (trichinosis encephalitis) may likewise affect the cerebrum or cerebellum. *Amniotic fluid* embolism is a possibility in the parturient patient.

PATHOLOGY

HEART DISEASE.—Cerebral infarcts secondary to auricular fibrillation or ventricular thrombus usually result from the occlusion of branches of large arteries. They are often multiple in location, hemorrhagic, conical in shape with base outward and liquefy in two to three days (Fig. 52). Vasoparalysis and stasis are found at a distance. When cerebral embolization results from rheumatic endocarditis, microscopic lesions of focal ischemia or necrosis are centered about a minute arteriole and are surrounded by "stars" of glial proliferation. These tiny infarcts are found almost exclusively in the cortex.

Intracranial emboli from bacterial endocarditis are distributed similarly but are much more numerous than the bland rheumatic counterparts, and infarction frequently progresses to suppuration which may attain the status of frank brain abscess (Fig. 53). In microscopic sections, bacteria may be seen plugging inflamed and necrotic small vessels, and polymorphonuclear leukocytes mingle with glial cells and fibroblasts. If an infected embolus rests in the bifurcation of a major artery, a mycotic aneurysm may result.

OTHER EMBOLIC DISEASES.—At autopsy, bubbles may be grossly visible in cerebral vessels after air embolism. Cerebral edema secondary to small vessel damage may be a late, fatal reaction (Masland). Sausages of fat in cortical capillaries feature the pathologic picture of fat embolism. The surrounding ischemic zones are ringed by hemorrhage. Venous emboli produce superficial, hemorrhagic infarcts which may be also suppurative if thrombophlebitis is the source.

Metastatic nodules in the brain, multiple or single, small or large, are the usual eventual manifestations of tumor emboli, which may also produce cerebral infarction acutely. Repeated superficial (meningeal) embolization with malignant cells results in arachnoidal changes grossly indistinguishable from meningitis. Parasitic invaders choke the cerebral capillaries, with attendant ischemia, hemorrhage and fibroglial response,

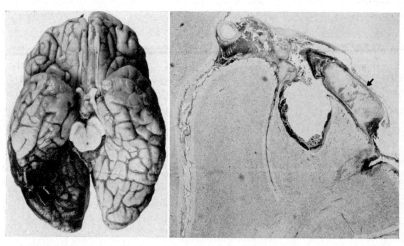

FIG. 52 *(left)*.—Embolic thrombosis of posterior cerebral artery. (George Washington University Laboratory of Neurology.)

FIG. 53 *(right)*.—Cortical arterial embolism (arrow). Subacute bacterial endocarditis. Cystic abscess in cortex.

or they proliferate to form granulomatous masses of various size and location, even intraventricular (choroid plexus). Many parasitic lesions calcify.

SYMPTOMS AND SIGNS

EMBOLISM FROM HEART DISEASE.—The onset of cerebral embolization from a cardiac source is usually sudden, without warning. The event may occur while the person is at rest or is active. A sharp drop in blood pressure signalizes cerebral embolism during cardiac surgery (Bailey *et al.*).

Previous embolic episodes are not uncommon, occurring in 32 per cent of patients reported by Merritt and Aring. Headache and vomiting are complaints of one third of patients. With a large embolus, coma supervenes rapidly, but the majority of patients remain awake. Peripheral systemic evidences of multiple embolization are common in endocarditis; conversely, evidences of cardiac disorder are almost invariably found in all patients in this group.

Neurologic signs are fulminating and correspond to the area of the brain involved (Fig. 39). Aphasia, hemiplegia and hemisensory deficit are common, since the middle cerebral arterial distribution is especially vulnerable. Although convulsions appear in less than 10 per cent of patients, multiple cortical embolization in endocarditis can result in intractable and fatal status epilepticus. Hemianopsia may be the sole consequence of plugging of the posterior cerebral artery. Nuclear palsies indicate rare embolic infarction of the brain stem. Brain abscess, a late result of an infected embolus, is revealed by the development of increased intracranial pressure and meningeal irritation, both rare with bland embolism.

OTHER EMBOLIC STATES.—Initial cerebral symptoms of air embolism are headache, vertigo and nausea. Apprehension and a shocklike condition appear, and vision is lost. Convulsions are followed by coma.

In fat embolism a lucid interval is followed by severe fever, tachycardia, irritability and other signs of central involvement, particularly decerebrate rigidity, which may mimic serious primary head injury. Ocular, cardiac and pulmonary phenomena indicate embolization elsewhere. Free fat is often present in the urine. Petechiae appear on the upper one half of the body during the third day of illness.

The clinical manifestations of venous, tumor and parasitic emboli develop late and are insidious in appearance. The neurologic deficit is combined with signs of increased intracranial pressure, and a nonspecific intracranial hypertension may be the only evidence of secondary intracranial dural sinus or venous occlusion. Small carcinomatous nodules are often associated with disproportionately severe cerebral edema. Again, multiple meningeal metastases may strongly suggest bacterial or virus meningitis. Cerebral malaria causes convulsions and coma. Other parasites may also produce an encephalitic syndrome or the clinical picture of brain tumor or of hydrocephalus in infants.

LABORATORY STUDIES

Leukocytosis and anemia accompany endocarditis, and the presence of red blood cells in the urine may indicate a renal infarct. The blood pressure corresponds to the cardiac status. If infarction is massive or an abscess has formed, x-rays of the skull may reveal displacement of the pineal gland. The lumbar cerebrospinal fluid pressure is usually normal but may sometimes be elevated above 300 mm. of water. The cerebrospinal fluid, though often clear, is xanthochromic or frankly bloody in 30 per cent of patients; turbid pleocytosis correlates with septic embolism.

If encephalography is performed, swelling of a part of a cerebral hemisphere with local ventricular collapse or shift may be seen with extensive lesions. With small infarcts air patterns are normal. Arteriography may demonstrate the exact site of vascular occlusion (Fig. 54). Neither of these surgical procedures is necessarily recommended in a

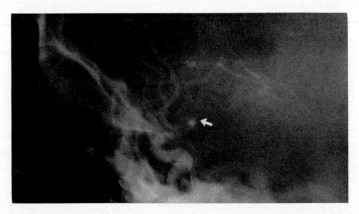

FIG. 54.—Embolic occlusion of middle cerebral artery in arteriogram. Rheumatic heart disease.

precarious situation in which the diagnosis may often be made by auscultation of the heart, for confirmation is academic unless drainage of an abscess is contemplated.

The electroencephalogram may be severely and generally abnormal due to multiplicity of embolic lesions. Low amplitude of alpha waves and focal slow activity are more common findings. Delta waves disappear by the third month after embolic infarction (Roseman *et al.*).

DIAGNOSIS

The diagnosis of cerebral embolism may be made when a sudden cerebral accident occurs in the presence of a verified source of embolic material, usually cardiac thrombosis or endocarditis.

DIFFERENTIAL DIAGNOSIS.—Chief differentiation is to be made from cerebral vasospasm, spontaneous cerebral infarction, intracerebral hemorrhage and ruptured congenital aneurysm. *Vasospastic* episodes are of brief duration and virtually without sequelae. The development of thrombotic *infarction* is gradual and premonitory symptoms are prominent. With thrombosis, the appearance of the cerebrospinal fluid is rarely bloody or turbid. Cerebral *hemorrhage* occurs in hypertensive patients. Symptoms and signs of intrinsic involvement of the brain are profound and the cerebrospinal fluid is grossly bloody.

Ocular palsies, frankness of meningeal signs and gross blood in the cerebrospinal fluid distinguish ruptured berry *aneurysm.* The course of *brain tumor* is one of slow progression, and pressure signs dominate. *Metabolic states* are recognized by alterations in blood chemistry and abnormal findings on urinalysis.

TREATMENT

Therapy in cerebral embolism is directed to the acute intracranial episode and the underlying responsible condition, usually cardiac.

TREATMENT OF ACUTE EPISODE.—Procaine injection of the stellate ganglion on the side of brain involvement is the emergency treatment of choice. This may relieve the angiospastic ischemia which accounts for much of the neurologic deficit. Neurologic results of stellate block are better in cerebral embolism than in cerebral thrombosis.

The use of pharmacologic antispasmodics is also in order: 0.065–0.13 Gm. of papaverine may be injected intravenously or intramuscularly. Histamine is given by slow intravenous drip to the point of facial flushing, 2.75 mg. of base being dissolved in 250 cc. of normal saline. Sublingual administration of nitroglycerin or inhalation of amyl nitrite is also of benefit. Caution must be observed not to lower systemic blood pressure too far, otherwise cerebral blood flow will be decreased and the desired purpose defeated. Inhalation of carbon dioxide in 5–7 per cent concentration is also used to increase cerebral vasodilation.

Embolization of the brain is almost the only type of cerebrovascular accident in which anticoagulant therapy is indicated. Here it is used principally to control or eliminate the source of emboli. Heparin, Dicumarol or other anticoagulant preparations may be used during the course of the cerebral illness or on a continual basis thereafter (auricular fibrillation). There is the danger of converting an anemic cerebral infarct into a hemorrhagic one, and drugs which interfere with the clotting mechanism are contraindicated if the cerebrospinal fluid is bloody. If stellate block is to be performed, it should be done before an anticoagulant regime is instituted to avoid a hematoma in the neck.

TREATMENT OF UNDERLYING DISORDER.—Bacterial endocarditis often responds to vigorous specific antibiotic treatment. The management of coronary occlusion with myocardial infarction is discussed in standard textbooks of medicine. Mitral stenosis and congenital cardiac defects are being corrected surgically. Bailey *et al.* report control of embolization during mitral commissurotomy by occlusion of the innominate and the left carotid arteries.

Laying the patient suffering from severe air embolism immediately on the left side may save his life. Cardiac embarrassment is thus minimized. The application of a tourniquet above the fractured extremity is recommended in fat embolism. If venous embolism is suspected, ligation of veins of the extremity or of the vena cava is indicated. Neurosurgical removal of metastatic tumor and parasitic masses has accomplished gratifying results in selected patients.

PROGNOSIS

Daley *et al.* reported a 49 per cent mortality in patients with cerebral embolism from rheumatic heart disease. However, the increasing use of stellate block and anticoagulant therapy is reducing the mortality rate of such intracranial accidents. Several investigators have described significant neurologic improvement in patients with cerebral embolism after stellate ganglion anesthesia. When stellate block succeeds, it usually does so rapidly and on the first occasion. The sustained administration of anticoagulants has permitted patients with chronic auricular fibrillation to carry on even after initial severe embolic episodes.

Forty per cent of patients with bacterial endocarditis used to die of intracranial complications. It would be impossible to estimate the mortality rate in this condition today when the use of antibiotics is being extended and improved.

If a patient with air embolism is going to die, he usually does so within one-half hour, although death due to cerebral edema may occur 24–48 hours later. When the critical period is past, recovery is rapid and usually complete. The incidence of mortality in fat embolism is high, but if the patient survives, slow recovery to almost a normal state may be anticipated.

The only type of malignant metastasis in which cure has been achieved by neurosurgery combined with removal of the primary tumor is hypernephroma. The prognosis in parasitic embolism is variable. Chemotherapy has occasionally been successful in patients with cerebral malaria. The course of trichina encephalitis may be self-limited, and surgical extirpation of helminthic granulomas has often been gratifyingly successful.

BIBLIOGRAPHY

Amyes, E. W., and Perry, S. M.: Stellate ganglion block in treatment of acute cerebral thrombosis and embolism: Report of 44 cases, J.A.M.A. 142:15-20, 1950.

Bailey, C. P., et al.: Technique for prevention of cerebral complications during mitral commissurotomy, J.A.M.A. 149:1085-1090, 1952.

Chase, W. H.: Cerebral thrombosis, hemorrhage and embolism: Pathologic principles, A. Res. Nerv. & Ment. Dis., Proc. 18:365-378, 1938.

Daley, R., et al.: Systemic arterial embolism in rheumatic heart disease, Am. Heart J. 42:566-581, 1951.

Gilbert, N. C., and deTakats, G.: Emergency treatment of apoplexy, J.A.M.A. 136:659-665, 1948.

Irish, C. W.: Cerebral vascular lesions in newborn infants and young children, J. Pediat. 15:64-74, 1939.

Kernohan, J. W.; Woltman, H. W., and Barnes, A. R.: Involvement of the nervous system associated with endocarditis, Arch. Neurol. & Psychiat. 42:789-809, 1942.

Loeb, C., and Sacchi, U.: Depression of the electrical cortical activity after experimental emboli, Proc. Soc. Italian di Elettroencefalog., April, 1951; reported in Electroencephalog. & Clin. Neurophysiol. 4:229, 1952.

Mackay, W. A., and Scott, L. D. W.: Treatment of apoplexy by infiltration of the stellate ganglion with novocaine, Brit. M. J. 2:1-4, 1938.

Madow, L., and Alpers, B. J.: Cerebral vascular complications of metastatic carcinoma, J. Neuropath. & Exper. Neurol. 11:137-148, 1952.

Masland, R. L.: Injury of the central nervous system resulting from decompression to simulated high altitudes, Arch. Neurol. & Psychiat. 59:445-456, 1948.

Merritt, H. H., and Aring, C. D.: Differential diagnosis of cerebral vascular lesions, A. Res. Nerv. & Ment. Dis., Proc. 18:682-695, 1938.

Naffziger, H. C., and Adams, J. E.: Role of stellate block in various intracranial pathologic states, Arch. Surg. 61:286-293, 1950.

Roseman, E.; Schmidt, R. P., and Foltz, E. L.: Serial electroencephalography in vascular lesions of the brain, Neurology 2:311-331, 1952.

Scheinker, I. M.: Medical Neuropathology (Springfield, Ill.: Charles C Thomas, Publisher, 1951).

Villaret, M., and Cachera, R.: Les embolies cerebrales (Paris: Masson & Cie, 1939).

CHAPTER 10

Cerebral Hemorrhage

SPONTANEOUS INTRACEREBRAL HEMORRHAGE was the third most frequent cause of death in the United States in 1948 and promises to be of increasing importance in view of the rising incidence of hypertensive cardiovascular disease. Heartening considerations are the growing interests in the therapy of high blood pressure and in the neurosurgical treatment of cerebral hemorrhage. Recognition of the hemorrhagic syndrome in young persons by means of angiography and other diagnostic aids has revealed that intracerebral bleeding is a not infrequent cause of cerebrovascular accident in the younger age groups and has thus led to the saving of many lives.

The relative frequency of hemorrhage, compared with that of cerebral infarction, is greater in patients who die of cerebrovascular accidents but is less among those who survive. Zimmerman found in 4,240 consecutive autopsies that 2.5 per cent of deaths followed cerebral hemorrhage and 1.7 per cent cerebral infarction. Merritt and Aring reported an incidence of 47 per cent hemorrhage and 43 per cent thrombosis in 245 autopsies of patients with strokes, whereas in patients clinically controlled diagnosis in 21 per cent was hemorrhagic apoplexy and in 66 per cent thrombotic brain disease. Cerebral embolism and spontaneous subarachnoid bleeding (ruptured intracranial aneurysm) are of much less frequent occurrence.

ETIOLOGY; PATHOGENESIS

HYPERTENSIVE CEREBRAL HEMORRHAGE

Although there is agreement on the cause of intracerebral bleeding in some diseases, the exact cause and pathogenesis of hypertensive hemorrhagic apoplexy, which represents 75 per cent of cases of cerebral hemorrhage, is doubtful. This is largely because it is so difficult to find the incontrovertible point of rupture at autopsy. It is no longer conceded that all cerebral hemorrhages, even those occurring in hypertensive patients, are of arterial origin; it is probable that many ingravescent cases in which intracerebral hematomas may be successfully evacuated are the result of venous bleeding.

Theoretic explanations.—The most popular theories explaining typical cerebral hemorrhage are the following.

1. Reduced perivascular consistency of tissue due to *preceding enceph-*

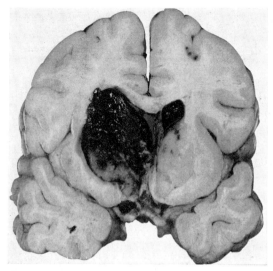

FIG. 55.—Typical hypertensive cerebral hemorrhage in internal capsule and basal ganglions. (AFIP #AMH 10524-E.)

alomalacia in the presence of elevated vascular tension was thought by Rouchoux (1844) to allow arterioles to perforate. This theory is upheld by Globus and Strauss. Several objections are apparent (Cobb): softened brain is hardly less supportive than normal cerebral tissue, since both are essentially fluids; the systolic arterial blood pressure is approximately 10 times the intracranial pressure normally; if lack of periarterial support is important, cerebral hemorrhage should occur most often from rupture of vessels of the circle of Willis lying free in the subarachnoid space, instead of from the interior arteries which are usually involved.

2. Minute *dissecting aneurysms* may form in the walls of small arteries or arterioles when vasa vasorum rupture, blood tearing through the adventitia to escape under high pressure into surrounding cerebral tissue

(Eppinger, 1888). Zimmerman found this to be the precise etiology of cerebral hemorrhage in 75 per cent of brains examined.

3. Charcot and Bouchard (1868) stated that they invariably found ruptured *miliary aneurysms* on smaller arterial branches, particularly the lenticulostriate arteries in hypertensive and arteriosclerotic apoplectic brains.

4. *Functional vascular disorder* (Ricker) could lead to angiospasm, hypoxia of small vessels, necrosis of their walls and tiny hemorrhages of venous origin which might pool together to form the large hematoma of familiar appearance. This deduction is championed by Aring who explains premonitory symptoms as being related to coalescence of blood and believes that cerebral hemorrhage is often of venous rather than arterial origin. Whereas this sequence of events may cause some intracerebral hematomas of subacute type, it is hard to believe that the hypertensive apoplexy characterized by obstinate bleeding against increasing intracranial pressure is not of arterial source.

Contributory factors.—Several additional factors bear upon the cause of typical cerebral hemorrhage. In cases confirmed at autopsy, patients almost invariably had a systolic blood pressure of at least 200 mm. The small arteries in the area where bleeding usually begins, that is, the basal ganglions and internal capsule, come directly off large parent vessels without a "stepping down" of systolic pressure, and at the points of derivation there are numerous defects in the spiral muscular coat of the media. Sclerotic changes increase the rigidity of the thick elastica of cerebral vessels to the point of brittleness, and disease of the vasa vasorum must contribute to weakening of the arterial wall. The high incidence of cerebral hemorrhage, compared with that of spontaneous ruptures into other organs, is undoubtedly due in part to the congenital poverty of the adventitia of cerebral arteries (Winternitz). Also, growth of arteriosclerotic plaques into a thinly muscular arterial media opens up avenues of potential perforation and intracerebral hemorrhage.

Emotional upheaval induced by sudden anger or other hostility may be followed, proverbially, by hemorrhagic apoplexy in the hypertensive plethoric patient.

Hemorrhage in Other Vascular Diseases

Arterial berry aneurysm may rupture largely or entirely into the brain instead of into the subarachnoid space (Fig. 68). An *arteriovenous anomaly,* such as angioma or cirsoid aneurysm, is one of the commonest causes of cerebral hemorrhage in youth or middle age. When of angiomatous and therefore usually venous origin, intracerebral hematoma tends to form rather more superficially than does the hypertensive type, in an area other than the internal capsule. The slow increase in size of the clot due to an increase in osmotic power from cellular breakdown often simulates brain tumor. On the other hand, the syndrome may be exactly that of hypertensive "blowout," but without hypertension. Tiny angiomatous lesions (Fig. 84) are often discovered in cerebral hemorrhage of otherwise unknown cause (Margolis *et al.*). Smooth-walled cavities are left when venous hematomas are removed.

Arteriosclerosis uncomplicated by high blood pressure rarely produces cerebral hemorrhage, but occasional instances do occur. Although cerebral infarction is more commonly the result of cardiac failure, there is thought to be a close association between spontaneous massive cerebral hemorrhage and *cardiovascular disease* (Rupp *et al.*). *Venous thrombosis* may cause major bleeding. Necrosis of arteries or veins in *inflammatory* vascular disease, for example, periarteritis nodosa, will allow major extravasations in the brain. In almost half the fatal cases of *eclampsia* there are parenchymal brain hemorrhages of varying degree, from petechiae to massive clots. Spontaneous, verified apoplexy has also occurred in *migraine*. The excessive hormonal activity of *pheochromocytoma* may result in cerebral hemorrhage.

BLOOD DYSCRASIAS; NEOPLASMS

Such bleeding or thrombotic diatheses as thrombocytopenic purpura, leukemia, polycythemia and sickle cell anemia are complicated by cerebral hemorrhage rather frequently. Cerebrovascular complications of blood dyscrasias are discussed in Chapter 17.

Primary intracranial tumor, as well as metastatic neoplasms, may first appear clinically as cerebral hemorrhage. In 3–4 per cent of gliomas spontaneous massive bleeding is a complication (Oldberg). Most such tumors are malignant. In six of 32 cases of secondary malignancy reported by Globus and Sapirstein, the cerebrospinal fluid was bloody. Malignant melanoma is particularly likely to bleed. Papanicolaou staining of a cerebrospinal fluid specimen may bring the true etiology of such cases to light.

HEMORRHAGE IN THE NEWBORN

The combination of birth trauma and prothrombin deficiency in newborn infants, especially if premature, often causes cerebral hemorrhages of variable magnitude. Erythroblastosis fetalis is almost always complicated by intracranial bleeding (see Chapter 17). Irish found 418 instances of brain hemorrhage in 1,000 autopsied cases of cerebrovascular accident in infants and young children. Numerous small centers of vascular rupture were characteristic lesions in 80 cases of intracranial hemorrhage in premature infants studied by Minkowski, who believes that vasodilatation and vascular fragility are of pathogenic importance.

Trauma

The role of trauma in the production of cerebral hemorrhage is a matter of conjecture and medicolegal interest. Ever since the description by Bollinger (1891) of delayed traumatic apoplexy (*Spätapoplexie*) in five patients who died suddenly of apoplectiform hemorrhage 12–50 days after head injury, there has been controversy over the relation of traumatic factors to hemorrhagic stroke. Langerhans (1903) considered vascular disease to be present in all such patients and felt that injury was simply a precipitating circumstance. Von Holder (1904) in microscopic studies found intimal tears in small vessels, aneurysmal dilatations and focal extravasations which may have resulted from trauma and which he believed paved the way for later and larger hemorrhages.

Syndromes of traumatic cerebral hemorrhage.—Three varieties of delayed traumatic cerebral hemorrhage are described by Symonds. (1) Early bleeding is thought to occur within a few weeks of injury as a result of weakening of an arterial wall. (2) Late hemorrhage may take place into a cyst which is the result of an earlier extravasation or is the residual of traumatic encephalomalacia, after an interval of months or years. (3) Chronic intracerebral hematoma may be present from the time of the cranial accident and resembles brain tumor in activity.

Craig and Adson reported two cases in which fresh clots present on the laminated base of previous, organized hemorrhage were successfully evacuated surgically; the head injuries had occurred six months and 19 months previously. Penfield described a 30 year old man in whom a fatal intracerebral hemorrhage originated from "a carpet of blood vessels" on the brain just beneath an old fracture of the occipital bone; the fracture had been sustained in childhood. An example of apparent bleeding into contused brain occurring suddenly nine days after the elevation of a compound, depressed skull fracture was reported by Jewesbury. The cerebrum was grossly normal at first operation; a large fresh intracerebral hematoma was removed at re-exploration.

Pathologic, medicolegal considerations.—Post-traumatic bleeding most often occurs beneath the poles of the frontal, temporal and occipital lobes, where bruising is likely to be extreme, and is usually superficial. When traumatic hemorrhage is central in location, the region of the external capsule is usually involved; thus, in 38 cases examined by Courville and Blomquist the internal capsule was spared. However, the problem is further complicated by Angrist and Mitchell's report of seven cases in which hemorrhage of obvious traumatic origin *did* involve the internal capsule.

It is hard to believe that trauma is responsible for hemorrhagic apoplexy when injury antedates the onset of symptoms by several months or even years and particularly when the degree of injury is trivial. If an absolute distinction between spontaneous and traumatic etiologies is necessary, as in a legal decision, it is wise to observe caution and to reject injury as the cause when (1) clearcut and definite evidences of severe trauma are lacking; (2) the time relationship between injury and onset of symptoms is not brief and direct; (3) the medical background of the patient is one predisposing to spontaneous hemorrhage, and (4) pathologic findings are more compatible with nontraumatic apoplexy.

PATHOLOGY

LOCATION OF HEMORRHAGE.—Over one third of all cerebral hemorrhages are located in the internal capsule and basal ganglions, the field of distribution of the ganglionic derivatives of the internal carotid, middle cerebral and posterior cerebral arteries (Fig. 55). Charcot believed that the lenticulostriate vessels were most often responsible and named them the arteries of cerebral hemorrhage. In a series reported by Zimmerman the frontal lobe and cerebellum were each involved in 13 per cent of cases; major extravasations were present in the calcarine areas in 8 per cent, in the occipital poles in 7 per cent, the ventricular system primarily in 7.5 per cent, the pons in 7 per cent, the centrum semiovale of the cerebral hemisphere in 6 per cent (Fig. 56) and the corpus callosum in 2 per cent. Hemorrhages are almost always unilateral in the cerebrum and cerebellum and occur on the right or left sides with equal frequency.

ACUTE, PROGRESSIVE HEMORRHAGE.—Arterial blood escapes under high pressure and a perivascular extravasation increases rapidly to a large hematoma. The size is limited only by the resistance of tissue planes and the tendency of the opening in the artery to be closed by spasm or external tamponade. As blood ploughs through the brain, traversing venules are torn; there results a mélange of arterial blood, venous blood and

pulpified brain. Flattening of gyri against the skull prevents venous outflow and adds tissue asphyxia.

The stumps of thrombosed veins may be seen in the lining of the
cavity from which a cerebral hemorrhage has been evacuated. Small ring
and ball extravasations are numerous in adjacent tissues. Death occurs
when the ventricular system is finally flooded, as happens in 47 per cent
of all cases, or when unilateral brain swelling results in downward herni-

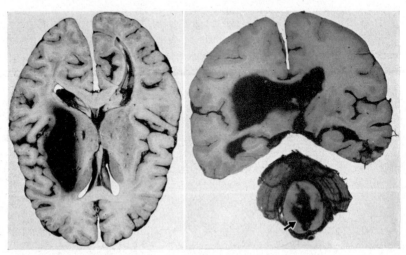

FIG. 56 *(left)*.—Hemorrhage in external capsule. (George Washington University
Laboratory of Neurology.)

FIG. 57 *(right)*.—Secondary hemorrhages in midbrain (arrow) due to hemorrhagic
cerebral apoplexy. (AFIP #AEC 284793.)

ation of the temporal lobe, compressing the arteries and veins supplying
the brain stem and leading to secondary hemorrhages in the mesencephalon and pons (Fig. 57).

Hemispheral cerebral hemorrhages of spontaneous origin usually per-
perforate the ependyma over the head of the caudate nucleus and enter the
anterior horn of the lateral ventricle. Extension to the superficial subarachnoid spaces is ordinarily sufficient only to color the cerebrospinal
fluid pink. Cortical hemorrhages of large size, especially if associated with
subdural hematoma, are almost always of traumatic origin.

SUBACUTE HEMORRHAGE; CHRONIC HEMATOMA.—When arterial
hemorrhage ceases soon after onset or when bleeding is primarily from
veins, the brain can often accommodate to the presence of an expansile
mass. The illness then becomes somewhat chronic in nature, and surgical

evacuation of the clot may cure before progressive edema causes late death (Fig. 58) or, in a few cases, the hemorrhage is actually absorbed. In the latter event, a chocolate cyst or a rust-stained cavity filled with glairy fluid is surrounded by a fibroglial wall; strands of connective tissue or remnants of projection systems cross the space like delicate cables, and glial phagocytes (*Gitterzellen*) are found in neighboring perivascular spaces. Hemosiderin-laden histiocytes appear five to six days after hemor-

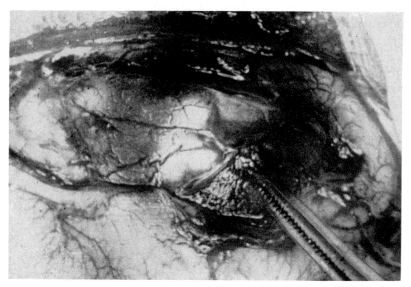

FIG. 58.—Chronic hematoma (forceps) of parietal lobe.

rhage, and hematoidin is visible after two weeks (Strassmann). In hemorrhages of venous origin, laminated clots in the wall of the hematoma membrane are indicative of repeated hemorrhagic episodes.

SYMPTOMS AND SIGNS

The average age of the patient with cerebral hemorrhage is between 40 and 70 years. The incidence is slightly higher in men than in women, but the predominance in men is not so disproportionate as in cerebral thrombosis. In two thirds of the patients onset is during the cold months of the year. In one-fifth, there have been previous cerebrovascular accidents. More episodes occur during the daytime than at night (Merritt and Aring). In some hypertensive persons, profuse nasal hemorrhage seems to ward off fatal apoplexy, at least temporarily.

Significant prodromes of hemorrhagic apoplexy in the hours or days preceding stroke include severe nuchal or occipital headaches, vertigo or syncope, motor or sensory neurologic disturbances, nosebleeds, retinal hemorrhages, mental disturbances and drowsiness. These complaints are uncommon in hypertensive patients in whom cerebral hemorrhage does not ultimately take place.

ACUTE INTERNAL CAPSULAR HEMORRHAGE.—There is no more dramatic clinical picture of sudden onset of devastating illness than that presented by spontaneous intracapsular hemorrhage. Characteristically, a hypertensive person at work or in a mood of anger or excitement complains of vertigo and a sense of oppression in the head. He then gives a sudden cry of pain, clutches at his temples and falls senseless to the floor or ground. Vomiting and convulsive seizures are not uncommon. Coma is deep and hemiplegia is profound from the outset. Breathing is rapid and stertorous, the respiratory cycle is Cheyne-Stokes, the pulse is slow and full, saliva drools from the corner of the mouth and the paralyzed cheek puffs out with each expiration.

Severe motor and sensory deficit is found on the side opposite that of the hemorrhage. The patient may be so deeply unconscious and generally flaccid that only total absence of a corneal reflex will indicate that the opposite cerebral hemisphere is the one affected, or the only lateralizing sign may be a difference in response to pinprick around the mouth. The paralyzed arm falls limply and heavily when dropped from an elevated position and the leg is turned outward. The face is flushed and covered with perspiration. Eyes and head are deviated to one side—"the patient looks at his stroke." The pupil is dilated ipsilaterally or contralaterally, or both pupils may be small, as with primary or secondary hemorrhages in the brain stem.

Stiff neck and Kernig's signs are present in over one-half the patients. Deep reflexes may be lost on one or both sides in the acute stage and are rarely exaggerated until hours or days have passed. The Babinski sign (upgoing toe) is frequently present on the side of paralysis or bilaterally. Loss or severe impairment of all forms of sensation, including vision, occurs on the side of paralysis. Agnosias and aphasia result from the involvement of the dominant (usually the left) parietotemporal areas. All types of retinal hemorrhages may be seen by ophthalmoscopy. Papilledema develops from massive intracranial hematoma and sometimes is recognizable in less than 12 hours. Fever is high, especially when the ventricular system is entered. Headache is severe in three fourths of conscious patients.

HEMORRHAGE ELSEWHERE IN THE BRAIN.—The foregoing descrip-

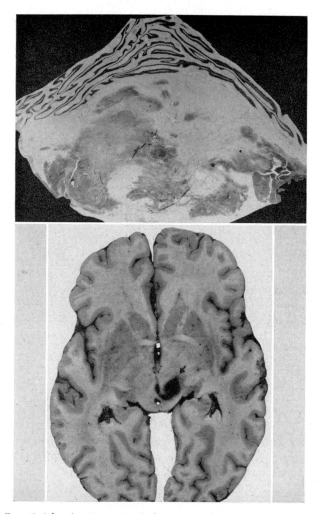

FIG. 59 *(above)*.—Hemorrhagic destruction of the pons (Nisslstain).

FIG. 60 *(below)*.—Hemorrhage into midbrain. (George Washington University Laboratory of Neurology.)

tion applies particularly to hemorrhage in the interior of the cerebral hemisphere. Paralysis is less, the farther the site of rupture from the internal capsule. When the *pons* is the locale of primary hemorrhage (Fig. 59), death may occur rapidly but never in less than one hour. Onset of symptoms is sudden, coma is deep, hyperthermia is common, the pupils are miotic and neurologic signs are bilateral. Decerebrate rigidity is often present. Spontaneous hemorrhage in the *mesencephalon* or *medulla oblongata* is rare. Weber's syndrome of unilateral oculomotor paralysis and contralateral hemiplegia is caused by hemorrhage in the former location (Fig. 60). In a remarkable case reported by Scoville and Poppen a hematoma was successfully removed from the cerebral peduncle. Bleeding in the lower bulb kills rapidly, with cardiac and respiratory oppression and signs of cranial nerve paralysis before death.

Cerebellar hemorrhage constitutes 10–15 per cent of all hemorrhagic cerebrovascular accidents. Although death may occur suddenly, the usual course is a chronic syndrome indicating an expanding clot in the hind-

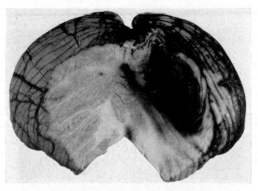

Fig. 61.—Spontaneous intracerebellar hemorrhage (AFIP #L6023-1.)

brain (Fig. 61) and resembling that of posterior fossa tumor. In a patient operated on by me, findings were those of bilateral pyramidal and extrapyramidal disease and of increased intracranial pressure; no cerebellar signs were present. When *intraventricular* hemorrhage is the end stage of parenchymal rupture, pyramidal signs become bilateral, the temperature mounts and coma deepens (Fig. 62).

LABORATORY STUDIES

A leukocyte count above 12,000 is an almost constant finding and a count of more than 22,000 in the peripheral blood is found in over one-half the patients with cerebral hemorrhage in the absence of infection. Urinary abnormalities consist of changes typical of primary or vascular nephritis, and sugar is found occasionally as a sequel of brain injury (Bernard's phenomenon).

Serum bilirubin concentration is frequently elevated and may remain so for several weeks (Furtado and Chichorro). Hyperglycemia and gly-cosuria may suggest diabetes mellitus. Serum nitrogen retention correlates with coincident renal failure.

The systolic *blood pressure* is almost always elevated above 200 mm., and the diastolic tension is high in patients with typical cerebral hemor-rhage. Both values rise still more as intracranial pressure is increased rapidly. Cardiac hypertrophy, left ventricular failure and other complica-

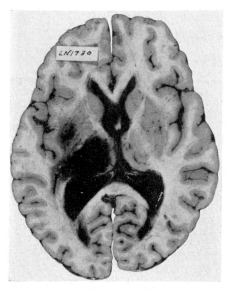

FIG. 62.—Rupture of thalamogeniculate artery with flooding of the ventricles. (George Washington University Laboratory of Neurology.)

tions of hypertensive cardiovascular renal disease may be present. In atypical (venous or aneurysmal) hemorrhage the blood pressure is not necessarily abnormal.

In most patients the *cerebrospinal fluid* pressure is greater than 200 mm. of water, and in at least 75 per cent of cases the fluid is frankly bloody. Xanthochromic or turbid fluids are found in an additional 10 per cent, and in 15 per cent of hemorrhages the cerebrospinal fluid may be clear inasmuch as blood may not have entered the ventricular system or subarachnoid spaces at the time of lumbar puncture. Erythrocytes are usually found microscopically in all specimens of fluid examined. Protein content is increased, and any type of colloidal gold curve may be evident.

X-rays of the skull may show lateral displacement of the pineal

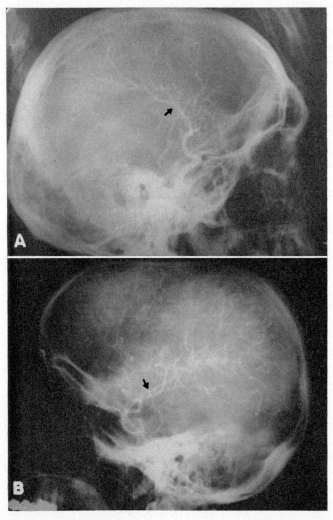

FIG. 63.—*A*, upward displacement of middle cerebral artery by temporoparietal hemorrhage. (Courtesy of S. W. Gross.) *B*, downward displacement of middle cerebral artery by frontal hemorrhage.

gland, often sufficient to verify the side of hemorrhage in subacute cases favorable for surgery. Very uncommonly, calcification of a chronic intra-cerebral hematoma may be seen. Air encephalography must be of the small type (Monrad-Krohn), but 10–15 cc. of air injected via the lumbar route may be safely tolerated and may disclose ventricular displacement. Ventriculography is better recommended because of high intracranial pressure but is a more complicated procedure in an unconscious or un-co–operative patient. The ventricle on the side of intrahemispheral hem-orrhage is collapsed, the contralateral chamber being slightly enlarged and shifted from the midline.

Carotid *angiography* may reveal an avascular mass (area) in the cerebral hemisphere in both arterial and venous phases (Fig. 63). In lateral views, the carotid siphon is uncoiled and displaced forward and the middle cerebral artery is narrowed and lifted up when hemorrhage extends into the temporal lobe. Both carotid and middle cerebral vessels are forced downward and backward by a hematoma in the posterior frontal lobe. In anteroposterior projections, the anterior cerebral artery is pushed to the opposite side of the midline by capsular hemorrhage.

Electroencephalograms in supratentorial hemorrhage consist of gen-eralized delta activity (very slow) if the patient is comatose, or focal slow waves are confined to one brain area or one hemisphere, alpha potentials being absent ipsilaterally. Brain shift results in bilateral hemi-spheral abnormalities (Fig. 64). The electroencephalogram is usually normal in lesions of the posterior fossa.

Radioactive fluorescein is said not to be concentrated in intracerebral hematoma (Ashkenazy *et al.*).

DIAGNOSIS

Diagnosis of typical spontaneous hemispheral intracerebral hemor-rhage may be made in a hypertensive individual, 40–70 years of age, in whom neurologic prodromes are followed by a sudden onset of severe headache, vomiting and often convulsive seizures terminating quickly in deep coma. The neck is stiff and Kernig's signs are present, the pulse is slow, respirations are stertorous and the temperature climbs. Either hemiplegia is profound or the body is generally flaccid. Either pupil is dilated or both are constricted, and the light reflex is absent bilaterally. Hemorrhages or papilledema are often visible in the optic fundi. The head and eyes are deviated toward the site of hemorrhage. The sign of Babinski is present on the hemiplegic side or in both feet. Focal paralyses progress over a period of 12–14 hours.

Leukocytosis is found. The lumbar cerebrospinal fluid pressure is elevated and the cerebrospinal fluid is usually bloody or xanthochromic. Serum bilirubin is increased. Glycosuria may be discovered. Skull films show lateral displacement of a calcified pineal gland with hemispheric lesions. Air studies reveal that one ventricle has collapsed from intracerebral bleeding and that the opposite ventricle is shifted laterally. Arteriography often demonstrates a straightened carotid siphon with an elevated middle cerebral artery or may show both displaced inferiorly. Electroencephalographic findings are those of general or focal slow waves

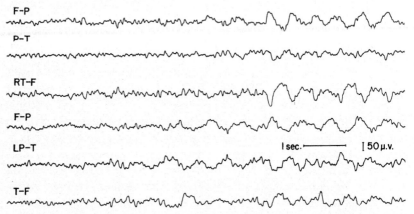

FIG. 64.—Bilateral delta activity in electroencephalogram associated with hematoma in left temporal lobe.

and absence of alpha activity at least homolaterally with the hemispheric hemorrhage.

DIFFERENTIAL DIAGNOSIS.—*Other cerebrovascular accidents.*—Principal differentiation must be made from cerebral thrombosis or infarction and from subarachnoid hemorrhage. The patient with cerebral thrombosis is more frequently normotensive and is older. The headache is less severe, convulsions are rare, consciousness is usually retained and neurologic disability is less profound. Most importantly, the cerebrospinal fluid pressure is not high and the fluid is clear.

In subarachnoid hemorrhage, coma is not as common or as profound as in cerebral hemorrhage. Cranial nerve signs predominate, and hypertension is not directly related. There is an elevated pressure of bloody cerebrospinal fluid which does not fall rapidly on the withdrawal of a small amount of fluid.

Cardiac disease usually sponsors cerebral embolism. In embolism, infarctive phenomena appear elsewhere, consciousness is not often lost and the cerebrospinal fluid is not grossly bloody. A gradual development of symptoms and signs, papilledema and high pressure of clear cerebrospinal fluid characterize brain tumor, although when glioma or metastatic malignancy is hemorrhagic differentiation is difficult.

Head injury.—In a patient with cerebral laceration, signs of severe head trauma are obvious. Subdural hematoma also results from head injury and is common in alcoholics. In subdural hematoma, neurologic and psychiatric symptoms and signs develop over a period of time. The cerebrospinal fluid typically is under moderately increased pressure, is faintly yellow but has a near-normal protein content. Epidural hematoma is of rapid progression after cranial injury. Temporal skull fracture is almost invariable, ipsilateral oculomotor paralysis is maximal, convulsive seizures begin in the face and decerebrate rigidity appears quickly.

Other conditions confused with cerebral hemorrhage are hypertensive encephalopathy, an epileptic attack, diabetic or uremic coma, drug poisoning, acute alcoholism, hysteria and nonspecific head injury. Each has peculiar features which permit differentiation.

TREATMENT

MEDICAL THERAPY.—Medical management is that of the seriously ill and unconscious patient who is at the complete mercy of his environment. Special attention must be given to the heart, lungs, temperature, bladder, bowel and skin (Chapter 19). There is no effective indirect method of stopping a continuing brain hemorrhage, either arterial or venous, although there is no real objection to the use of icebags to the head and neck or to venesection, especially if hypertensive cardiac failure impends. The parenteral use of coagulants is a futile gesture.

SURGICAL THERAPY.—Neurosurgical evacuation of the intracerebral clot is the only measure which affords direct and effective control of hemorrhage and the increasing intracranial pressure. This implies ability to localize the site of bleeding and proper selection of cases. Although first reported by Heusner in 1888 and advocated by Cushing in 1903, operative removal of spontaneous cerebral hematoma has not been a procedure attractive to neurosurgeons until fairly recently. With more time and interest now devoted to the treatment of hemorrhagic apoplexy, reported results in small series of cases are most encouraging.

There is general agreement that the syndrome favorable to surgery consists of sudden onset of signs and symptoms of hemorrhage, the preservation or quick regaining of consciousness and slow progression of neurologic signs and increase of intracranial pressure. Surgery is usually performed in the subacute or chronic stage of hemorrhage, days or weeks after the attack. Insistence that this sequence of events be present before exploration eliminates the hopeless, brain-destroying and ventricle-flooding, massive, hypertensive "blowouts" and avoids the almost certain death attendant on operations on patients in coma. Few surgeons have had any success with attempts to aspirate fresh blood or newly softened brain through a ventricular cannula as an emergency procedure.

Localization, removal of clot.—Because most hemorrhages amenable to surgery tend to occur in certain areas of the brain, notably the paracapsular and deep temporo-occipital regions, visible displacement of the pineal gland is considered sufficient objective proof of the site of bleeding by many surgeons. Others advise routine use of ventriculography or angiography for localization. Each case must be weighed individually as to the risk of possible complications of air or Diodrast studies in a patient with acute cerebrovascular disease, compared with the possibility of missing the position of hemorrhage at operation. Either bur-hole drainage or evacuation through a craniectomy opening or bone flap is effective in dealing with the clot. Reported operative mortality has ranged from 12 to 28 per cent. In cerebellar hemorrhages recognition and evacuation have been as effective as in the more common cerebral type.

Not only does surgery offer the only logical hope of successful treatment, but so often does chronic intracerebral hematoma resemble advanced intrinsic brain tumor that refusal to investigate such a theoretically inoperable patient (glioma) may allow him to die of a treatable condition (hemorrhage). Naturally, destroyed brain cannot be replaced by surgery, and the fundamental underlying process remains. It is remarkable, however, how often high blood pressure is reduced after a major stroke.

PROGNOSIS

Cerebral hemorrhage has a high incidence of rather rapid fatality but does not cause immediate death. First day mortality in tabulated groups has varied from 30 to 80 per cent. The shortest period of survival is one to two hours, in contrast to subarachnoid hemorrhage which may kill in minutes. Brain stem extravasations, either primary or secondary to transtentorial herniation of the temporal lobe, cause death soon after appearance. Cerebellar hemorrhages are often tolerated for surprisingly long periods. Of 107 fatalities from hemorrhage in all locations studied by Zimmerman, 87 per cent of the patients died within five weeks. The average survival period after cerebral thrombosis is 15 times as long as that after cerebral hemorrhage. Accessory causes of death are aspiration pneumonia, cardiac failure, uremia, diabetes and pulmonary infarct.

These gloomy figures are in the process of being revised favorably by greater interest in the differential diagnosis of cerebrovascular accidents and the use of surgery in more and more favorable cases. The hypertensive capsular "blowout" which quickly floods the ventricular system occurs all too commonly, however, and still defies therapeutic efforts in any direction.

BIBLIOGRAPHY

Angrist, A., and Mitchell, N.: Traumatic hemorrhage of the internal capsule, Arch. Surg. 46:265-276, 1943.

Aring, C. D.: Vascular diseases of the nervous system, Brain 68:28-55, 1945.

Ashkenazy, M.; Davis, L., and Martin, J.: An evaluation of the technic and results of the radioactive diiodofluorescein test for the localization of intracranial lesions, J. Neurosurg. 8:300-314, 1951.

Cobb, S.: Cerebral circulation: A critical discussion of the symposium, A. Res. Nerv. & Ment. Dis., Proc. 18:719-750, 1938.

Courville, C. B., and Blomquist, O. A.: Traumatic cerebral hemorrhage, Arch. Surg. 41:1-28, 1940.

Craig, W. M., and Adson, A. W.: Spontaneous intracerebral hemorrhage: Etiology and surgical treatment with report of nine cases, Arch. Neurol. & Psychiat. 35:701-716, 1936.

Furtado, D., and Chichorro, V.: Diagnostic différentiel des hémorragies et des thromboses cérébrales établi sur une valeur de laboratoire, Arch. internat. pharmacodyn. 78:229-235, 1949.

Globus, J. H., and Sapirstein, M.: Massive hemorrhage into brain tumor: Its significance and probable relationship to rapidly fatal termination and antecedent trauma, J.A.M.A. 120:348-352, 1942.

Globus, J. H., and Strauss, I.: Massive cerebral hemorrhage, Arch. Neurol. & Psychiat. 18:215-239, 1927.

Irish, C. W.: Cerebral vascular lesions in newborn infants and children, J. Pediat. 15:64-74, 1939.

Jewesbury, E. C. O.: Atypical intracerebral hemorrhage, Brain 70:274-303, 1947.

Margolis, G.; Odom, G. L.; Woodhall, B., and Bloor, B. M.: Role of small angiomatous malformations in production of intracerebral hematomas, J. Neurosurg. 8:564-575, 1951.

Merritt, H. H., and Aring, C. D.: The differential diagnosis of cerebral vascular lesions, A. Res. Nerv. & Ment. Dis., Proc. 18:682-695, 1938.

Minkowski, A.: Involvement of small vessels in neonatal hemorrhages, Sang 22:701-712, 1951.

Oldberg, E.: Hemorrhage into gliomas, Arch. Neurol. & Psychiat. 30:1061-1073, 1933.

Penfield, W.: The operative treatment of spontaneous intracerebral hemorrhage, Canad. M. J. 28:369-372, 1933.

Rupp, C.; Riggs, H., and Stratemeyer, W.: Acute cerebral apoplexy, Tr. Am. Neurol. A. 73:20-23, 1948.

Scoville, W. B., and Poppen, J. L.: Intrapeduncular hemorrhage of the brain, Arch. Neurol. & Psychiat. 61:688-694, 1949.

Strassmann, G.: Formation of hemosiderin and hematoidin after traumatic and spontaneous cerebral hemorrhages, Arch. Path. 47:205-210, 1949.

Symonds, C. P.: Delayed traumatic intracerebral hemorrhage, Brit. M. J. 1:1048-1051, 1940.

Winternitz, M. C.: Personal communication.

Zimmerman, H. M.: Cerebral apoplexy: Mechanism and differential diagnosis, New York J. Med. 49:2153-2157, 1949.

Subarachnoid Hemorrhage; Intracranial Aneurysm

SUBARACHNOID HEMORRHAGE IS the disease syndrome in which sudden flooding of the subarachnoid fluid spaces with arterial blood commonly produces a clinical picture of spectacular intracranial vascular accident in which the prominent signs are both meningeal and cerebral and are of grave character. Bleeding is usually due to the rupture of a congenital arterial aneurysm of the circle of Willis. The first or a subsequent attack may strike without warning in a person, often young, who has been in perfect health, and may kill in a matter of minutes.

On the other hand, if favorable circumstances permit the tiding of the patient through the initial critical period, treatment of the condition and prevention of recurrence by surgical means can be a gratifying experience. Amenability to operative therapy and prognosis after surgery are often better in cases of ruptured intracranial aneurysm than in brain tumor, and the outlook after control of the lesion is also superior to that for hemorrhagic cerebral apoplexy.

ETIOLOGY; PATHOGENESIS

Congenital Arterial Aneurysm

Although arterial dilatations of basal trunks are sometimes the end stage of syphilitic or arteriosclerotic processes, the saccular or berry variety of aneurysm which ruptures and is responsible for the greatest number of subarachnoid hemorrhages almost always is of developmentally aberrant origin (Fig. 1, B). Syphilitic or arteriosclerotic aneurysms seldom rupture and manifest their presence in other ways.

Morgagni (1761) was the first pathologist to describe intracranial arterial aneurysm at autopsy, and Biumi (1778) recognized ruptured aneurysm as a cause of subarachnoid hemorrhage. Virchow (1851) called attention to the frequent occurrence of small saccules on the circle of Willis, which Charcot and Bouchard named "miliary aneurysms." What

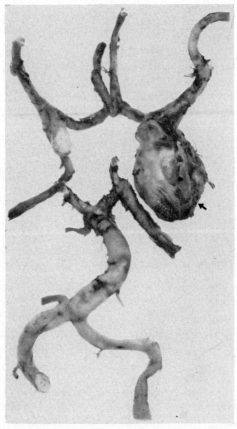

FIG. 65.—Typical congenital aneurysm of the circle of Willis. (Courtesy of P. M. Levin.)

was probably the first diagnosis of saccular arterial aneurysm in a living patient was made by Hutchinson (1875). The descriptive label of "berry aneurysms" was attached to these lesions by Richardson and Hyland. Hamby estimated that intracranial aneurysm occurs in 0.5–1 per cent of the general population. Familial incidence has been reported.

Embryologic deviations.—Finger-like and morular aneurysmal sacs which depend or project from narrow necks arising from arteries of the circle of Willis (Fig. 65) are probably the vestiges of primitive supernumerary vessels which should have disappeared but have been retained into adult life (Padget). Fusiform and globular aneurysmal enlargements with broad, sessile bases attached to the forked clefts of branching arteries are best accountable to lack of proper growth of the arterial media (Forbus; Bremer). The points of bifurcation of the middle cerebral and basilar arteries were studied by Richardson and Hyland in seven adult brains of various ages without grossly visible aneurysm and in an-

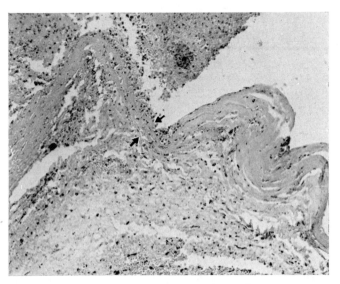

FIG. 66.—Necrosis in wall of ruptured carotid aneurysm.

other with a congenital sac on one major artery; in five, medial defects were evident, and in two microscopic aneurysms were found. Failure of accurate fusion of coalescing vascular anlagen is yet another error of nature; a bulge at the line of division of the basilar trunk into the two posterior cerebral vessels was seen by Bremer in an embryo of 42 weeks.

Further pathologic changes.—Vestigial saccules are partially or totally devoid of both media and elastica to begin with. The intima then gradually proliferates to form a fibrous plaque at the site of attachment to the parent artery, the internal elastic membrane degenerates and finally disappears, and the further enlarged pouch either thromboses and becomes organized or, more often, perforates as arterial pressure beats upon the atrophic and eventually necrotic wall (Forbus). Studies of serial sections of aneurysms led to the conclusion that the degenerative and necrotizing changes of atherosclerosis superimposed on the initial malformation account for the break in the wall and rupture (Carmichael). Thus, many supposedly arteriosclerotic sacs are actually congenital at basis, particularly if they bleed. The vasa vasorum in the neck of an aneurysm must be very deficient, and nutrition of the sac is consequently poor.

It may be stated positively that all aneurysms which rupture do so through a point of necrosis in the internal elastic membrane. This is often at the neck of the sac, a fact of importance surgically (Fig. 66). It is no wonder that fresh bleeding often starts when a metal clip is applied to the attachment of the saccule to its artery. This observation has further bearing medicolegally when an attempt is made to relate subarachnoid hemorrhage to industrial hazard or activity. As a matter of fact, in many cases of ruptured aneurysm, intracranial hemorrhage occurs while the patient is under no physical strain.

Rarely, the construction of the lesion is that of a dissecting aneurysm in the arterial wall.

Arterial pressure effects.—Black and German studied the destructive effect of systolic blood pressure on the wall of aneurysmal sacs. They observed that differences in velocity of flow vary in terms of the square of the velocity, that pulsatile variations may have a water-hammer effect in the interior of an aneurysm and that the jet action of passage of blood through the orifice of the sac can cause internal turbulence. Elevation of blood pressure which may result from unusual physical activity, such as sexual intercourse, undoubtedly can precipitate rupture. Vibration of the vessel bearing the sac must also contribute to fragility of the aneurysmal stalk. The progressive enlargement of vestigial aneurysms is probably due largely to atrophic changes in the internal elastic membrane induced by arterial pulsations.

Mycotic and Neoplastic Aneurysms

Mycotic aneurysm may develop when an infected embolus, usually from bacterial endocarditis, lodges in an intracranial artery, often at a fork or in a small branch. The suppurative process destroys the vessel wall and rupture results. Because of the predominance of rheumatic and endocarditic disorders in the younger age group, mycotic embolism and aneurysm formation are rare over the age of 50. Fungi, yeasts and molds may also be responsible (McKee).

Tumor emboli can likewise be arrested at arterial forks or can produce aneurysm by metastatic growth. A classic episode of subarachnoid hemorrhage in an elderly woman seen by me was traced to cancer metastasis only by Papanicolaou examination of the cerebrospinal fluid. In another, younger woman a tumor embolus from an ovarian carcinoma resulted in a carotid-cavernous fistula with pulsating exophthalmos.

OTHER ETIOLOGIES

Head injury is the most common cause of bloody cerebrospinal fluid. *Cerebral hemorrhage* is at least as frequently responsible for the appearance of blood in the cerebrospinal fluid as is ruptured arterial aneurysm. *Cerebral infarction* of the hemorrhagic variety, due to arterial or venous thrombosis, usually is followed by bleeding into the subarachnoid space. Repeated episodes of intracranial hemorrhage characterize *arteriovenous anomaly*. Massive subarachnoid leakage occurs sometimes in the hemorrhagic *blood dyscrasias*. Virtually all types of *inflammatory* vascular disease cause meningeal hemorrhage on occasion. *Eclampsia* is often featured by subarachnoid bleeding. *Meningitis* may be a source, owing to rupture of infected vessels. Intracranial hemorrhage has also been observed in *encephalitis* and with *venous* or *sinus thrombosis*.

Metallic and other *poisons* may injure pial vessels to the point of perforation and extravasation. Focal arterial necrosis with hemorrhage, a toxic or hyperergic reaction, has occurred after surgical operations (Kernohan and Woltman). Primary intracranial *neoplasms,* such as gliomas, meningiomas and pituitary adenomas, and metastatic malignant tumors in the brain may be manifested by bloody cerebrospinal fluid. Neoplasm of the cauda equina can bleed into the dural sac and produce signs of generalized subarachnoid hemorrhage (Fincher), as do *vascular malformations* of the *spinal cord* and meninges. In at least one authenticated case, *laceration* of a cerebral artery by a spicule of bone from a basal skull fracture caused a traumatic aneurysm which later ruptured, causing death. Severely *sclerosed* basilar or carotid arteries may split with fatal hemorrhage thereafter. Subarachnoid hemorrhage may follow insulin or electric *shock therapy* or *pneumoencephalography.*

PATHOLOGY

Diffusion of subarachnoid blood from the site of rupture of an arterial aneurysm is rapid because the circle of Willis is suspended in a large fluid space. At autopsy, the entire brain is dusky red externally. Masses of fresh

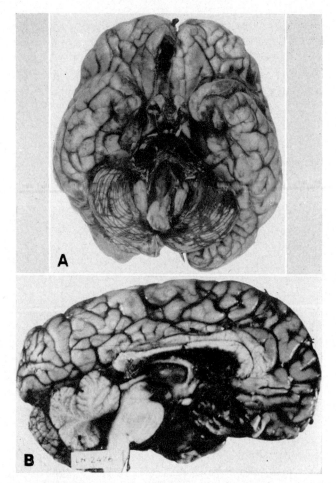

FIG. 67.—Blood in basal cisterns, *A*, and ventricular system, *B*, after fatal subarachnoid hemorrhage. (*A*, AFIP #AC 158606-821; *B*, George Washington University Laboratory of Neurology.)

blood clog the sulci and arachnoid cisterns and form clots in the fissures of the cerebrum, cerebellum and brain stem. The fourth ventricle may be entered in retrograde fashion from the cisterna magna, blood passing upward through the foramens of Luschka and Magendie (Fig. 67).

When cerebral parenchyma is immediately adjacent to an aneurysm and especially in the sylvian fissure, perforation of a congenital sac through previously softened brain results in intracerebral hematoma (25

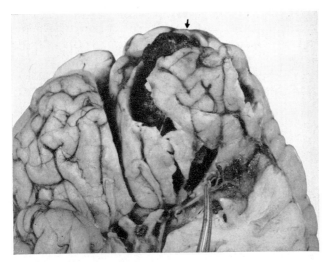

FIG. 68.—Intracerebral hematoma (arrow) in frontal lobe. Hemostat on ruptured aneurysm. (AFIP #11609-B.)

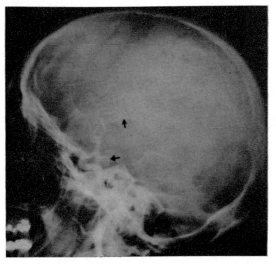

FIG. 69.—Elevation of middle cerebral artery (upper arrow) by hematoma in temporal lobe due to rupture of carotid aneurysm (lower arrow).

205

per cent of cases), a frequent cause of death. This occurs in the frontal and temporal lobes from aneurysms on the anterior circle, and although it is perfectly possible for rupture to take place into the brain without a trace of meningeal leak, intrinsic and extrinsic bleeding are usually combined (Figs. 68 and 69). When an aneurysm or its internal hemorrhage erodes into a regional ventricle, death results from ventricular flooding (Fig. 74,*I*).

An abutting cerebral gyrus can and frequently does seal off the point

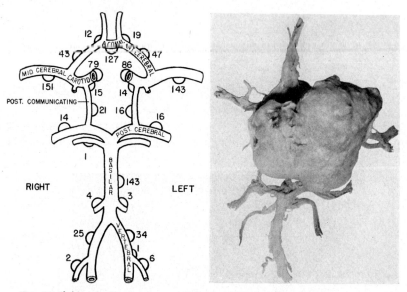

FIG. 70 *(left)*.—Incidence of congenital intracranial arterial aneurysms. (After McDonald and Korb.)

FIG. 71 *(right)*.—Enormous aneurysm which destroyed the hypothalamus. (Courtesy of J. T. B. Carmody.)

of perforation, a lifesaving circumstance that must be remembered in retracting the brain during surgical exposure of aneurysmal lesions. In rare instances, subdural hematoma may be a result of aneurysmal rupture, intracerebral or subarachnoid extravasation breaking through the arachnoid membrane and allowing blood to pass into the subdural space (Bassett and Lemmen; Golden *et al.*).

MENINGEAL REACTION.—The inflammatory process which accompanies subarachnoid bleeding terminates in fibroblastic organization, a reparative action which tends to prevent secondary rupture. Connective tissue growth from both the vascular adventitia and arachnoid is first evident on the third day after rupture and is later replaced by collagen (Alpers and Forster). Organization is usually imperfect, patchy, mild and does not invade the brain. The ventriculoarachnoid pathways remain partially open, although subarachnoid hemorrhage is often followed by internal or communicating hydrocephalus. Absorption of blood is effected largely by the passage of intact erythrocytes through the meninges (Simmonds).

LOCATION AND SIZE OF ANEURYSMS.—McDonald and Korb collected 1,125 cases of aneurysm, 77 per cent of which had ruptured (Fig. 70). Forty-eight per cent were located on the internal carotid or middle cerebral arteries and 15 per cent on the anterior communicating artery; 28 per cent arose from vessels posterior to the carotid, particularly the basilar trunk (7 per cent of all). Aneurysms occur on all components of the circle of Willis and other major arteries. Rupture of anterior aneurysms is three times as common as that of posterior lesions.

Aneurysmal sacs are usually of millimeter dimensions, often are 1 cm. wide, but may attain huge size, at times becoming as large as a duck egg or a small orange, especially when originating from the carotid or basilar arteries (Fig. 71). Because these congenital anomalies enlarge during life, they are encountered more often in the middle aged than in youths or children. Multiple aneurysms are not uncommon (10–20 per cent of cases) and one or several arteries may be implicated (Figs. 74, G and 128).

ASSOCIATED ABNORMALITIES.—The combination of a congenital berry aneurysm and an arteriovenous angioma on the same or on different intracranial vessels occurs rarely; hemorrhage is more apt to come from the aneurysmal sac (Fig. 72). Additional evidence that aneurysm formation may result from a general cerebral vascular dysplasia is found in the construction of the circle of Willis in the presence of such malformation: there is not only a higher than normal incidence of absent arteries, but arterial communications are often larger than usual (Padget). Atheromatous change in the cerebral vessels of children, adolescents and young adults with congenital aneurysmal lesions is remarkably frequent (McDonald and Korb).

The presence of congenital anomalies elsewhere in the body also suggests a fundamental systemic dysplasia. Eppinger (1888) first noted the concurrence of coarctation of the aorta and cerebral aneurysm. Aortic stenosis or renal malformation should be thought of when the young aneurysm patient is also hypertensive. The association of polycystic kidneys with congenital intracranial arterial disease is not uncommon; Brown

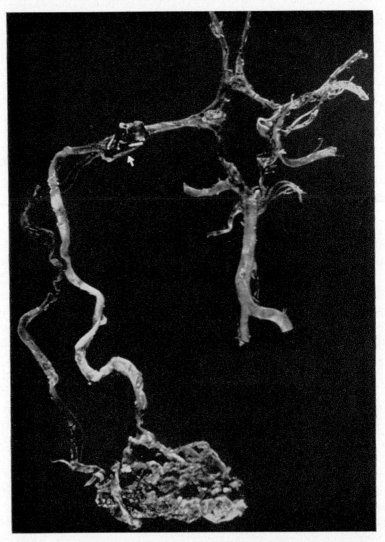

FIG. 72.—Perforated congenital aneurysm (arrow) and arteriovenous malformation, both arising from the middle cerebral artery. (George Washington University Laboratory of Neurology.)

found the combination in 4 per cent of aneurysm patients and in 16.6 per cent of patients with polycystic kidney in a series of 11,245 autopsies.

SYMPTOMS AND SIGNS

The time of life in which spontaneous subarachnoid hemorrhage may occur ranges from birth to old age. Richardson and Hyland in 118 cases of intracranial aneurysm found the average age at time of first rupture to be 46 years. The incidence by sex is about equal, with a slight preponderance in females. Of 110 patients seen by Poppen, 74.5 per cent had previous episodes of intracranial bleeding. In 90 per cent of 150 cases reviewed by Magee, rupture occurred when the patient was believed to be under no physical strain, and in 28 per cent the accident took place in bed or a chair. Clinical experience suggests that the initial history as given at the time of hospitalization may be erroneous; repeated questioning often reveals that hemorrhage actually was initiated during sexual intercourse and not in quiet sleep. Bleeding commenced during labor in only four of 28 pregnant women who had subarachnoid hemorrhage (Conley and Rand). In 14 it began prepartum and in 10 after delivery.

Hemorrhage may be brought on by intercourse, micturition, defecation or other temporary physical strain. There seems to be a seasonal incidence of subarachnoid bleeding with somewhat greater frequency in spring and fall.

The Acute Episode

The attack usually comes on with lightning rapidity, as the proverbial "bolt from the blue," but may be so gradual in development as to suggest even a nonorganic condition such as hysteria. The clinical syndrome most commonly is one of catastrophic intracranial accident and is featured by headache, meningeal irritation and cranial nerve signs which are usually oculomotor or ocular in type. The finding of bloody cerebrospinal fluid on lumbar puncture confirms the diagnosis of subarachnoid hemorrhage. Premonitory or chronic symptoms before major hemorrhage include bouts of head pain, atypical facial neuralgia, ophthalmoplegia or paresis, diminished vision, nausea, dizziness, syncopal attacks and vague aches in the back of the neck and extremities.

Headache.—The headache of subarachnoid hemorrhage is of high intensity. The patient sometimes relates it correctly to "something snapping in the head." Although usually of agonizing, refractory painfulness, headache may be mild or absent in the elderly. Pain is almost always maximal in the back of the cranium and in the upper neck, is often referred to the forehead or eye or may be generalized from the outset. Cephalalgia is accentuated by flexing the head on the neck. When aneurysm of the internal carotid or immediate branches is responsible for hemorrhage, pain may be felt in the ipsilateral frontal and orbital region only. The distribution of headache can assist in the localization of the source of arterial rupture, but flooding of the subarachnoid spaces often confuses such an attempt.

High-intensity headache in patients not treated surgically persists for seven to 10 days and then tapers off to leave entirely at the end of two months. Migraine and periodic headaches of other character occur in a significant percentage of persons sustaining subarachnoid hemorrhage. Aneurysmal headache is often unilateral, as in migraine, but this does not necessarily mean that the latter is due to enlargement of the sac; both conditions may exist separately in the same patient. Wolff has suggested that recurrent vasomotor changes associated with periodic headache may weaken the walls of a congenital aneurysm, leading to rupture.

Meningeal and systemic signs.—Meningeal and cranial or spinal nerve root irritation may be so severe as to render the patient opisthotonic. The neck is stiff and Kernig's signs are present. With slow leakage of blood there may be complaints of diffuse facial pain and stiffness and aching of the neck and extremities.

Fever and leukocytosis parallel the intensity of meningeal signs. The temperature is usually high at the beginning of the illness, may drop for two or three days and then rise again to diminish by lysis in one or two weeks. Recrudescence may indicate repeated bleeding. Rise of the polymorphonuclear concentration in a total white blood cell count of 20,000–30,000 may, in the presence of fever and a stiff neck, lead to the mistaken diagnosis of meningitis. Vomiting and photophobia accompany the febrile illness. Twenty-five per cent of patients lapse into coma at the onset of hemorrhage and an additional 25 per cent become unconscious soon thereafter.

Eye signs.—Small, flame- or splinter-shaped retinal hemorrhages often appear near the optic disk. Subhyaloid hemorrhage, a large preretinal extravasation lying between the hyaloid membrane of the vitreous chamber and the retina and usually seen in the region of the macula, is a variable but characteristic lesion and often indicates associated subdural hematoma. It has a round outline below and straight edge above. These extravasations absorb slowly and often leave white or pigmented scars; there may be subsequent impairment of sight. Papilledema of various degree is a late development in about 20 per cent of ruptured aneurysm cases. When present, swelling of the optic nerve head should suggest the possibility of associated intracerebral or intraventricular hemorrhage, hypertension, brain tumor or sinus thrombosis.

Optic atrophy which is indicative of chronic impairment of the second cranial nerve due to aneurysmal pressure is seen in 10 per cent of patients. Complete blindness is uncommon but does occur. Constriction of the visual fields accompanies papilledema, and various hemianoptic field

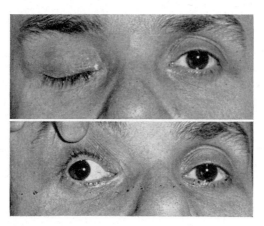

FIG. 73.—Oculomotor paralysis from aneurysm of the terminal carotid.

defects are produced by pressure of the aneurysm on the optic nerve, chiasm or tract or result from injury of the visual projections by hematoma or hemorrhagic infarction of the brain.

Cranial nerve signs.—The oculomotor, abducens, trochlear and trigeminal nerves are frequently involved because of their close grouping in the cavernous sinus and superior orbital fissure, immediately adjacent to the carotid siphon and its terminal branches where the greater percentage of aneurysms occur. Seventy per cent of all aneurysm patients have some form of ocular palsy. *Oculomotor* paralysis (ptosis, pupillary dilatation, external strabismus) is the single most common cranial nerve sign (Fig. 73). Any cranial nerve may be involved either by hemorrhage into its sheath or by aneurysmal pressure.

Motor and sensory phenomena.—The reported incidence of convulsive seizures with subarachnoid hemorrhage due to aneurysm varies from 10 to 25 per cent. Epileptic attacks are thus somewhat less common than with arteriovenous anomaly. Convulsions may be generalized or may be focal, particularly if intracerebral hematoma exists. Decerebrate attacks of tonic rigidity are characteristic of aneurysms of the basilar artery. Seizures may coincide with the onset of bleeding or may take place in the next few days.

Hemiplegia is of sudden onset in 10 per cent of patients. It is caused by rupture into the brain, dissection of blood in massive quantity over the cortical motor area, thrombosis of the vessel from which the aneurysm arises or, rarely, subdural hematoma. The sign of Babinski is often bilateral with meningeal inundation; even if unilateral, its presence is not necessarily of localizing or even of lateralizing significance.

Sensory loss is much less common but may result from extrinsic or intrinsic injury to the spinothalamic projections and thalamoparietal system. Aphasia associated with hemorrhage or infarction in the left cerebral hemisphere may be either motor or sensory.

Mental phenomena.—The mental reaction in acute subarachnoid hemorrhage is frequently that of delirium or symptomatic psychosis. The patient often presents a picture of un-co-operative aggression, wild excitement and childish behavior entirely incompatible with the premorbid personality. Hallucinations and severe organic depression may be late sequelae. Psychosis is most likely to develop after rupture of an anterior aneurysm or from pressure on the base of the brain by a large sac or clot. Korsakoff's syndrome of confusion, loss of memory, confabulation, *Witzelsucht* and euphoria is not uncommon.

Miscellaneous signs.—*Exophthalmos* occasionally results from erosion of the sphenoid wing or optic canal by large arterial sacs, more often is due to rupture of an aneurysm into the cavernous sinus, in which case the eyeball pulsates visibly. *Cranial bruit,* of uncommon occurrence, is audible to the patient and examiner locally or generally and is caused by the rapid rushing of arterial blood either from artery to vein or through the stenosed orifice of an aneurysmal sac. *Herpes simplex* sometimes comes on in the subacute stage of subarachnoid hemorrhage; the trigeminal skin field is usually involved. A patient of Beadles' had a profuse *nasal hemorrhage* due to rupture of a large aneurysm in the middle fossa through an irregular communication into the nasopharynx.

ANEURYSMAL SYNDROMES

Internal carotid artery

In almost 50 per cent of all cases of intracranial aneurysm the sac arises from the terminal internal carotid or its middle cerebral division.

Carotid aneurysms may lie in the cavernous sinus, in which instance they often represent fusiform enlargements of the artery, or may originate from the supracavernous carotid, when they usually are bottle-shaped sacs of vestigial origin.

CAVERNOUS ANEURYSM.—With an aneurysm of the carotid in the cavernous sinus (Fig. 74, A), the patient, often a middle-aged woman, complains of pain in the eye and forehead. Subarachnoid hemorrhage is rare since the lesion is extradural. There is partial or complete paralysis of the oculomotor nerve, evidenced in ptosis of the upper lid, dilatation and failure of the pupil to respond to light and external strabismus. The trochlear or abducens nerves may be involved instead of the oculomotor or in addition to it. Associated sympathetic paralysis (pericarotid plexus) may further modify the pupil. Regeneration of the injured oculomotor nerve leads to abnormal associated eye movements. Levin found neuromas on the oculomotor nerve trunk in such a case. The combination of unilateral frontal headache and ocular palsies from cavernous aneurysm may lead to a mistaken diagnosis of ophthalmoplegic migraine (Bull, 1877).

Trigeminal nerve involvement depends on the exact location of the aneurysm in the cavernous sinus. If it lies anteriorly, pain and hypalgesia are found in the domain of the ophthalmic division innervating the forehead and eye. Aneurysm in the middle of the sinus injures the ophthalmic and maxillary branches, and a posterior or very large sac presses on all three derivatives of the fifth cranial nerve (Jefferson). Very large cavernous aneurysms can destroy the sella turcica and produce bitemporal hemianopsia, an effect similar to that of pituitary neoplasm, and hypophyseal destruction may result in Simmond's disease. A vestigial aneurysm of the primitive trigeminal artery arising from the carotid siphon may bleed directly into the surrounding cavernous sinus, causing pulsating exophthalmos.

SUPRACAVERNOUS CAROTID ANEURYSM.—Finger-like vestigial aneurysms arising from the carotid artery just after its emergence from the sinus may project in any direction (Fig. 74, B and C). Anterior aneurysms may be mistaken for sacculations of the anterior communicating artery; posterior sacs are confused with aneurysms of the posterior communicating artery. Bulging enlargements due to medial defect occur at points of arterial bifurcation, and the carotid-posterior communicating junction is a particularly favorite site. From all these locations, hemorrhage is subarachnoid and is much more liable to be fatal than is rupture of a sac within the dural sinus.

If the aneurysm points toward or is attached to the oculomotor or abducens nerves, ocular palsies result. Pressure on the optic nerve, chiasm or tract will produce appropriate homolateral blindness or field defects, usually homonymous in type. Progressive amaurosis in middle-aged or elderly patients can result from fusiform dilatation of the intracranial carotids; there is concentric reduction of the visual fields, especially in the

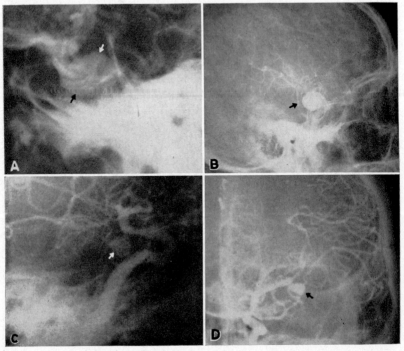

FIG. 74.—Congenital intracranial arterial aneurysms visualized during angiography or at autopsy. *A,* cavernous carotid artery (dilatation); *B,* supracavernous carotid artery (paracarotid) (V.A. Hospital, Washington, D. C., neg. 5032-1693); *C,* carotid siphon; *D,* middle cerebral artery (courtesy of O. Sugar).

lower halves, and pituitary adenoma or sellar meningioma is usually thought to be responsible for symptoms.

Ophthalmic artery

Ophthalmic aneurysm, extremely rare, causes optic atrophy, progressive blindness and enlargement of the optic foramen of the skull. Since the artery is usually superior to the nerve, visual loss begins in the lower fields. Fusiform arteriosclerotic dilatation may affect the ophthalmic vessels and cause loss of vision. The rich collateral circulation from the external carotid through the angular artery serves to protect the optic nerve if thrombosis of the ophthalmic artery occurs. Heimburger *et al.* removed an intraorbital aneurysm of the lacrimal artery, a branch of the

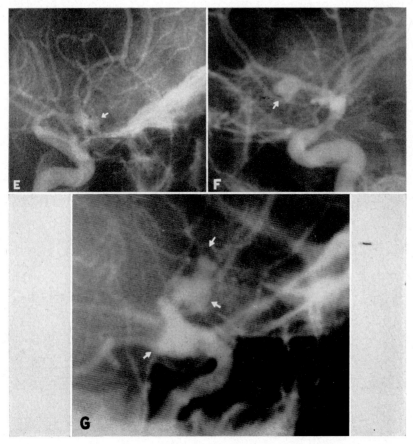

FIG. 74 *(cont.).—E,* anterior communicating artery; *F,* anterior cerebral artery; *G,* carotid, anterior communicating and anterior cerebral arteries (multiple aneurysms).

ophthalmic. The clinical syndrome was that of unilateral exophthalmos without pulsation, increased intraocular tension and failing vision.

Middle cerebral artery

Aneurysms of the middle cerebral artery cause no extraocular paralyses because they are remote from the second to sixth cranial nerves (Fig. 74, *D*). Jacksonian or generalized seizures are not uncommon. Hemiplegia develops quickly if the lesion ruptures into the sylvian fissure. It is less sudden in appearance when thrombosis extends peripherally in the artery from the aneurysmal sac and is of only gradual progression if slow expansion of the aneurysm results in pressure atrophy of the motor

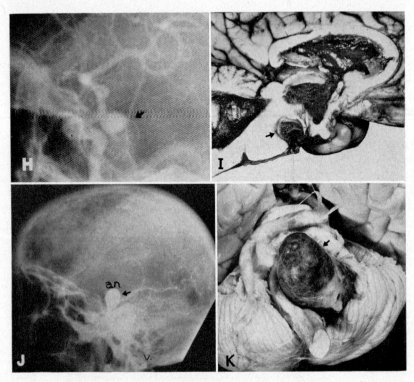

FIG. 74 *(cont.).*—*H,* posterior communicating artery; *I,* posterior cerebral artery (George Washington University Laboratory of Neurology); *J,* basilar artery (courtesy of O. Sugar); *K,* vertebral artery (courtesy of M. Bushard *et al.*). .

areas or projections. Bruit was audible in one of my patients who had a bulbous lesion at the origin of the middle cerebral artery, but this should not be regarded as a typical finding.

Anterior communicating artery

Approximately 15 per cent of all aneurysms are found on the anterior communicating artery (Fig. 74, *E*). There may be no regional neurologic signs whatever. If the lesion is large enough to impinge on the optic chiasm from above, defects will appear in the lower halves of the visual fields. Mental symptoms are frequently severe after rupture occurs and the patient may seem to have had a prefrontal lobotomy. The organic confusional syndrome can persist for some time thereafter.

Anterior cerebral artery

Aneurysms arising from the origin of the anterior cerebral artery may press on both olfactory and optic nerves, causing unilateral loss of vision and anosmia. Aneurysm formation above the chiasm may lead to the same visual field alterations (lower altitudinal hemianopsia) as occasionally result from sacculation of the anterior communicating artery (Fig. 74, F). Rupture into the frontal lobe will produce contralateral hemiplegia, and hemorrhage between the medial hemisphere and falx or thrombosis of aneurysm of the terminal anterior cerebral artery will cause paralysis of the opposite leg. Mental changes may resemble those of the postlobotomy state, owing to injury of the infrafrontal or medial frontal cortex.

Anterior choroidal artery

Temporary hemiplegia can be the result of rupture of an aneurysm of the anterior choroidal artery, since a portion of the internal capsule is supplied by this vessel. Poppen and others have reported instances of fistulous communication between the anterior choroidal artery and the vein of Galen, with audible cranial bruit.

Posterior communicating artery

Aneurysms of the posterior communicating artery are extremely rare (Fig. 74, H). With such aneurysms, paralysis of the oculomotor and abducens nerves may develop. In an elderly patient with a dilatation of the posterior communicating artery, only the eye signs of cavernous aneurysm were found, but the cerebrospinal fluid was bloody. The differentiation between aneurysm of the internal carotid and aneurysm of the posterior communicating artery is very difficult.

Posterior cerebral artery

Another pathologic rarity, aneurysm of the posterior cerebral artery may cause quadrantal or complete hemianopsia, Weber's syndrome or, if large, may produce additional hemiplegia, bulbar signs and mental defect (Fig. 74, I). Since the third cranial nerve emerges from the brain stem between the posterior cerebral and superior cerebellar arteries, oculomotor paralysis may develop. Boldrey and Miller described two patients in whom large arteriovenous fistulas were formed by the posterior communicating and posterior cerebral arteries and the galenic venous system.

Basilar artery

UNRUPTURED ANEURYSM.—Failure of fusion of the two primitive longitudinal neural arteries in the embryo accounts for the formation of bulging aneurysm in the midline of the basilar trunk (Fig. 74, J). Fifty per cent of lesions which do not bleed disclose their presence by evidences of compression of the brain stem. Cranial nerve, motor and sensory signs depend on the degree of pressure atrophy of the midbrain, pons and medulla, and a most complex mixture of neural and tract deficits results. Compression of the aqueduct and fourth ventricle from below by large aneurysms will add hydrocephalus. The differential diagnosis in such circumstances is usually from tumor in the posterior fossa. Campbell and Keedy reported two cases of basilar aneurysm which produced both tic douloureux and hemifacial spasm.

RUPTURED ANEURYSM.—Headache is usually occipital in location. Perforation of the basilar trunk and bleeding cause severe opisthotonos and attacks of tonically rigid decerebration. Quadriplegia with difficulty in swallowing, talking and breathing is a frequent sequel of hemorrhage and infarction in the pons. The prognosis for life with congenital basilar aneurysms is very poor and little can be done to afford relief, nothing to effect cure.

Vertebral artery

Aneurysms of the vertebral artery are quite unusual (Fig. 74, K). Attacks of vertigo and regional headache with progressive neurologic deficit resembling the Wallenberg syndrome of posterior inferior cerebellar artery occlusion form the clinical picture in reported cases. The patient seen by von Monakow and Ladame had ipsilateral deafness, tinnitus, ataxia, dysphagia, dysarthria and heterolateral hemianesthesia. The pulse was irregular and episodes of bleeding occurred. Bushard et al. described a patient who was troubled by intermittent headaches and had developed a peripheral facial paralysis 40 years before. Vomiting, vertigo and weakness of the right arm and leg preceded death caused by an enormous aneurysm of the left vertebral artery.

Cerebellar arteries

Proximal enlargement of the *superior* cerebellar artery will cause oculomotor paralysis. *Anterior inferior* cerebellar dilatations have been implicated in both trigeminal neuralgia and Ménière's disease (Dandy). *Posterior inferior* cerebellar aneurysms, if peripheral in location, will be evidenced in the syndrome of the cerebellopontile angle, with ipsilateral ataxia, facial sensory loss and paralysis, tinnitus and loss of hearing, late dysphagia and dysarthria. There may be no vicinity symptoms at all and the clinical picture can be only that of an expansile, bleeding lesion in the posterior fossa.

LABORATORY STUDIES

Leukocytosis may accompany the febrile illness, and the total leukocyte count may rise as high as 20,000–30,000 per cu. mm. Rarely, transient glycosuria and albuminuria have been found in urinalysis. The blood pressure is not related etiologically, but coarctation of the aorta or polycystic kidney disease may coexist with aneurysm. Moreover, the incidence of hypertension in patients with these congenital arterial malformations is higher than in corresponding groups in the general population (Black and Hicks). Severe subarachnoid hemorrhage itself can raise both systolic and diastolic arterial tensions to hypertensive levels, and slowing of the pulse is concomitant. Cardiac murmurs are usually present when hemorrhage is from a mycotic aneurysm.

CEREBROSPINAL FLUID.—The cerebrospinal fluid is uniformly and grossly bloody in fresh subarachnoid hemorrhage, and erythrocyte counts may range as high as 3,500,000 per cu. mm. of fluid. However, if lumbar puncture is performed within two hours of aneurysmal rupture, the specimen occasionally may be clear and colorless when leakage has occurred directly into the brain substance. The initial lumbar fluid pressure is usually greater than 300 mm. of water and does not fall rapidly after withdrawal of 10 cc. unless intracerebral hematoma is present.

The supernatant fluid becomes xanthochromic within four to six hours, at which time crenated erythrocytes are visible microscopically. The yellow color is intensified during the next 10 days. Xanthochromia, uniformity of admixture of blood with cerebrospinal fluid and failure of clotting in the samples withdrawn distinguish spontaneous hemorrhage from a traumatic spinal tap. The number of leukocytes in the lumbar fluid is proportionate to that of the peripheral blood in first specimens, but leukocytosis and pleocytosis increase as meningeal irritation proceeds.

The protein concentration is high, sugar and chlorides are normal or slightly reduced and the gold curve is abnormal.

ROENTGENOLOGY.—Plain x-rays of the skull may show erosion or destruction of the sella turcica or optic foramen ipsilateral with an anterior aneurysm. There may be visible calcification of the wall of the sac (Fig. 75) or of its contents (Sosman and Vogt).

Encephalographic alterations are usually minimal and are evidenced only in encroachment on the basilar cisterns and the anterior third ventricle by aneurysms arising from the circle of Willis. Posterior lesions may distort the aqueduct and fourth ventricle. A certain degree of hydrocephalus is present in patients who have had repeated hemorrhages. Rarely, a large aneurysm may be seen projecting into a part of the ventricular system (Fig. 75). Large quantities of air should not be injected when there is fresh bleeding, but 10–15 cc. may be tolerated and partial encephalography may be combined with angiography. Withdrawal of large amounts of cerebrospinal fluid, particularly if aneurysm is present in the vertebrobasilar system, may be dangerous. Either encephalography or ventriculography may be necessary to demonstrate intracerebral or intraventricular hematoma.

Angiography.—Moniz' introduction of arteriography into clinical neurology in 1927 has been largely responsible for present-day accuracy in diagnosis, localization and successful therapy of subarachnoid hemorrhage due to ruptured aneurysm and of neurologic disability caused by unruptured arterial sacs. Today, no patient with meningeal bleeding can be said to be managed properly without angiography, unless the hemorrhage is evidently caused by blood dyscrasia, embolism or some other condition much rarer than congenital vascular anomaly.

The percutaneous method of injecting the carotid or vertebral artery with Diodrast (iodopyracet) is preferred (pp. 372-376). It is usual to wait for the patient's condition to become stabilized before intra-arterial examination, but many surgeons have no hesitancy in undertaking the procedure immediately, even in the face of active bleeding. It has been shown that intracarotid pressures at some distance above the point of needle insertion are not increased by the rapid injection of 10 cc. of fluid. Bilateral carotid angiograms are usually advisable because of the possibility of multiple malformations, but unilateral visualization may be sufficient with lesions of obvious location.

While angiography is not infallible in the verification of aneurysm, carotid arteriography will reveal approximately 75 per cent of all such anomalies, although Hamby believes that in fact less than 50 per cent of these arterial lesions are actually verified in this manner. The posterior cerebral artery will appear in 25 per cent of cases with the usual 2–8 film exposure method, but to see the vertebrobasilar circulation for certain, vertebral arteriograms must be made. Since the technic of the latter is more difficult and the risks somewhat greater, one must decide

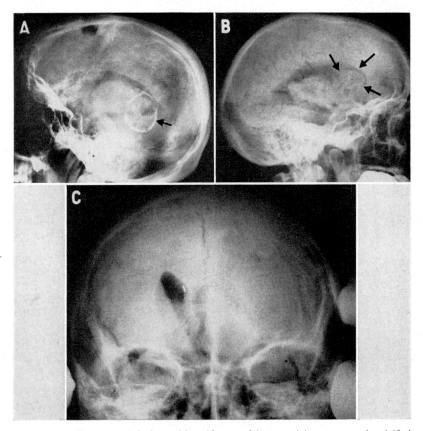

FIG. 75.—Pneumoventriculographic evidences of intracranial aneurysm. *A,* calcified aneurysm sac (courtesy of D. Oscherwitz and L. M. Davidoff); *B,* aneurysm extending into anterior horn of lateral ventricle (courtesy of D. H. Echols and H. D. Kirgis); *C,* ventricular shift due to enormous carotid aneurysm.

whether visualization of arteries below the tentorium will be of practical value. Few aneurysms in this location are amenable to surgery. A general survey of the entire circle of Willis and other major arteries by five injections performed through one carotid artery, as described by Ecker, may be an efficient compromise.

ELECTROENCEPHALOGRAPHY.—The   electroencephalogram   as   a means of lateralizing and localizing the aneurysmal source of subarachnoid hemorrhage is believed to be of dependable accuracy by some investigators but is considered by most clinical neurologists to be not entirely reliable as an exclusive diagnostic test. When a striking abnormality of the electroencephalogram is confined to one side or area of the cerebrum, this evidence can be of material assistance in proceeding with further diagnostic confirmation and surgical therapy (Fig. 76). Large anterior arterial lesions which hollow out the cerebral hemisphere act as

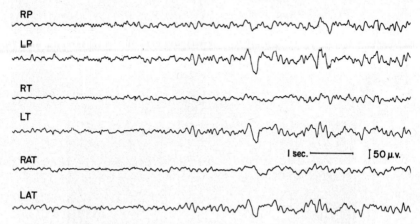

FIG. 76.—Slow wave focus from left hemisphere in electroencephalogram after subarachnoid hemorrhage, right hemiparesis.

any space-consuming mass and electrical alterations are evident in the border zone of tissue destruction. Aneurysms below the tentorium cerebelli are electrically silent.

Rupture of an aneurysm situated anterior to the basilar trunk may produce recognizable and significant changes in the electroencephalogram. Abnormalities were found in 95 cases of aneurysm with subarachnoid hemorrhage by Roseman et al. on records taken within two weeks of the initial rupture. Decrease in amplitude of potential, delta wave foci and a slowing of alpha activity were present homolateral with the arterial lesion. Amplitude asymmetry was frequently notable and persisted longest. High-voltage, slow delta waves indicated intracerebral hematoma, spasm or thrombosis of parent arteries of the anterior circle of Willis. Millar found major abnormality and low amplitude in the electroencephalogram to occur on the side of bleeding in 11 of 13 patients with ruptured aneurysm. Delta activity of high amplitude was chiefly frontal in appearance. The electroencephalogram lateralized cerebral lesions in two patients with anterior cerebral-anterior communicating aneurysm reported by Elvidge and Feindel.

Lambert Rogers first suggested use of the electroencephalogram to determine tolerance for carotid ligation in the surgery of aneurysm. When carotid ligation is uncomplicated, the record usually remains normal; when hemiparesis appears, delta foci often develop and may persist for three months. These observations, unfortunately, are not invariable and do not permit complete reliance on the electroencephalogram to predict safety of carotid ligature.

Focal abnormalities resembling those occurring as late sequelae of head injury were found by Walton in the 12.5 per cent of 120 patients surviving subarachnoid hemorrhage who had epileptic manifestations in later life.

DIAGNOSIS

The sudden onset of severe occipito-frontal headache, frank signs of meningeal irritation and the finding of bloody cerebrospinal fluid in a middle-aged or young patient is the basic clinical pattern of subarachnoid hemorrhage. Rupture of a congenital arterial aneurysm, usually of the anterior circle of Willis, is the commonest cause and is often indicated by cranial nerve palsies, chiefly oculomotor and trigeminal. Coma or stupor develop rapidly or subacutely in 50 per cent of patients, and convulsive seizures occur in 20 per cent. Babinski's signs are often bilateral. Hemiplegia or a unilateral Babinski reaction may appear on the side opposite the source of bleeding. Retinal and subhyaloid intraocular hemorrhages are characteristic. The acute illness is typically febrile, and vomiting and photophobia are common. X-rays of the skull may rarely show intracranial calcification or erosion of the sella turcica or optic foramen. Electroencephalographic changes often are at least homolateral with the arterial lesion if not focal; they consist of a reduction in amplitude of electrical potential and delta wave activity.

Accurate etiologic diagnosis is most frequently and always most reliably made by means of arteriography.

DIFFERENTIAL DIAGNOSIS.—*Traumatic* intracranial bleeding is associated with a history and physical evidences of head injury. In *cerebral hemorrhage* the patient is hypertensive, hemiplegia is the rule and coma is profound. *Arteriovenous malformation* bleeds, as does aneurysmal anomaly, but the episodes are less catastrophic and convulsive seizures are more usual. The cerebrospinal fluid in *cerebral embolism* is usually only faintly bloody, and it is clear in *cerebral thrombosis* and *cerebral vaso-spasm*.

Hemorrhaging primary or metastatic *brain tumor* is a rare cause of sub-arachnoid bleeding. *Blood dyscrasias* are recognized by hematologic studies, and *metabolic coma* should offer no problem of distinction. In the latter, the cerebrospinal fluid is never bloody. The diagnosis of *hysteria* has often been made in patients with subarachnoid hemorrhage, even by experi-enced psychiatrists; lumbar puncture should never be withheld in ques-tionable cases.

TREATMENT

In 1902, Sir Victor Horsley ligated the right common carotid artery when he found a large aneurysmal sac in the parasellar region at crani-otomy and verified its arterial origin by the application of a sterilized stethoscope. Cure was substantiated by a long term follow-up. The first planned intracranial attack on a ruptured aneurysm was undertaken by Dott in 1931; he packed muscle fragments around a saccular enlarge-ment of the bifurcation of the internal carotid. German was first to excise an intracranial aneurysm, of the posterior cerebral artery, in 1938. In the same year Dandy clipped and fulgurated a congenital sac arising from the supraclinoid carotid, became interested in arterial aneurysms and may be said to have been instrumental in bringing the problem of treatment of subarachnoid hemorrhage to the attention of neurosurgeons. Today it would be difficult to state how many patients with ruptured aneurysm have been and are being managed successfully and how many have been cured by surgical means, but the number is large and is growing.

CONSERVATIVE MANAGEMENT

Indications.—Medical therapy is indicated when (1) the origin of subarachnoid hemorrhage is not a bleeding vascular anomaly; (2) a sus-pected aneurysm cannot be located arteriographically and characteristic regional neurologic signs are absent; (3) an aneurysmal sac is intimately attached to or incorporated in an indispensable or inaccessible major vessel, such as the middle cerebral artery or basilar trunk; (4) multiple aneurysms are present on the intracranial arteries bilaterally; (5) inade-quacy of collateral circulation through the circle of Willis, determined by preliminary carotid compression, precludes any surgical approach, or (6) arteriosclerotic dilatations or sacculations are accompanied by few or no symptoms.

General measures.—Strict bed rest is most important in the nonoperative care of subarachnoid hemorrhage and must be maintained at least four to six weeks after the cessation of active bleeding. Rutin and vitamins C and K should be supplied if deficiencies are suspected. The bowels must be kept open and all forms of straining avoided. In the convalescent stage, the patient should be managed as though he were recovering from an attack of pulmonary tuberculosis or rheumatic fever. Return to work or usual duties should not be permitted for three months after discharge from the hospital.

The question of the frequency of spinal puncture is moot. Many neurologists advise no further taps after the first diagnostic examination, whereas others advocate repeated withdrawal of fluid to keep headache at a minimum and to prevent excessive arachnoid scarring by removal of blood breakdown products. It is unlikely that cerebrospinal fluid in any quantity can be withdrawn without a slight sag or shift of the brain, and this may be just far enough to tear away filmy adhesions binding the site of arterial rupture to adjacent brain. One will never be congratulated on the reappearance of bleeding coincident with lumbar tap. Spinal puncture is best performed only for diagnosis, for relief of intolerable headache or when new symptoms and signs develop.

The control of headache, anxiety and restlessness, so necessary to prevent the patient from exhausting himself or initiating a secondary rupture, requires much pharmacologic support. Oral administration of aspirin or aspirin-phenacetin-caffeine compound with additional codeine may be sufficient but is ineffectual in the presence of vomiting. Hypodermics of 65 mg. of codeine every three or four hours are often needed; if this is not enough to keep the patient as quiet as is essential, 11 mg. of morphine may be substituted. Subarachnoid hemorrhage is the only intracranial condition associated with increased intracranial pressure in which the use of morphine is permitted; the advantages of relieving headache and attaining quietude outweigh the disadvantages of medullary depression.

For sedation, 0.065–0.1 Gm. Luminal sodium may be given every four hours instead of or with codeine or morphine. Paraldehyde is useful by mouth or rectum in amounts of 15–20 cc. Barbiturates orally at night will ensure a restful sleep.

CAROTID LIGATION

Application.—Since most congenital berry aneurysms are situated on the intracranial carotid or its immediate branches and attachments, ligation of the carotid artery in the neck is of benefit in preventing secondary rupture and allowing thrombosis of many of these arterial lesions. The circle of Willis functions as a cross-cerebral anastomosis, and proximal carotid ligation may materially reduce the head of arterial pressure playing upon the weakened walls of an aneurysm and permit thrombosis in the sac without rendering distal cerebral tissue ischemic to the point of infarction when collateral connections through the arterial circle are open.

Proximal, cervical carotid ligation is most applicable to aneurysms arising from the terminal, intracranial carotid (Dott). Concerning distal congenital arterial lesions, opinion as to the efficacy of cervical ligature is divided. Cervical ligation, in my opinion, is preferable to intracranial clipping of aneurysms of the communicating, proximal anterior and middle cerebral arteries which fill from one side only in carotid angiography. Distally placed lesions of the anterior, middle and posterior cerebral arteries are probably best approached directly. Bilateral carotid closure may be as effective as and safer than intracranial clipping of aneurysms of the anterior communicating artery fed from both carotids if preliminary compression reveals that this radical procedure will be tolerated by the brain. The common carotids and not the internal carotids should be ligated.

Naturally, carotid ligation will have no effect on congenital lesions of the vertebrobasilar circulation. Nor will it relieve intracerebral hematoma, which must be evacuated before any type of surgery directed at the aneurysm is carried out. It is also necessary that the patient be in a favorable operative state; "heroic" emergency ligations in the presence of active bleeding in a comatose patient do nothing but speed the patient to his death.

Determination of the usefulness of cervical vertebral ligation in the management of the 25 per cent of aneurysms which lie below the carotid circulation must be made in the presence of such lesions. Analogies as to possible success cannot be drawn from occasional cases in which one vertebral artery has been ligated to control operative hemorrhage during neurosurgical procedures in the posterior fossa or upper cervical spine. Possibly the proximal, indirect approach to vertebrobasilar aneurysms will prove of greater value than anticipated, although preliminary studies by Bakay and Sweet revealed no significant drop in pressure in the vertebral or posterior inferior cerebellar arteries distal to occlusion of one vertebral artery at the atlas.

Results.—Carotid ligation has a much lower rate of mortality than intracranial clipping of aneurysm, but a disadvantage is the lack of absolute certainty of control of the lesion. Ligature of the common carotid is attended by many fewer fatal and neurologic complications than closure of the internal carotid and is permissible in the patient age 50 or older. Closure of the common carotid lowers tension in both large and small cerebral arteries to about the same extent as ligation of the internal carotid and reduces systolic and pulse pressures in peripheral arterial derivatives almost as much as does direct clipping of major vessels intracranially (Bakay and Sweet). The arterial pressure in intracranial vessels above the site of cervical carotid ligature is undoubtedly restored to normal within days after surgical occlusion. However, this does not negate the

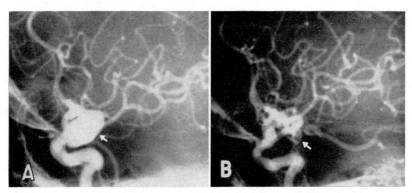

FIG. 77.—*A*, preoperative and *B*, postoperative arteriograms showing paracarotid aneurysm apparently thrombosed by ligation of common carotid artery. (Courtesy of A. D. Ecker and P. A. Riemenschneider.)

therapeutic effect of carotid ligation, because induced thrombosis in an aneurysm of the circle of Willis must occur within a period of hours to be efficacious. Restoration of distal arterial circulation thereafter can only be beneficial even when due to late recanalization of the ligated carotid.

Thrombosis of aneurysms of the carotid tree following ligature of the common carotid artery has been verified by postoperative arteriography (Fig. 77) (Ecker and Riemenschneider; Jefferson). Long term followups have been reported by Black and German in patients with both intracavernous and cerebral aneurysms derived from the carotid branches who were treated by ligation of either the common or internal carotid in the neck. The common carotid was ligated in patients age 40 or over, either the internal carotid or the common carotid being ligated in younger patients. Twenty-seven of 35 patients are living one to 16 years after surgery. Six deaths occurred in 20 patients with actively bleeding supra-clinoid saccular aneurysms treated with carotid ligature by Krayenbühl; five deaths were due to massive destruction of brain substance by hemor-rhage rupturing into a ventricle. The other 14 patients were benefited.

Gross has encountered no recurrences of subarachnoid hemorrhage and no neurologic complications in a large group of aneurysm patients treated by carotid ligation over more than 15 years. He ligates the com-mon carotid artery and divides it, as does Rogers, whose long term expe-rience has been similarly satisfactory. Rogers believes that ligature of the common carotid is less likely to eventuate in propagating thrombus than is internal occlusion. On the other hand, re-rupture of aneurysm after carotid ligation has occurred in the experience of many other neuro-surgeons.

Complications.—In a series of 88 ligations of the internal carotid artery performed by Dandy for aneurysm, there were a 5 per cent surgical mortality and a slightly higher incidence of nonfatal neurologic compli-cations. Poppen has recorded 101 ligations with three deaths, one the direct result of ligature, and eight instances of hemiplegia. Voris' experi-ence has not been so fortunate; he reported an incidence of 17 per cent mortality and 25 per cent hemiplegia and other neurologic disability in a group of 40 patients treated by ligation of the internal carotid. On the other hand, Gross and Rogers have observed no surgical deaths or serious neurologic consequences of ligation of the common carotid artery.

Serious complications from carotid ligation for intracranial aneurysm include: (1) hemispheric ischemia and infarction due to inadequacy of cross-circulation through the circle of Willis; (2) cerebral vasospasm; (3) thrombosis beginning in the aneurysmal sac and extending into the brain; (4) thrombosis commencing at the site of cervical ligation and propagating superiorly into the cerebral circulation beyond the terminal carotid; (5) intracranial embolism from a thrombus in the cervical ca-rotid, and (6) late, fatal erosion of a sclerosed artery at the point of liga-tion. Neurologic disability from the first two untoward developments—collateral inadequacy and vasospasm—is reversible if appropriate therapy is instituted early enough. Other postligation intracranial accidents are apt to be permanent in their effect.

Re-rupture of aneurysm following carotid ligation is an additional possibility of rare occurrence. Autopsy examination in such cases has shown that fatal hemorrhage is frequently due to perforation of another, unsuspected congenital sac rather than to failure of control of the known lesion.

Intracranial Surgery of Aneurysm

Six methods of intracranial treatment of congenital berry aneurysm were suggested by Dandy (Fig. 78): (1) application of a silver (or tantalum) clip to the neck of the sac; (2) trapping the lesion between an intracranial clip above its origin and a ligature in the patient's neck; (3) isolation of the aneurysm between two clips; (4) excision of the

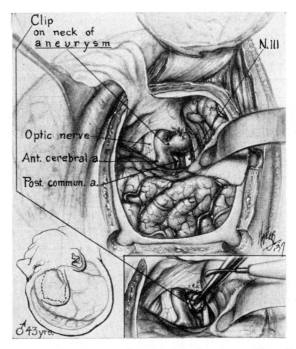

FIG. 78.—Intracranial clipping and coagulation of aneurysm. (From Dandy.)

berry sac and closure of the entering vessel; (5) insertion of muscle into the aneurysm and coagulation of the whole mass; (6) turning the saccule backward or to one side and coagulation of the neck and lesion proper. The packing of muscle fragments around aneurysms has been undertaken many times, with variable results. Encasement of these lesions with cellophane or liquid latex may prove fruitful in the future.

Intracranial intervention, if successful, is superior to indirect reduction of the arterial pressure-head in that the aneurysmal lesion is directly controlled and propagation of thrombosis into the brain is less probable. However, surgical mortality in the best hands to date averages 25 per cent or more (Hamby). The lesion may bleed again during surgery, cerebral edema may be uncontrollable or clip occlusion of a major artery may cause fatal cerebral infarction. So often rupture occurs just at the time the aneurysm is exposed or the first clip is applied, as the sealing cerebral tissue is retracted or the necrotic arterial wall gives way and tears again. Planned, deliberate hypotension by venesection, spinal anesthesia or intravenous administration of hexamethonium has permitted control of hemorrhage and the clipping of actively bleeding lesions. However, controlled hypotension is not without deleterious effect in the precipitation of thrombosis in the heart, brain, spinal cord and kidney. The emergency intracranial surgery of ruptured aneurysm is attended by an immediate mortality of 75 per cent, indicating the need for at least preliminary watchful waiting. New statistics on direct surgery for aneurysm will be forthcoming as induced hypotension is adopted generally.

Direct clipping of aneurysm may be combined with proximal ligation of the carotid when another episode of subarachnoid hemorrhage occurs after ligature or when continuing local pain indicates that the aneurysm is not securely thrombosed. If intracranial surgery is planned to follow occlusion of the cervical carotid, the procedures may be staged days apart or, if preliminary carotid compression indicates adequate anastomotic potential, ligation may be safely combined with clip-isolation of the aneurysm at the same session.

ANEURYSMS IN SPECIFIC LOCATIONS

Carotid artery.—Cavernous sinus. Cervical ligation is followed by the application of a clip to the artery above the sinus, trapping the aneurysm. The ophthalmic circulation ordinarily does not suffer because of collateral supply from the external carotid, but homolateral blindness has followed such a "trap" operation (Matson and Woodhall).

Terminal carotid. Isolation of the pathologic segment between the cervical and intracranial ligatures is advised, with an additional clip on the neck of aneurysm if possible.

Carotid bifurcation. Cervical ligation alone is advocated by Poppen. Dandy warned of possible inclusion of the posterior communicating artery in the lesion, in which case direct attack will seriously compromise collateral supply through the circle of Willis. Atherosclerotic and necrotic changes in the neck of even long, pedunculated aneurysms will often prevent successful application of a clip, and ligature in the neck is usually preferable in such cases.

Anterior communicating artery.—The sessile and incorporative nature of aneurysms of this artery, which is only a few millimeters in length, makes difficult the isolation of the sac without sacrifice of one or both anterior cerebral arteries. Nonetheless, Krayenbühl and others prefer the intracranial approach to these lesions. After clipping of an aneurysm of the anterior communicating artery, Elvidge and Feindel noted freedom from recurrent hemorrhage during a long follow-up period, although the patient was disabled intellectually.

In addition to the danger of rupture of the sac which lies in a relatively inaccessible position between and below the frontal lobes, the procedure is further complicated by the possibility of metabolic death or paraplegia and the chronic lobotomy syndrome if both anterior cerebral arteries must be sacrificed. Poppen has applied clips above and below an aneurysm of the communicating artery to a unilaterally feeding anterior cerebral artery when the other anterior cerebral was patent. Tonnis advocates the placing of muscle packs around the arterial wall to reinforce its strength; the systolic arterial pressure must be reduced to 60–80 mm. Hg if the muscle fragments are to remain in place and not be washed away (Elvidge). Norlén and Barnum have reported an impressive series of cases in which aneurysm of the anterior communicating artery was cured by direct surgical ligation.

Anterior cerebral artery.—Both Dandy and Poppen advise excision or isolation of aneurysms of this artery. Successful treatment has been reported of congenital lesions of the anterior cerebral, proximal (Elvidge and Feindel) and distal in location on the vessel (Sugar and Tinsley). Extreme caution must be exerted to preserve adequate blood pressure and oxygenation if the artery is to be occluded at its origin.

Middle cerebral artery.—Direct attack on this most important cerebral vessel is fraught with great risk to life and health, and Dandy cured no patients with aneurysms on the main trunk by intracranial surgery. If compression of the cervical carotid can be performed without additional neurologic disability, ligation in the neck is preferable. Small lesions on peripheral branches in the anterior frontal or temporal areas may be isolated without serious deficit. Successful removals of several sizeable aneurysms arising from the middle cerebral artery were reported by Campbell and Burklund. They emphasize temporary occlusion (three minute periods) of the vessel proximal to the sac by a silk noose while the lesion is being excised. Resection of the tip of the temporal lobe permits adequate visualization. The ostium of the aneurysm is closed with fine suture.

Posterior communicating artery.—Excision or trapping of aneurysms truly of the posterior communicating artery is ill advised, in the opinion of both Dandy and Poppen, because of the necessity of collateral circulation through this artery. Jaeger as well as Madow and Alpers reported removal or isolation of several arterial lesions here. Many finger-like aneurysms thought to be of the posterior communicating artery are really posterior vestigial derivatives of the internal carotid.

Posterior cerebral artery.—German's report of excision of an aneurysm of this vessel is widely quoted as an example of the proper approach to congenital sacs on the posterior cerebral artery. Certainly the indirect method of proximal ligature does not have much hope of safety or success.

Basilar and vertebral arteries.—Aneurysms of these arteries are better left alone. Unilateral vertebral ligation has been suggested, but there are no reports of effective treatment of congenital lesions of the vertebrobasilar system by this method. Schwartz excised a parabasilar vestigial aneurysm producing the cerebellopontile angle syndrome, with an excellent postoperative result.

Cerebellar arteries.—Rizzoli and Hayes successfully clipped a large aneurysm of the distal posterior inferior cerebellar artery which had ruptured and was causing internal hydrocephalus and other signs of expansile mass in the posterior fossa. If diagnosable, the rare aneurysms of the cerebellar arteries should be handled in this manner if it is certain that the lesion lies beyond the intrinsic supply of the brain stem.

Multiple aneurysms involving the internal carotid and middle cerebral arteries of the same side were clipped at open operation by Bassett (Fig. 128). I treated an exactly similar case by common carotid ligation, with a hemorrhage-free six year follow-up. If multiple aneurysms are bilateral in location, surgery has little to offer.

PERSONAL EXPERIENCES.—Either the indirect or direct surgical methods of treating intracranial arterial aneurysms may be effective. Therapy in each case must be individualized. The potential risks in any event are considerable, but subarachnoid hemorrhage is a serious and eventually lethal disease. Dandy called cervical carotid ligation a "shot in the dark," but no procedure can be more blind than frantic groping around in a faucet-like stream of arterial blood to place a silver clip on an aneurysm which has just re-ruptured during intracranial exploration.

Proximal ligation of the cervical carotid artery has proved a simple, effective and relatively secure procedure for control of arterial aneurysmal lesions arising from the anterior circle of Willis. There is actually little risk if the operation is planned carefully and there is little difference in protective effect if either the common carotid or the internal carotid is ligated, whereas in my experience and from the reports of other surgeons fatal and serious neurologic complications are more common after occlusion of the internal carotid.

I have treated 19 patients (five operated on by Dr. Garrett M. Swain) with congenital aneurysms of the terminal carotid, the anterior and middle cerebral and the anterior and posterior communicating arteries by ligation of the common carotid artery alone. All but one had sustained subarachnoid hemorrhage. In every instance but one, progressive compression of the common carotid before permanent ligation was undertaken by means of digital or mechanical external occlusion or gradual closure of a metal clamp on the artery. Seventeen of the 19 patients are alive and well four years to six months after surgery.

Fatal secondary hemorrhage from a vestigial aneurysm of the carotid took place in one patient on the seventh postoperative day, as she strained over a bedpan. In another patient with re-rupture six weeks after surgery, autopsy showed the aneurysm to involve the origin of the posterior cerebral artery and not the internal carotid, as had been diagnosed from angiograms. In one patient, in whom compression was not done before surgery, hemiplegia developed 30 hours after ligation. Since the cerebrospinal fluid was not bloody, it was supposed that intracerebral propagation of thrombosis began in a large paracarotid aneurysmal sac.

Ligation was combined with intracranial surgery in three other patients. One aneurysm in the cavernous sinus was trapped between a ligature below and a clip on the terminal carotid. An aneurysm of the anterior cerebral artery re-bled during craniotomy and could only be packed with Gelfoam; carotid ligation was undertaken later for safety. Occlusion of the cervical carotid did not cause cessation of bleeding from a congenital vascular malformation involving the middle cerebral arterial circulation and galenic venous drainage. The lesion was extirpated from the temporal lobe.

Two other patients were treated by intracranial clipping alone. One case was that of a bottle-shaped sac arising from the internal carotid in a woman, 62; she has remained well for four years. Carotid clipping has controlled a cavernous aneurysm in a 41 year old woman for three years. However, I believe that if intracranial surgery is to be used in the treatment of aneurysm arising from the anterior circle of Willis, craniotomy is best preceded by carotid ligature in the neck, unless Campbell's method of temporary occlusion of the parent cerebral artery will allow actual firm closure of the neck of the sac with suture material.

As noted by Woodhall *et al.,* intra-aneurysmal tension is the important factor relating to re-rupture of the sac, and aneurysms can be said to be cured only when isolation or destruction of these lesions or increasing the local resistance of the arterial wall to intravascular pressure eliminates the potential danger of persisting tension. The mortality rate following direct surgical therapy has ranged as high as 50 per cent or more in reported series; carotid ligature has been proved to reduce distal intra-arterial tensions to safe limits. There is no subject of greater current neurosurgical controversy than that of how to treat intracranial arterial aneurysms.

PROGNOSIS

INITIAL SUBARACHNOID HEMORRHAGE.—The first attack of spontaneous subarachnoid hemorrhage has a high incidence of fatality, the mortality rate varying from 30 to 50 per cent. The initial mortality is high because many aneurysmal sacs fail to seal off and continue to pour forth blood; intracerebral hematomas form or large areas of brain may be destroyed. Hamby found intracerebral hematomas in 52 per cent of 44 fatal cases.

Subarachnoid bleeding accounts for about 5 per cent of all sudden deaths (Helpern and Rabson), and ruptured intracranial aneurysm is responsible for approximately 25 per cent of fatalities due to diseases of the nervous system. Of immediate, spontaneous deaths in young soldiers, 75 per cent were found to be associated with hemorrhage from aneurysm (Moritz and Zamchek). Whereas patients with hypertensive cerebral hemorrhage rarely die in less than a matter of hours, subarachnoid inundation may be fatal in 30 minutes or less. Unfavorable prognostically are a history of previous attacks, multiple hemorrhages while the patient is in the hospital, mental disturbances, unconsciousness and convulsive seizures.

RECURRENCES.—Cessation of hemorrhage is often temporary and re-rupture may occur, usually from the seventh to twenty-first day after the original episode. A second major hemorrhage has been fatal in 75 per cent of cases in some series reported. About 25 per cent of patients have minor leakages before the first serious hemorrhage. Many such mild attacks are recognized only in retrospect and may have been diagnosed as "migraine" or "influenza." Minor ruptures usually precede the major and often fatal hemorrhage by months or a year or so; in two verified instances the intervals between frank subarachnoid hemorrhages were 18 and 27 years.

Hamby found a 72 per cent mortality from second hemorrhage, but Hyland maintains that patients who live through the initial episode have an 80 per cent chance of carrying on for years without recurrence. Walton reported a 45 per cent mortality in the first eight weeks of illness in 312 patients treated conservatively. An additional 11 per cent subsequently died of repeated hemorrhage, but 25 per cent of the patients were fully employed many years after initial rupture. Walton advises his patients to resume full activities after a rest period of appropriate length in order to prevent the development of a hypochondriac state and because he is not convinced of the relationship of re-rupture to exertion.

WITH SURGICAL THERAPY.—In a large series of cases of subarachnoid hemorrhage collected by Mount, the over-all mortality rate in 752 patients treated medically was 48 per cent; in 469 patients treated surgically it was 14 per cent, less than one-third as great. Every patient with spontaneous subarachnoid hemorrhage presumably or actually due to ruptured intracranial aneurysm should be offered the benefits of surgery if at all possible. Although most patients will have to be supported through the primary accident before operation can be undertaken, in more and more ruptured aneurysms exploration is being undertaken during the acute phase of bleeding. In any patient who survives the initial episode there is the possibility of intracerebral hematoma or of re-rupture within a few days. No matter how well the individual may come through the acute illness, the uncontrolled lesion must be looked on as a tiny volcano, smoldering more or less silently but with the potentiality of erupting again at any time and place.

CAROTID-CAVERNOUS ANEURYSM (FISTULA)

ETIOLOGY; PATHOGENESIS; PATHOLOGY

The intracranial terminal portion of the internal carotid artery lies extra- or intradurally just before its bifurcation and is enveloped by the cavernous sinus. This anatomic peculiarity of an artery being surrounded by a vein is unique in the body. When the wall of the intracavernous carotid siphon is lacerated or breaks, arterial blood spurts into the sinus with every heart beat and passive congestion of the veins of the orbit results. Deleterious effect on the brain is negligible at first because of the paucity of cerebral venous drainage into the cavernous sinus. Systemic evidences of major arteriovenous fistula—wide pulse pressure, cardiac hypertrophy —are rare because of the restricted nature of carotid-cavernous shunt.

Trauma accounts for 75 per cent of cases. The usual type of injury is a shearing basal skull fracture of the sphenoid bone, overriding fragments lacerating the wall of the carotid at the foramen lacerum or just above. Knife wounds have also caused carotid-cavernous fistula. The other 25 per cent arise *spontaneously* from the rupture of a vestigial aneurysm of the primitive trigeminal artery (Sugar) or simply from a crack in the wall of a sclerosed carotid artery. Malignant or bacterial *metastasis* to the terminal carotid is an unusual cause of leaking carotid aneurysm in the cavernous sinus. I have seen fistula develop in the course of metastasizing ovarian carcinoma and in a patient dying of bacterial endocarditis.

SYMPTOMS AND SIGNS

Onset of aneurysm.—The evidences of head injury and basal skull fracture, including bleeding from the nose, ears and mouth, orbital hematoma, otorrhea and rhinorrhea, are usually present when trauma is the cause of carotid-cavernous aneurysm. However, rupture of artery into vein has occurred after falls from a height, with the patient landing on his feet. The signs and symptoms of fistula may be slow to develop after basal skull fracture, but the condition is usually manifest within one month. With spontaneous rupture of the intracavernous carotid, the condition may become apparent immediately in the sudden appearance of a crashing noise or machinery murmur in the head. Most patients with non-traumatic carotid-cavernous aneurysm are in middle age or late life and generalized arteriosclerosis is advanced, although Beadles reported spontaneous carotid shunt in a woman, aged 22.

Eye signs.—Pulsating exophthalmos is the most striking external evidence of carotid-cavernous fistula (Fig. 79). Veins in the orbit, eyelids and conjunctiva become engorged, and chemosis may develop to a degree that dewlaps of mucous membrane droop on the lower lids. The retina is cyanotic, venules are distended and throbbing, hemorrhages appear and papilledema develops. All these changes remain homolateral with the perforated carotid in two thirds of the patients, but they become bilateral in one-third as arterial blood forces its way into the opposite cavernous sinus through the circular venous connections around the pituitary. Rarely, exophthalmos is entirely contralateral, due to unequal patency of the two cavernous sinuses.

Ocular and frontal headache is dull and constant, and the patient becomes nauseated and feels ill. With progression of exophthalmos, extraocular palsies involving the abducens, oculomotor and trochlear nerves in that order are seen, as is trigeminal sensory loss, and in the end the second to sixth cranial nerves may all be implicated.

Cranial bruit.—Bruit is systolic and diastolic and may be faint at first or loud from the beginning. It is usually but not necessarily constant and is accentuated by emotion or attention. The hemic souffle is audible

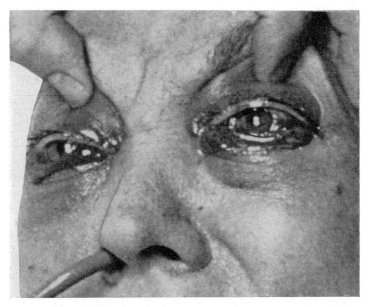

Fig. 79.—Bilateral pulsating exophthalmos and chemosis due to carotid-cavernous fistula, left.

to the patient and examiner on the side of carotid fistula or throughout the head, and it is best heard with a stethoscope over the affected eye, maxillary sinus or ipsilateral temple. The sound can be reduced or eliminated by compression of the cervical carotid.

DIAGNOSIS

Cranial bruit and pulsating exophthalmos coming on after basal skull fracture or in an arteriosclerotic person characterize carotid-cavernous aneurysm. To be considered in the differential diagnosis are cavernous sinus thrombosis, orbital tumors, defects in the roof of the orbit, arterial aneurysm of the carotid artery or ophthalmic vessels and congenital arteri-ovenous malformations. In no other disease is the combination of frank bruit and pulsating exophthalmos invariably present. When a carotid-cavernous fistula is overlooked, it is usually because a stethoscope was not applied to the head. Angiography will confirm the diagnosis (Fig. 80).

TREATMENT

Carotid ligation.—Proximal closure of the cervical carotid artery has been the treatment of choice in carotid-cavernous fistula since 1809, when

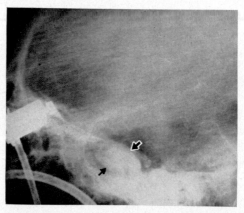

FIG. 80.—Carotid-cavernous aneurysm. (Courtesy of G. M. Swain.)

Travers recognized the origin of pulsating exophthalmos and cured the condition by ligating the common carotid artery in the neck. Of 130 reported cases of carotid arteriovenous aneurysm surveyed by Locke, 68 per cent of patients treated by common carotid ligature were cured or greatly improved, with 7 per cent operative mortality; interruption of the internal carotid resulted in cure or benefit in 87.5 per cent of patients, with a surgical fatality rate of 9 per cent. When bilateral carotid ligation was thought necessary, incidence of relief of pulsating exophthalmos was 62 per cent and the mortality 14 per cent. Of course, fistulas in the last group were refractory to unilateral ligation. Dandy stated that only one third of patients are amenable to complete or partial cervical liga-ture, that in one-third additional clipping of the internal carotid within the skull is required and that in the rest, in whom bruit and pulsation continue, the ophthalmic artery should be occluded in addition, as sug-gested originally by Adson. This last procedure ordinarily does not cause blindness because of the accessory circulation through the external angular artery.

In a significant majority of patients with carotid-cavernous fistula, ligation of the common carotid artery after preliminary testing of the brain's tolerance of ischemia by arterial compression will usually be effective. Partial or fractional closure may be employed in elderly persons. If this is not sufficient to stop the bruit and exophthalmos, either or both external or internal carotids may be tied off or ligated and divided seven to 10 days later. Should symptoms and signs persist thereafter, one may then consider intracranial occlusion of the terminal carotid below the bifurcation, clipping of the ophthalmic artery or vein or ligature of the opposite common or external carotid.

Other methods of therapy.—Occasionally (5–10 per cent) the fistula will thrombose and close spontaneously when the patient is kept at complete rest for a long period and the carotid is compressed externally. Usually, however, this is at the price of severe residual ocular paralysis or blindness. A few carotid-cavernous aneurysms have been treated successfully by surgical occlusion of the ophthalmic veins alone.

BIBLIOGRAPHY

Adson, A. W.: Surgical treatment of vascular diseases altering the function of the eyes, Tr. Am. Acad. Ophth. (1941) 46:95-111, 1942.

Alpers, B. J., and Forster, F. M.: The reparative processes in subarachnoid hemorrhage, Tr. Am. Neurol. A. 70:110-112, 1944.

Bakay, L., and Sweet, W. H.: Cervical and intracranial pressures with and without vascular occlusion: Their significance in treatment of aneurysms and neoplasms, Surg., Gynec. & Obst. 65:67-75, 1952.

Bassett, R. C.: Multiple cerebral aneurysms, J. Neurosurg. 8:132-133, 1951.

Bassett, R. C., and Lemmen, L. J.: Subdural hematoma associated with bleeding intracranial aneurysm, J. Neurosurg. 9:443-450, 1952.

Beadles, C. F.: Aneurysms of the larger cerebral arteries, Brain 30:285-336, 1907.

Black, B. K., and Hicks, S. P.: The relation of hypertension to arterial aneurysms of the brain, U.S. Armed Forces M. J. 3:1813-1818, 1952.

Black, S. P. W., and German, W. J.: Treatment of internal carotid artery aneurysms by proximal arterial ligation, J. Neurosurg. 10:590-601, 1953.

Boldrey, E., and Miller, E. R.: Arteriovenous fistula (aneurysm) of the great cerebral vein (of Galen) and the circle of Willis, Arch. Neurol. & Psychiat. 62:778-783, 1949.

Bremer, J. L.: Congenital aneurysm of the cerebral arteries: An embryologic study, Arch. Path. 35:819-831, 1943.

Brown, R. A. P.: Polycystic disease of kidneys and intracranial aneurysm, Glasgow M. J. 32:333-362, 1951.

Bushard, M.; Yuhl, E., and Barris, R. W.: Vertebral artery aneurysm, Neurology 2:356-359, 1952.

Campbell, E., and Burklund, C. W.: Aneurysms of the middle cerebral artery, Ann. Surg. 137:18-28, 1953.

Campbell, E. H., and Keedy, C.: Hemifacial spasm: Note on etiology in two cases, J. Neurosurg. 4:342-347, 1947.

Carmichael, R.: Pathogenesis of noninflammatory cerebral aneurysms, J. Path. & Bact. 62:1-19, 1950.

Conley, J. W., and Rand, C. W.: Spontaneous subarachnoid hemorrhage occurring in noneclamptic pregnancy, A.M.A. Arch. Neurol. & Psychiat. 66:443-463, 1951.

Dandy, W. E.: Results following ligation of the internal carotid artery, Arch. Surg. 45: 521-533, 1942.

Dandy, W. E.: *Intracranial Arterial Aneurysms* (Ithaca, N. Y.: Comstock Publishing Co., Inc., 1944).

Dandy, W. E.: *Surgery of the Brain* (Hagerstown, Md.: W. F. Prior Co., Inc., 1945).

Dott, N. M.: Intracranial aneurysms, Edinburgh M. J. 40:219-234, 1933.

Ecker, A. D.: *The Normal Cerebral Angiogram* (Springfield, Ill.: Charles C Thomas, Publisher, 1951).

Ecker, A. D., and Riemenschneider, P. A.: Deliberate thrombosis of intracranial arterial aneurism by partial occlusion of carotid artery with arteriographic control, J. Neurosurg. 8:348-353, 1951.

Elvidge, A. R., and Feindel, W. H.: Surgical treatment of aneurysm of anterior cerebral and of anterior communicating arteries, diagnosed by angiography and electroencephalography, J. Neurosurg. 7:13-32, 1950.

Fincher, E. H.: Spontaneous subarachnoid hemorrhage in intradural tumors of the lumbar sac: A clinical syndrome, J. Neurosurg. 8:576-584, 1951.

Forbus, W. D.: On the origin of miliary aneurysms of the superficial cerebral arteries, Bull. Johns Hopkins Hosp. 47:239-284, 1930.

German, W. J.: Intracranial aneurysm: A surgical problem, Zentralbl. Neurochir. 3:352, 1938.

Golden, J.; Odom, G. L., and Woodhall, B.: Subdural hematoma following subarachnoid hemorrhage, A.M.A. Arch. Neurol. & Psychiat. 69: 486-489, 1953.

Gross, S. W.: Personal communication.

Hamby, W. B.: *Intracranial Aneurysms* (Springfield, Ill.: Charles C Thomas, Publisher, 1952).

Hamby, W. B.: The aneurysmal origin of nonfatal subarachnoid hemorrhage, J. Neurosurg. 10:35-37, 1953.

Heimburger, R. F.; Oberhill, H. R.; McGarry, H. I., and Bucy, P. C.: Intraorbital aneurysm: A case of aneurysm of the lacrimal artery, Arch. Ophth. 42:1-13, 1949.

Helpern, M., and Rabson, S. M.: Sudden and unexpected natural death: III. Spontaneous subarachnoid hemorrhage, Am. J. M. Sc. 220:262-271, 1950.

Hyland, H. H.: Prognosis in spontaneous subarachnoid hemorrhage, Arch. Neurol. & Psychiat. 63:61-78, 1950.

Jaeger, J. R.: Personal communication.

Jefferson, G.: Compression of the chiasma, optic nerves and optic tracts by intracranial aneurysms, Brain 60:444-497, 1937.

Jefferson, G.: Personal communication.

Kernohan, J. W., and Woltman, H. W.: Postoperative, focal, nonseptic necrosis of vertebral and cerebellar arteries: With rupture and subarachnoid hemorrhage, J.A.M.A. 122:1173-1177, 1943.

Krayenbühl, H.: Immediate and late results of carotid ligature in intracranial aneurysms, Schweiz. med. Wchnschr. 76:908-914, 1946.

Krayenbühl, H.: Personal communication.

Levin, P. M.: Intracranial aneurysms, A.M.A. Arch. Neurol. & Psychiat. 67:771-787, 1952.

Locke, C. E.: Intracranial arteriovenous aneurism or pulsating exophthalmos, Ann. Surg. 80:1-24, 1924.

Madow, L., and Alpers, B. J.: Aneurysm of the posterior communicating artery, A.M.A. Arch. Neurol. & Psychiat. 70:722-732, 1953.

Magee, C. G.: Spontaneous subarachnoid hemorrhage, Lancet 2:497-500, 1943.

Matson, D. D., and Woodhall, B.: Intracranial and cervical trap ligation of the carotid artery complicated by blindness of the homolateral eye, J. Neurosurg. 5:567-571, 1948.

McDonald, C. A., and Korb, M.: Intracranial aneurysms, Arch. Neurol. & Psychiat. 42: 298-328, 1939.

McKee, E. E.: Mycotic infection of the brain with arteritis and subarachnoid hemorrhage: Report of a case, Am. J. Clin. Path. 20:381-384, 1950.

Millar, J. H. D.: The EEG in cases of subarachnoid hemorrhage, Electroencephalog. & Clin. Neurophysiol. 4:253, 1952.

von Monakow, C., and Ladame, P.: Nouv. iconog. de la Salpetriere 13:1, 1900.

Moritz, A. R., and Zamchek, N.: Sudden and unexpected deaths of young soldiers, Arch. Path. 42:459-494, 1946.

Mount, L. A.: Treatment of spontaneous subarachnoid hemorrhage, J.A.M.A. 146:693-698, 1951.

Norlén, G., and Barnum, A. S.: Surgical treatment of aneurysms of the anterior communicating artery, J. Neurosurg. 10:634-650, 1953.

Padget, D. H.: The development of the cranial arteries in the human embryo, Contrib. Embryol. 32:205-262, 1948.

Poppen, J. L.: Diagnosis of intracranial aneurysms, Am. J. Surg. 75:175-186, 1948.

Poppen, J. L.: Specific treatment of intracranial aneurysms: Experiences with 143 surgically treated patients, J. Neurosurg. 8:75-103, 1951.

Richardson, J. C., and Hyland, H. H.: Intracranial aneurysms, Medicine 20:1-83, 1941.

Rizzoli, H. V., and Hayes, G. J.: Congenital berry aneurysm of the posterior fossa: Case report with successful operative excision, J. Neurosurg. 10:550-551, 1953.

Rogers, L.: Carotid ligation for intracranial aneurysm, Brit. J. Surg. 32:309-311, 1944-45.

Roseman, E.; Bloor, B. M., and Schmidt, R. P.: The electroencephalogram in intracranial aneurysms, Neurology 1:25-38, 1951.

Schwartz, H. G.: Arterial aneurysm of the posterior fossa, J. Neurosurg. 5:312-316, 1948.

Simmonds, W. J.: Absorption of blood from cerebrospinal fluid in animals, Australian J. Exper. Biol. & M. Sc. 30:261-270, 1952.

Sosman, M. C., and Vogt, E. C.: Aneurysms of the internal carotid artery and circle of Willis from a roentgenologic viewpoint, Am. J. Roentgenol. 15:122-134, 1926.

Sugar, O.: Pathologic anatomy and angiography of intracranial vascular anomalies, J. Neurosurg. 8:3-22, 1951.

Sugar, O., and Tinsley, M.: Aneurysm of terminal portion of anterior cerebral artery, Arch. Neurol. & Psychiat. 60:81-85, 1948.

Sweet, W. H.; Sarnoff, S. J., and Bakay, L.: A clinical method for recording internal carotid pressure: Significance of changes during carotid occlusion, Surg., Gynec. & Obst. 90:327-334, 1950.

Tonnis, W.: Treatment of intracranial aneurysms, Deutsches med. J. 3:1-4, 1952.

Voris, H. C.: Complications of ligation of the internal carotid artery, J. Neurosurg. 8: 119-131, 1951.

Walton, J. N.: The late prognosis of subarachnoid hemorrhage, Brit. M. J. 2:802-808, 1952.

Walton, J. N.: The electroencephalographic sequelae of spontaneous subarachnoid hemorrhage, Electroencephalog. & Clin. Neurophysiol. 5:41-52, 1953.

Wolff, H. G.: *Headache and Other Head Pain* (New York: Oxford University Press, 1948).

Woodhall, B.; Odom, G. L.; Bloor, B. M., and Golden, J.: Studies on cerebral intravascular pressure, J. Neurosurg. 10:28-34, 1953.

CHAPTER 12

Vascular Tumors; Arteriovenous Malformations of the Brain

VASCULAR TUMORS and malformations of the brain are coming to increasing clinical attention as more and more patients with convulsive seizures and intracranial hemorrhage are being investigated with the procedure of angiography. Angiomatous anomalies and neoplasms represented 2 per cent of Cushing and Bailey's series of intracranial tumors reported in 1928. Twenty years later, Olivecrona and Riives found these vascular lesions to have an incidence seven times as great in a similar but larger group of intracranial tumors.

Surgical interest in arteriovenous lesions has developed because of the increasing knowledge of their characteristics and the improvement in hemostatic technics. Whereas Cushing, Bailey and Dandy advised extreme caution and conservatism in the handling of arteriovenous malformations, Olivecrona and Riives reported removal of 43 such vascular anomalies, with a surgical mortality of 9.3 per cent.

ETIOLOGY; PATHOGENESIS

All vascular malformations and tumors of the brain and meninges are of developmental origin. Embryologic rests may take on features of autonomous growth in later life. The *hemangioblastoma,* arising almost always in the cerebellum, is undoubtedly derived from one or several anlagen of retained angioblastic syncytium. *Hemangiomas* and *cavernous angiomas,* most often found in the interior of the cerebrum and brain stem, represent arrest in the second embryologic period of differential growth of arteries and veins.

Arteriovenous malformations, which are largely superficial in location, also result from failure of complete definition of afferent from efferent vascular channels, as do the more rare pial *telangiectasias*. Wedge-shaped or pyramidal arteriovenous malformations extending from the scalp or pia to the ventricle are most common in the sylvian fissure, since lateral meningeal growth is least likely to meet dorsal vascular trunks and accomplish separation of the three circulations of the head (scalp, dura, pia) during intrauterine life. Arteriovenous fistulas between the choroidal arteries and galenic veins probably are due to partial arrest of intracranial vascular development at the 20 mm. stage of the human embryo (Padget).

Sturge-Weber disease (encephalotrigeminal angiomatosis) also represents persistence of primitive vascular systems, undifferentiated plexuses of vessels remaining in the skin of the face and eye and on the surface of the sensory cortex.

Lichtenstein considers angiomas and vascular malformations of the brain to be local manifestations of a hemangiomatous dysplasia which is a part of a generalized neurocutaneous syndrome, related to such heredo-congenital diseases as neurofibromatosis and tuberous sclerosis. The frequency of related developmental abnormalities elsewhere in the head and in other parts of the body supports this contention. Hereditary tendencies to the development of angiomatous lesions of the central nervous system are strong.

PATHOLOGY

HEMANGIOBLASTOMA (ANGIORETICULOMA).—True hemangioblastomas are uncommon intracranial tumors. They usually arise in the cerebellum but may be found rarely in the cerebral hemispheres or lateral ventricles (Fig. 81). Neoplastic activity is shown by the hemangioblastoma which enlarges in size and recurs if the tumor is not completely removed at operation. There is almost always an increase of intracranial pressure since the growth usually is present in the posterior fossa. The combination of a vascular nodule, which may be tiny, in the wall of an incorporating cyst is present in most cases. The cyst may be composed of leptomeningeal fibrosis if the hemangioblastoma lies in the cerebellopontile angle or is an expansion of the cerebellar hemisphere or vermis.

Approximately one-fifth the hemangioblastomas are entirely solid and these occasionally are attached to the floor of the fourth ventricle from which successful removal is difficult. Mixed solid-cystic forms are more common; the firm portion of the growth may be present on the surface of the cerebellum or as a mural nodule in the cyst wall. Solid hemangioblastoma is red-brown in color, extremely vascular and may be evidenced externally by convergence of thin-walled and enlarged vessels. When the disease is of hereditary predisposition, multiple cerebellar angioblastic tumors are found in a single patient.

Microscopically, fat-containing, plump cells of endothelial derivation resembling the cellular unit of a xanthoma or hypernephroma line fluid-filled spaces and are interspersed in cords with innumerable capillaries. A rich connective tissue reticulum envelopes all. Mitoses are not uncommon. Staining of the reticular fibers by silver impregnation is pathognomonic (Fig. 82).

Lindau's disease.—Associated lesions elsewhere in the body are believed to result from mesodermal aberrations during the third month of

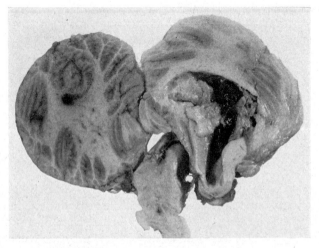

FIG. 81.—Hemangioblastoma of cerebellar hemisphere. (George Washington University Laboratory of Neurology.)

intrauterine life. Lindau (1926) first noted the concurrence of von Hippel's angiomatosis of the retina and cerebellar hemangioblastoma (von Hippel-Lindau disease). In many cases of Lindau's disease intraspinal hemangiomas are also found. Pericranial sinus is considered to be a member of the Lindau complex. Cystic, angiomatous or neoplastic lesions often reside in the lung, liver, kidney, pancreas and epididymis (Fig. 83). Polycythemia vera complicates 9 per cent of primary and 63.6 per cent of recurrent cerebellar hemangioblastomas for unknown reasons (Cramer and Kimsey) and may disappear after complete removal of the tumor.

The fundamental histologic formula for all pathologic changes in Lindau's disease is the formation of endothelium-lined spaces and the pro-

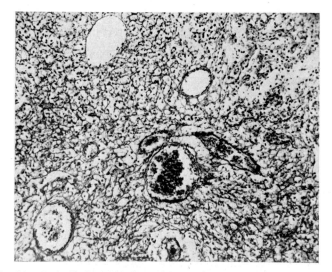

FIG. 82.—Reticulin formation in cerebellar hemangioblastoma (silver stain).

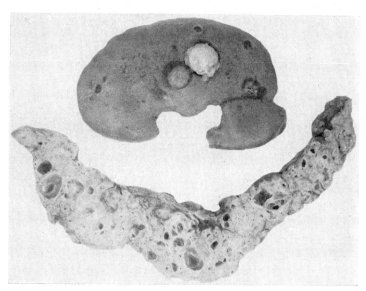

FIG. 83.—Lesions in kidney and pancreas. Lindau's disease. (Courtesy of H. O. Tonning *et al.*)

liferation of reticulum cells, with a lack of integration between blood vessels and their field of supply. This leads to the development of cysts during fetal growth and of neoplasms in later life (Lichtenstein; Tonning *et al.*).

HEMANGIOMAS; CAVERNOUS ANGIOMAS.—Cavernous angiomas (Fig. 84) may be formed in any part of the brain, but location in the brain

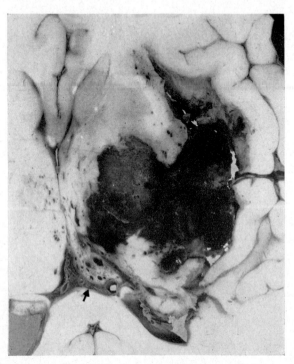

FIG. 84.—Angioma of hypothalamus (arrow) with intracerebral hemorrhage. (Courtesy of N. Antoni.)

stem is common (Virchow). Here these lesions are almost entirely venous, probably because the posterior primitive plexus of veins persists the longest in embryologic life and the vascular beds of the third and fourth ventricles are especially rich. Elsewhere, hemangiomas may be arteriovenous in nature. The absence of nervous parenchyma between vessels is thought to classify these angiomas as true neoplasms, but they certainly are not new growths even in the same sense as the hemangioblastoma.

Grossly, the large blood and colloid cysts are really enormously di-

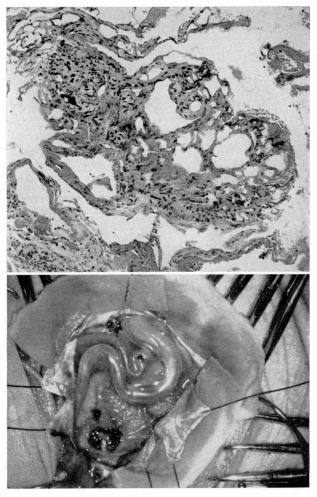

FIG. 85 *(above)*.—Sclerosing vascular changes in cerebral hemangioma.
FIG. 86 *(below)*.—Enormous cerebral arteriovenous malformation exposed at craniotomy. (Courtesy of J. R. Jaeger.)

lated vessels, essentially of a venous type but malformed and degenerate.
Calcification and thrombosis are common, as is rupture of thinning sinuses.
These vascular rests may be multiple. Mesencephalic and pontile cavern-
omas may encroach on and occlude the aqueduct of Sylvius or fourth
ventricle. Bailey and Ford called attention to the sclerosing nature of
cavernous angiomas (Fig. 85). The presence of phagocytes containing

fat and hemosiderin distinguish these lesions from hemangiomas outside the nervous system.

ARTERIOVENOUS MALFORMATIONS.—Arteriovenous malformation, which is rarely telangiectatic, purely arterial or entirely venous, is the commonest type of intracranial vascular anomaly next to saccular arterial aneurysm. Arteriovenous malformations usually lie on the surface of the cerebral hemisphere (Fig. 86) or in the centrum semiovale, in relation to major arterial or venous channels. A single lesion may extend through the whole thickness of one hemisphere as an inverted cone with a pial base and an apex near the ventricle. The covering arachnoid is thickened and rusty from hemorrhages and exudation. Interposed and underlying gyri are atrophic and yellow, soft or fibrogliotic. The truly enormous size of these lesions and their arterial, venous or arteriovenous makeup are best realized from a study of clinical angiograms. Communicating hydrocephalus and local brain atrophy are the results of arachnoidal fibrosis and cerebral ischemia due to drainage of incoming blood into the vascular lesion and away from the nerve parenchyma (Askenazy et al.).

It is difficult to tell arteries from venous channels, even microscopically, and the spectrum of vascular pathologic change runs from leiomyomatous nodules in the media of arteries to arteriosclerosis. Glial tissue is found between arterial coils. The striking feature of all lesions is an overgrowth of intima in the form of loose areolar tissue which will actually occlude vessels. Thromboses are also found. Rupture of overfilled and imperfect veins occurs. "Arteriolized" veins may attain fantastic proportions. Calcification is found in the walls of the vessels or in intervening nerve tissue.

Telangiectasias are rare and are composed of thin-walled plexuses resembling venules (Fig. 2). Exclusively venous malformations are likewise uncommon and resemble telangiectasias except for greater size and slightly sturdier composition of vessels. Arterial types, seldom seen, are made up of imperfect arterioles and arteries, thick and thin.

Physiologic changes.—The pathophysiologic effect of intracranial arteriovenous malformations is similar to that of any large vascular shunt elsewhere in the body. There are increase in local cerebral blood flow and decrease of cerebrovascular resistance (Bessman et al.), increase of cardiac output and heart size and decrease in diastolic blood pressure. The oxygen content of jugular venous blood is greatly augmented, a determination of diagnostic significance (Horton et al.; Logan et al.). Whereas congenital arteriovenous fistula in an arm or leg will often increase its growth, intracranial arteriovenous anomalies "steal" blood from the brain, so that increased cerebral blood flow through the lesion only results in diminished rather than increased cerebral nutrition and eventual cerebral atrophy.

Associated vascular abnormalities.—In 20–33 per cent of cases, similar lesions are present in other organs. In particular, angiomas are also found in the esophagus and urinary bladder (Geschickter and Keasbey). The combination of congenital heart defect and intracranial arteriovenous malformation is seen rarely in children (Padget). Intracranial berry aneurysms may accompany angiomas (Figs. 72 and 96).

STURGE-WEBER DISEASE.—The rare Sturge-Weber syndrome differs

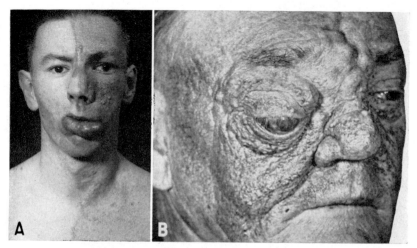

FIG. 87.—*A,* Sturge-Weber disease (courtesy of A. D. McCoy and H. C. Voris). *B,* variant of Sturge-Weber syndrome; glaucoma, right.

from all the preceding types of vascular malformations. In Sturge-Weber disease there is telangiectasia of the face and sometimes forequarter of the body and angiomatosis of the posterior cerebral pia with calcification of the underlying cortex. Wyburn-Mason attributes the strange pattern of the complex to retention into adult life of the close association of primitive ophthalmic and brain stem vessels at the 4 mm. stage of the embryo. Nevi are present in the distribution of the trigeminal nerve, especially of its ophthalmic division which has a recurrent branch to the falx and superior leaf of the tentorium.

Port-wine stains are seen on the forehead or upper cheek or may be spread unilaterally over the entire head, neck, chest and ipsilateral arm (Fig. 87, *A*). Angiomatous change may be present in the choroid of the retina (with or without glaucoma), the nose, ear, intestines or genitalia (Fig. 87, *B*). All angiomas may enlarge progressively (Danis). Cranio-facial hemihypertrophy has included bones as well as soft tissues. Neuro-

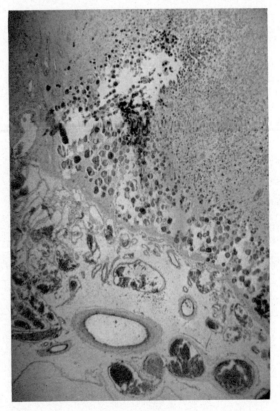

FIG. 88.—Calcospherites in occipital cortex, Sturge-Weber disease. (Courtesy of J. R. Green *et al.*)

cutaneous features of tuberous sclerosis and Recklinghausen's disease have also been encountered.

Pial telangiectasia is usually of the occipital lobe but may extend into or be present alone in the superficial layers of the parietal, temporal or frontal lobes. Cortical capillaries and neurons are calcified in laminar fashion and calcospherites besprinkle the ground substance of the gray mantle (Fig. 88).

SYMPTOMS AND SIGNS

HEMANGIOBLASTOMA.—The basic clinical picture of hemangioblastoma is that of any space-consuming lesion of the cerebellum or posterior fossa. Occipitocervical headache radiates frontally, and papilledema, nystagmus, ataxia, tremor, hypotonia, nausea and vomiting appear as pressure increases below the tentorium. Hemorrhage into or rapid enlargement of a cyst in the tumor will make the syndrome acute. Onset of intracranial symptoms has often followed trauma.

Retinal vascular malformations are visible only with wide dilatation

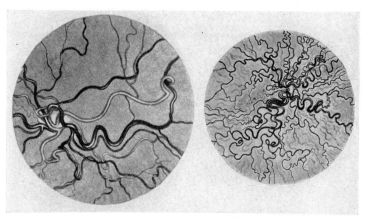

FIG. 89.—Retinal angiomas in von Hippel-Lindau disease. (Courtesy of P. Danis.)

of the pupil (Fig. 89). Intraspinal hemangiomas are manifest in the syndrome of cord compression. Cystic and neoplastic changes in lung, kidney, pancreas and liver may be evident or only suspected. Polycythemic plethora may be apparent.

HEMANGIOMA, CAVERNOUS ANGIOMA.—Cavernous angiomas of the midbrain, pons and medulla oblongata produce acute episodes of partial or complete decerebration accompanied by pupillary and other ocular palsies, nystagmus and dysarthria, pyramidal and cerebellar signs, psychotic behavior and sudden loss of consciousness (Jefferson). Subarachnoid hemorrhage from the lesion often precipitates such an attack. Chronically, closure of the aqueduct of Sylvius or fourth ventricle results in internal hydrocephalus. Non-neoplastic, cirsoid angiomatosis of the retina is seen at least as often as with cerebellar hemangioblastomas, and progressive, permanent impairment of the pupils and extraocular muscles develops. Combined retinal and midbrain vascular anomalies are often associated with intellectual and psychic changes (Wyburn-Mason). Hemangiomas also occur elsewhere in the brain (thalamus, basal ganglions). They are a not uncommon cause of intracranial hemorrhage in the young (Fig. 90).

ARTERIOVENOUS MALFORMATIONS.—Arteriovenous malformations or cirsoid aneurysms of the surface and interior of the cerebral hemispheres are evidenced in the syndrome comprised of: (1) convulsive seizures, usually jacksonian in type because of the frequency of location

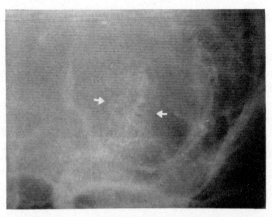

FIG. 90.—Hemangioma or choroidal-galenic malformation of thalamus (arrows). Anteroposterior arteriogram: anterior cerebral artery to left, middle cerebral artery to right.

of anomalies in the sylvian fissure; (2) progressive hemiparesis or hemisensory loss, and (3) episodes of subarachnoid hemorrhage, unlikely to be severe or fatal since the source of bleeding is usually venous. Subdural hematoma may result.

Onset of symptoms is usually in the third or fourth decade. Pulsating exophthalmos is observed rarely on the side of the lesion; optic atrophy has been reported. Enlargement of the extracranial vascular supply is not infrequent. Cutaneous nevi may be evident on the scalp, face or neck. A cranial or ocular bruit is sometimes heard on auscultation of the head, and the noise may increase during excitement or intellectual activity. Cardiac enlargement and a low diastolic blood pressure are due to arteriovenous shunt.

Formal neurologic signs may be frank, meager or entirely absent even with sizeable lesions. The cerebral deficit depends on the location of the malformation. Mental dulness is a result of pressure atrophy of the brain or of cerebral malnutrition consequent to the draining of blood through the lesion. Seizures are particularly difficult to control, even after definitive surgery. Bleeding into the brain may be crippling or fatal.

Arteriovenous malformations involving the galenic venous circulation are characterized by the early appearance of symptoms, particularly hydrocephalus and visual disturbances.

STURGE-WEBER DISEASE.—The clinical triad of Sturge-Weber syndrome is: (1) facial vascular nevus or port-wine stain, usually on the forehead or cheek but sometimes more extensive; (2) focal epileptic attacks of inveterate nature in over one-half the cases, and (3) mental deficiency, with or without psychosis. Ipsilateral glaucoma is not uncommon. Vascular lesions elsewhere in the body have been described. One-half the head may be hypertrophied. Associated cutaneous manifestations of tuberous sclerosis or neurofibromatosis have been found. Many patients show brain involvement in hemianopsia, contralateral sensory impairment or hemiparesis according to the location of pial angioma. As a *forme fruste,* some persons born with facial nevus flammeus apparently are without accompanying cerebral defect.

LABORATORY STUDIES

Polycythemia is often found in a patient with cerebellar hemangioblastoma. Urinalyses or pyelography may disclose an associated hypernephroma. The blood pressure will reveal low diastolic tension when arteriovenous cross-communication is extensive.

CEREBROSPINAL FLUID.—The lumbar fluid pressure is elevated if a vascular anomaly is causing hydrocephalus by impinging on ventricular pathways. The cerebrospinal fluid is bloody, xanthochromic or cellular after recent hemorrhage, and the protein content and gold curve are abnormal if chronic cerebral tissue destruction is taking place or thrombosis has occurred.

ROENTGENOLOGY.—X-rays of the skull reveal changes due to increased intracranial pressure when posterior fossa hemangioblastoma is of chronic nature. Widening of the middle meningeal groove and enlargement of diploic channels suggest but are not in themselves diagnostic of large arteriovenous anomaly. Almost 50 per cent of all intracranial vascular malformations are calcified to some degree (Fig. 91). This is particularly true of the cerebral pathologic change in the Sturge-Weber

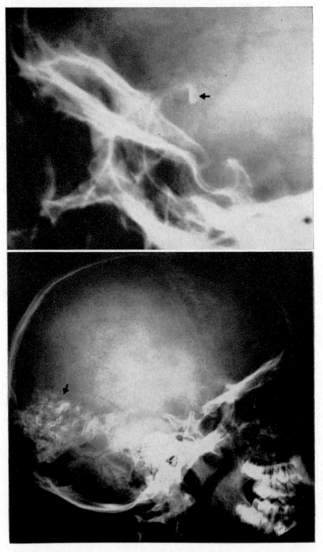

FIG. 91 *(above).*—Calcifying hemangioma of middle cerebral artery.
FIG. 92 *(below).*—Intracranial occipital calcification. Sturge-Weber syndrome. (Courtesy of J. R. Green *et al.*)

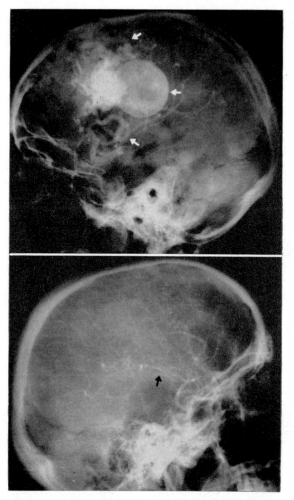

FIG. 93 *(above)*.—Arteriovenous malformation between ascending frontoparietal branch of middle cerebral artery and vein of Trolard. False aneurysm sac.

FIG. 94 *(below)*.—Elevation of middle cerebral artery (arrow) due to arteriovenous malformation involving choroidal artery and vein of Galen, later removed surgically.

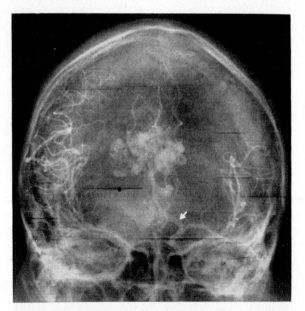

FIG. 95.—Midline arteriovenous angioma arising from anterior cerebral artery (arrow). (Courtesy of J. W. Watts.)

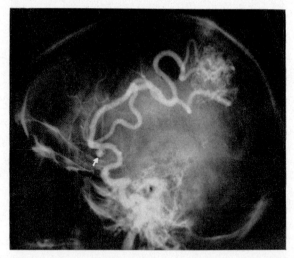

FIG. 96.—Arteriovenous malformation and arterial aneurysm (arrow), arising from middle cerebral artery. (Courtesy of J. M. Williams.)

syndrome, in which calcium deposits in the pia and cortex, usually of the occipital lobe, are almost always visible (Fig. 92). Vascular hamartomas may also calcify (Alexander).

Ventriculograms in a patient with cerebellar hemangioblastoma disclose dilatation of the superior ventricular system and enlargement of the aqueduct of Sylvius with rostral bending of its caudal end. The fourth ventricle is not seen. Aqueductal blockage with hydrocephalus may be produced by a midbrain angioma. Encephalography often reveals cortical atrophy underneath an arteriovenous anomaly. Ventricular encroachment of the lesion may be evident or intraventricular clots may be disclosed.

Angiography is the most valuable, revealing and accurate diagnostic aid (Figs. 93–96). In some extensive lesions both carotids and one vertebral artery must be injected to visualize the entire source of supply and drainage. However, since most surgical arteriovenous anomalies involve the carotid system, bilateral or unilateral carotid injection is usually sufficient. Three components of cirsoid aneurysms are outlined: the afferent artery, an abnormally enlarged "capillary" network and efferent veins. Moniz described a peculiar arteriographic finding with arteriovenous angiomas of the carotid zone, in which arterial blood passes rapidly into the superior longitudinal sinus through a large anastomosing vein (Fig. 93). Curtis emphasized the time factor in visualizing anomalies; in one of his cases, a parietal angioma, the lesion did not opacify until $6\frac{2}{3}$ seconds after injection, when normally all dye has left the head, and was not completely filled until three seconds later.

Dilatation of feeding vessels may be shown as far down as the cervical carotid. Of special interest is the frequent failure of the normal cerebral circulation to fill, indicating that the great bulk of blood bypasses the brain and flows through the vascular anomaly. After removal of these lesions, reinjection of contrast mediums may visualize the natural cerebral arterial supply and the carotid is reduced to original size (Fig. 97) (Norlén). Pathologically increased cerebral blood flow and decreased cerebrovascular resistance also return to normal after excision of arteriovenous malformations (Bessman *et al.*).

ELECTROENCEPHALOGRAPHY.—Electroencephalography is of little diagnostic assistance unless bleeding has occurred into the brain. The electroencephalogram is often entirely normal or reveals only local spiking even with large cirsoid aneurysms. Silver *et al.* observed mixed frequencies and delta formation with large cerebral arteriovenous malformations, but neither change was as prominent as with tumor. Parietal and parieto-occipital angiomas cause suppression of alpha activity. In the Sturge-

Weber complex, a focus of dysrhythmia with high amplitude bursts is usual in the occipital region, particularly when epilepsy and mental deficiency are severe.

DIAGNOSIS

A family history of congenital cerebrovascular anomalies or associated lesions is helpful in diagnosing any one of the various types of intra-

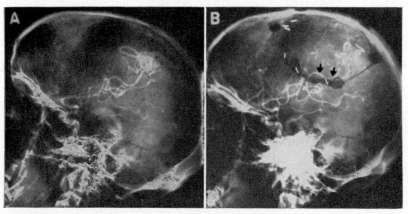

Fig. 97.—*A,* preoperative and *B,* postoperative angiograms showing restoration of normal carotid circulation after excision of arteriovenous malformation. (Courtesy of G. Norlén.)

cranial vascular malformation, particularly the Lindau complex. External, vascular "birthmarks" may be seen elsewhere on the body.

Hemangioblastoma of the cerebellum typically appears as a posterior fossa tumor in a young or early middle-aged adult in whom abnormality of the retinal vasculature is evident. Polycythemia may be present. Cavernous angioma usually produces the midbrain or pontile syndrome, with episodes of subarachnoid hemorrhage, psychic disturbance and ocular choroidal vascular anomaly. An intracranial calcium deposit may indicate the site of hemangioma of the brain.

Focal convulsions, progressive hemiparesis and repeated intracranial hemorrhages are diagnostic of arteriovenous malformation or cirsoid aneurysm. Plain x-ray films of the skull may show calcification of the lesion, which will usually appear in an angiographic survey. A cranial bruit may be audible, the carotid artery is sometimes enlarged, the heart may be hypertrophied, the diastolic blood pressure is low and the oxygen content of the jugular blood is increased.

Sturge-Weber disease is evidenced in a facial port-wine stain, intractable focal epilepsy and mental deficiency. Choroidal angioma may be seen in ophthalmoscopy. Calcification of the occipital lobe is found, and a focus of electroencephalographic abnormality is present. Cerebral involvement may appear in abnormal neurologic signs.

DIFFERENTIAL DIAGNOSIS.—The only reliable means of distinguishing vascular anomalies from other intracranial processes is by arteriography. Two other conditions are much more common causes of subarachnoid bleeding. *Cerebral hemorrhage* ordinarily occurs as a complication of the hypertensive cardiovascular syndrome, and coma and profound hemiplegia are the usual results. Rupture of a *congenital berry aneurysm* of the circle of Willis produces a more severe subarachnoid hemorrhage, often fatal, and neurologic signs, if present, are ordinarily confined to unilateral ocular palsies. Convulsive seizures are less common with berry aneurysm than with arteriovenous malformation.

Brain tumor, primary or metastatic, is usually accompanied by increased intracranial pressure, which is rare in cerebral vascular anomaly. Subarachnoid bleeding from true neoplasm is very unusual. However, cavernoma of the brain stem and hemangioblastoma of the cerebellum are often indistinguishable from gliomas. *Inflammatory* and other diseases of the brain are rarely accompanied by bleeding phenomena.

TREATMENT

The principal therapy of vascular anomalies, when possible, is surgery. Medical management is confined largely to the control of epileptic seizures, and this may be difficult even if definitive surgery has been undertaken. X-ray therapy has been advocated to reduce the size of these lesions by its endarteritic and thrombotic effect. Roentgen irradiation should be undertaken if definitive surgery is impossible. Some vascular malformations tend to calcify after x-ray treatment.

Suboccipital craniectomy is mandatory once a diagnosis of *hemangioblastoma* of the cerebellum has been made because of the life-endangering nature of posterior fossa tumors. It is not sufficient to drain a xanthochromic cyst; the mural nodule must be removed. After any partial extirpation, recurrent growth may be expected. Solid lesions attached to the large venous sinuses or diffuse vascular growths may be impossible to remove and are best treated with radiation. A generous bony decompression should be left, in any case. Cystic hemangioblastoma is a type of cerebellar tumor very amenable to cure by surgery.

Cavernous angiomas of the brain stem cannot be removed; procedures, such as Torkildsen's, designed to reroute cerebrospinal fluid from the ventricular system to the subarachnoid spaces, avoiding the blocked aqueduct, will reduce internal hydrocephalus. Roentgen therapy may be directed to the midbrain. Elsewhere in the brain *hemangiomas* may be removable unless major and indispensable vessels are incorporated. The evacuation of complicating intracerebral hematoma is mandatory.

Arteriovenous malformations (cirsoid aneurysms) of the cerebrum are attacked in two ways: indirectly, with carotid ligation, and directly, by radical extirpation. Each method has its adherents. Olivecrona states that carotid ligation is valueless and may be dangerous; Krayenbühl considers ligation frequently to be the procedure of choice. Opinion as to the value of additional x-ray therapy is also divided. The effect of carotid occlusion on convulsive seizures is capricious, and the principal aim of ligation is to prevent further hemorrhagic episodes. It is hard to contemplate intracranial removal of a cirsoid aneurysm when the patient presents no neurologic findings, has had mild attacks of subarachnoid bleeding and harbors a lesion involving important areas of the brain in a relatively inaccessible place. Rich collateral circulation usually permits carotid ligation which, in my experience, is indicated in this special circumstance. In a patient treated by cervical arterial ligation, a bulging decompression receded and the patient became conscious.

Radical removal has the advantage of complete and definitive control of the lesion but the disadvantages of the risk of surgical mortality or of postoperative deficit such as hemiplegia. Pilcher recommended total removal of cirsoid aneurysms and had a high degree of success in selected cases. Olivecrona and Riives reported 43 cases so treated; one-third were entirely well and one-third had minor defects postoperatively. The surgical mortality rate was 9.3 per cent. New methods of induced hypotension during surgery permit removal of cirsoid aneurysms with greater ease, but the risk of thrombosis in heart, brain or elsewhere must be calculated. Total extirpation of cerebral arteriovenous malformations, if uncomplicated, is the ideal method of treatment of these lesions.

Extirpation of pial angiomas and calcified cortex in the *Sturge-Weber syndrome* has been effective in the elimination of epilepsy (Lund; Green et al.).

PROGNOSIS

In untreated cerebellar hemangioblastomas mortality will be almost total. Surgery offers a high percentage of cure. Forty-two of 64 patients operated on by Olivecrona over a period of 28 years are well and working. In patients with cavernous angiomas of the brain stem, procedures designed to relieve hydrocephalus will prolong life, but fatal outcome from intraventricular hemorrhage or mesencephalopontile destruction is inevitable. Approximately one-half the patients with arteriovenous malformations die of intracranial bleeding when untreated, and the rest are incapacitated by psychic or neurologic disability. There is a significantly high percentage of improvement and cure by direct or indirect surgical methods. Patients with Sturge-Weber syndrome should be treated by a resection of the cerebral lesion unless seizures are easily managed.

BIBLIOGRAPHY

Alexander, W. S.: Calcified vascular hamartoma with epilepsy, J. Neurosurg. 10:69-74, 1953.

Askenasy, H. M.; Herzberger, E. E., and Wijsenbeek, H. S.: Hydrocephalus with vascular malformations of the brain, Neurology 3:213-220, 1953.

Bailey, O. T., and Ford, R.: Sclerosing hemangiomas of the central nervous system, Am. J. Path. 18:1-27, 1941.

Bessman, A. N.; Hayes, G. J.; Alman, R. W., and Fazekas, J. F.: Cerebral hemodynamics in cerebral vascular disease, M. Ann. District of Columbia 21:422-425, 1952.

Cramer, F., and Kimsey, W.: Cerebellar hemangioblastomas, A.M.A. Arch. Neurol. & Psychiat. 67:237-252, 1952.

Curtis, J. B.: Rapid serial angiography, J. Neurol., Neurosurg. & Psychiat. 12:167-182, 1949.

Cushing, H., and Bailey, P.: *Tumors Arising from the Blood Vessels of the Brain: Angiomatous Malformations and Hemangioblastomas* (Springfield, Ill.: Charles C Thomas, Publisher, 1928).

Danis, P.: Ophthalmologic aspects of angiomatosis of nervous system, Acta neurol. et psychiat. belg. 50:615-679, 1950.

Geschickter, C. F., and Keasbey, L. E.: Tumors of blood vessels, Am. J. Cancer 23:568-591, 1935.

Green, J. R.; Foster, J., and Berens, D. L.: Encephalotrigeminal angiomatosis (Sturge-Weber syndrome) with particular reference to roentgenologic aspects before and after neurosurgery, Am. J. Roentgenol. 64:391-398, 1950.

Horton, B. T.; Ziegler, L. H., and Adson, A. W.: Intracranial arteriovenous fistula: III. Diagnosis by discovery of arterial blood in jugular veins, Arch. Neurol. & Psychiat. 33:1232-1234, 1935.

Jefferson, M.: Altered consciousness associated with brain stem lesions, Brain 75:55-67, 1952.

Krayenbühl, H.: Personal communication.

Lichtenstein, B. W.: *A Textbook of Neuropathology* (Philadelphia: W. B. Saunders Company, 1949).

Logan, M., *et al.*: Arterialization of internal jugular blood during hyperventilation as aid in diagnosis of intracranial vascular tumors, Ann. Int. Med. 27:220-224, 1947.

Lund, M.: On epilepsy in Sturge-Weber's disease, Acta psychiat. et neurol. scandinav. 24:569-586, 1949.

Moniz, E.: Arteriovenous angiomas of brain, Arq. neuro-psiquiat. 9:303-323, 1951.

Norlén, G.: Arteriovenous aneurysms of the brain, J. Neurosurg. 6:475-494, 1949.

Olivecrona, H.: The cerebellar angioreticulomas, J. Neurosurg. 9:317-330, 1952.
Olivecrona, H., and Riives, J.: Arteriovenous aneurysms of the brain, Arch. Neurol. & Psychiat. 59:567-602, 1948.
Padget, D. H.: Personal communication.
Pilcher, S.: Vascular anomalies of the brain, in Bancroft, F. W., and Pilcher, C. (eds): *Surgical Treatment of the Nervous System* (Philadelphia: J. B. Lippincott Company, 1946).
Silver, M. L.; Taft, G. H., and Tennant, J. M.: The electroencephalogram in some angiomatous malformations, Electroencephalog. & Clin. Neurophysiol. 4:245, 1952.
Tonning, H. O.; Warren, R. F., and Barrie, H. J.: Familial hemangiomata of the cerebellum, J. Neurosurg. 9:124-132, 1952.
Wyburn-Mason, R.: Arteriovenous aneurysm of midbrain and retina, facial naevi and mental changes, Brain 66:163-203, 1943.

CHAPTER 13

Intracranial Venous Disease; Venous Sinus Disease

ALTHOUGH NEITHER as spectacular nor as common as diseases of the cerebral arterial system, processes of thrombosis and thrombophlebitis involving the intracranial veins and venous sinuses similarly produce neurologic disability, general morbidity and death. Indeed, more diffuse and extensive brain damage may result from phlebothrombosis or venous inflammation than from arterial occlusions. The chief consequences of intracranial venous and venous sinus diseases are cerebral tissue destruction from infarction, transmission and spread of infection and an increased intracranial pressure due to passive congestion of the cerebrum.

ETIOLOGY; PATHOGENESIS

Etiologic factors in intracranial venous diseases are those associated with blood dyscrasias, other changes in the composition of the circulating blood, central extension of infection from the skull and soft tissues of the head and neck, metastatic and diffuse inflammatory vascular conditions and trauma.

HEMATOLOGIC FACTORS.—Thrombosis of cerebral veins and dural sinuses may complicate the course of leukemia, polycythemia vera, sickle cell anemia, thrombocytopenic purpura or other blood dyscrasia. The vessels may actually be plugged with clumps of pathologic cells or may be simply thrombosed.

Marantic thrombosis, seen in infants and children, has become a clinical rarity since the maintenance of adequate fluid balance and use of antibiotics have become routine in pediatrics. In young patients, injury to the endothelium of the intracranial venous sinuses by circulating toxins can result in aseptic thrombosis, particularly when or solely because the

263

blood is concentrated by severe dehydration. Puncture of the sagittal sinus for transfusion may initiate the process.

Puerperal intracranial venous or sinus thrombosis is either related to normal maternal hematologic changes following delivery, such as thrombocytosis, increase of fibrinogen or "stickiness" of the blood, or results from emboli coming from pelvic veins via the vertebral system. Sinus stasis produced by increased abdominal tension and forced expiration during parturition favors the intracranial vascular complication.

Chronic or acute cardiac failure, especially that associated with congenital heart disease and its secondary polycythemia or of rheumatic or other origin, may result in thromboses of cerebral sinuses or veins. Hemoconcentration and arterial hypotension favor intravenous clotting.

REGIONAL INFLAMMATORY PROCESSES.—Uncontrolled pyogenic infections of the soft tissues of the face, orbit, nose and paranasal sinuses, the ear and mastoid, scalp, skull and neck can extend intracranially through retrograde thrombophlebitis of the diploic or emissary vessels to inflame and occlude the cerebral sinuses and veins. Furuncle of the upper lip or naris may involve the anterior facial vein, from which infection travels via the angular vessel at the inner canthus of the eye and the communicating ophthalmic vein to reach the *cavernous sinus*. Cavernous thrombophlebitis may also result from orbital inflammation, paranasal sinusitis, pharyngitis, otitis or petrositis, emissary channels and the carotid venous plexus transmitting the infection.

The more common *transverse (lateral) sinus* thrombosis almost always follows infection of the middle ear, mastoid or petrous bone, which causes emissary thrombophlebitis or perisinal abscess. From the sigmoid or transverse sinus, thrombotic change may extend to other dural channels and to the bulb of the jugular vein (two-thirds of cases). Infections of the neck may involve the jugular vein primarily and the lateral sinus secondarily by retrograde thrombosis.

Petrosal sinuses are also attacked by otogenic disease; from the petrous tip, the cavernous may be reached via the superior petrosal sinus, and from the middle ear the jugular veins can be infected through the inferior petrosal sinus.

Infections of the scalp, skull and paranasal sinuses may be transmitted to the *superior sagittal sinus* by diploic vessels. The thrombotic process then extends readily to the important superior cerebral veins if the anterior sagittal sinus is involved. Occlusion of the essential rolandic vein results in infarction of the motor area. The lateral, straight and cavernous sinuses may become involved secondarily through anastomotic channels.

Carbuncles of the neck will rarely continue interiorly to the *occipital sinus* and sigmoid dural vessels.

SYSTEMIC VASCULAR DISEASE.—Generalized inflammatory disease of the veins may involve intracranial venous vessels. Syphilis, rheumatic fever, other collagen disorders and thromboangiitis obliterans have been implicated in primary cerebral thrombophlebitis (Smith). An idiopathic, recurrent, systemic phlebitic disease has resulted in retinal and cerebral cortical thromboses and subdural hematoma (Bucy and Lesemann). In a patient followed by Wright, a chain of repetitive major venous occlusions was initiated by a trivial injury to the leg; intracranial thromboses rendered her psychotic 10 years later.

EMBOLI.—Pelvic and abdominal conditions associated with venous stasis may be sources of intracranial metastases. Bland or septic clots from pulmonary thrombosis or phlebitis accompanying intrathoracic suppuration or chronic passive congestion may reach the brain and often cause the cerebritis and cerebral abscess which so frequently complicate lung abscess, bronchiectasis, empyema and congenital heart disease. The vertebral veins transport emboli to the brain from the chest, abdomen and pelvis. The heart is by-passed and fragments of thrombi are carried directly from vein to vein.

HEAD INJURY.—Trauma to the head may cause thrombosis of intracranial sinuses when dural venous channels are perforated by spicules of bone or surgical instruments or when infection develops at the site of injury. Shearing of the skull in difficult or premature obstetric deliveries sometimes tears the tentorium cerebelli and the straight or transverse sinuses. If death does not occur from subdural hematoma in the posterior fossa, thrombosis of the vein of Galen may result. Depressed fracture of the vertex of the skull posteriorly may, by compressing the superior sagittal sinus, cause an acute increase of intracranial pressure without actual thrombosis.

PATHOLOGY

Cerebral or cerebellar venous thrombosis produces local or general passive congestion of the brain, single or multiple red infarctions, parenchymal and arachnoidal hemorrhages and scarring. Phlebitis adds an acute or chronic inflammatory reaction, depending on the stage of disease, which involves the vessels and regional parenchyma, perivascular spaces and meninges. Cerebritis or brain abscess may be the end result. Cystic, gliotic or demyelinating changes in the fields of drainage of specific veins are end stages of inactive phlebothrombosis or healed phlebitis. Axis cylinders may or may not be preserved in microscopic fields of perivascular demyelination ("leukoencephalopathy"). Status marmoratus of the internal capsules and basal ganglions, the pathologic substrate of one type of spastic choreoathetosis of childhood, is the late result of thrombosis of the veins of Galen at birth.

In sinus thrombosis, the process beginning in one dural venous sinus (Fig. 98) often extends to other connecting sinuses and is propagated in retrograde fashion into contributing veins. In the latter event, multiple parenchymal infarctions are produced. If the process is confined to the

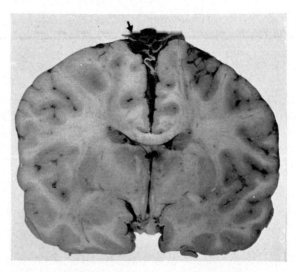

FIG. 98.—Thrombosis of the superior sagittal sinus. (AFIP #ACC 293226-27127.)

sinuses alone, tributary veins are congested and enlarged and internal and external anastomotic channels are opened. In superior sagittal sinus occlusion, transcerebral veins running from vertex to base may be demonstrated in the living patient (Fig. 100). Brain edema is general or local depending on the importance of the sinus or sinuses involved. General tissue hypoxia eventuating in cerebral atrophy is one final result of thrombosis of the sagittal sinus, marantic or otherwise, and is a cause of cerebral hypogenesis in childhood (Bailey). A subdural hygroma or hematoma may develop acutely or chronically as in meningitic phlebitis (Guthkelch). Tortuosity of the veins of the scalp and subcutaneous edema are seen over the vault of the skull when the superior sagittal sinus is thrombosed and behind the ear when the transverse sinus is occluded.

When sinus phlebitis is the pathologic process destructive changes in the vessels and neighboring parenchyma of the brain are more serious and extensive. Intrasinal thrombi are purulent and friable and pus cells infiltrate the adventitial coats of sinus and tributary veins. Subdural empyema may be a complication, though meningitis is more common, and cerebritis terminating in brain abscess is not infrequent. Systemic pyogenic seeding is a mode of death in infected sinus thrombosis. Inflammatory necrosis of the pituitary has been found at autopsy in cavernous sinus thrombosis (Walsh).

SYMPTOMS AND SIGNS

VENOUS THROMBOSIS; PHLEBITIS.—*Polyvascular venous occlusions* produce widespread brain destruction and a confusing clinical picture resembling that of multiple intracranial tumors (Keschner and Davison). Local cerebral tissue involvement is revealed by focal palsies and convulsize seizures. The rich anastomoses between the superficial and deep venous drainage pathways in the cerebrum may compensate for one or several occlusions if these develop gradually.

Passive congestion of the brain causes symptoms resembling those of cerebral anemia or anoxia. Sleeplessness or drowsiness, vertigo, headache, mental confusion, excitability, depression, delirium, convulsions and coma are common. Some elderly patients with chronic cardiac or pulmonary disease must sleep sitting up to avoid hallucinations which appear when they lie flat.

All clinical phenomena are accentuated in the presence of *phlebitis,* in which suppurative necrosis is added to infarction and complications such as cerebritis, subdural empyema and multiple abscess formation arise. Spiking fever, severe headache, repeated jacksonian attacks, coma and paralyses result. The mortality rate is high.

Puerperal venous thromboses develop four to 21 days after delivery and are manifested in headache, seizures, paralyses, papilledema and subarachnoid hemorrhage (Hyland). Signs may be bilateral. The mortality rate is 30–56 per cent. Thrombosis of the veins of the hypophyseal-portal system is probably responsible for some cases of postpartum pituitary necrosis (Sheehan's disease). Premature separation of the placenta predisposes to intracranial venous clotting.

Acute infantile hemiplegia, in the opinion of Mitchell, is most frequently due to cortical or intracerebral venous thrombosis. The affected child is usually under 6 years of age. Onset of the syndrome occurs with

268   CEREBROVASCULAR DISEASE

convulsive seizures, which terminate in coma. On regaining consciousness the child is hemiplegic, and this condition may be permanent.

Venous syndromes (Bailey).—Occlusion of the *great vein of Galen* produces hyperpyrexia and coma, rapid pulse and respiration, decerebrate rigidity and exaggerated tendon reflexes. Hyperemia and hemorrhages in the brain stem, basal ganglions and adjacent white matter occur after experimental occlusion of the galenic system (Schlesinger). Obstruction of the *superior cerebral vein* of Trolard causes infarction of the motor area and severe hemiplegia, or paraplegia if thrombosis is bilateral. *Middle cerebral vein* ligation results in facial palsy and epileptic attacks which begin in the throat and face; aphasia is added if the left hemisphere is involved. *Lateral occipital* venous thrombosis is associated with visual hallucinations and aphasia(left). *Medial, posterior occipital* vein ligation causes hemianopsia. Clipping the *petrosal vein* in exposure of the cerebellum or pontile angle sometimes destroys the dentate nucleus, and severe cerebellar disturbances follow.

DURAL SINUS THROMBOSIS; PHLEBITIS.—Clinical phenomena are of two types. Interference with drainage of blood from the brain causes increased intracranial pressure and stagnant cerebral anoxia. The infective process, if present, is manifested in irregularly high temperature, chills, malaise, prostration and septicemia.

Superior sagittal sinus.—Thrombosis of the superior sagittal sinus (Fig. 98) may occur in debilitated and anemic infants 8–9 months of age (marantic thrombosis). Coma, convulsive seizures, meningeal irritation, bulging of the fontanel, subgaleal edema and swelling of scalp veins (caput medusae) reveal sinus occlusion. In older children and adults the clinical syndrome is often called pseudotumor cerebri. Papilledema, vomiting, slow pulse and impairment of consciousness without focal neurologic signs mimic unlocalized brain tumor. Jacksonian convulsions begin in the leg when the superior cerebral veins become involved by extension, and hemiplegia or paraplegia may develop.

When occlusion proceeds slowly, intracerebral anastomotic veins will drain blood that is normally intended for the sagittal sinus inferiorly into the galenic system and the transverse, cavernous and petrosal sinuses. Externally, blood may escape into the veins of the eye, face and occipitovertebral plexus through emissary channels. This collateral drainage permits subsidence of cerebral edema if the patient with major sinus thrombosis can be tided over the critical period of acute passive congestion. Resection of the anterior sagittal sinus has been accomplished successfully when the vessel has been obstructed slowly by invading meningioma.

Cavernous sinus.—Acute cavernous sinus thrombosis is recognized in the syndrome of deep-seated pain about the eye, orbital congestion, lacrimation, conjunctival swelling, edema of the lids, ptosis, exophthalmos and a septic temperature (Fig. 99). Papilledema and retinal hemorrhages develop rapidly and vision may be lost. Extraocular palsies are common in the acute or chronic state. In 50 per cent of patients both cavernous sinuses become involved as the disease spreads contralaterally through the circular sinus and pterygoid plexus. Before use of the antibiotics, death was due to septicemia, meningitis, brain abscess or pituitary necrosis.

Transverse sinus.—Thrombosis of the transverse (lateral) and sigmoid sinus produces edema and engorgement around the mastoid process

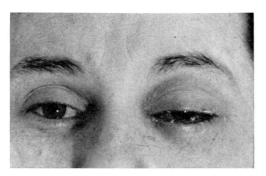

Fig. 99.—Cavernous sinus thrombophlebitis, *right.*

and jugular vein, tenderness behind the ear and in the neck and palsies of the glossopharyngeal, vagus and accessory nerves if the jugular bulb is occluded. Pressure on the jugular vein will not congest the homolateral eye as it does normally. In 75 per cent of cases not controlled by antibiotics there are intracranial complications such as meningitis or perisinal, subdural, cerebral or cerebellar abscess. Intracranial hypertension develops if the dominant sinus (which may be either right or left) is obstructed. This syndrome is sometimes referred to as otitic hydrocephalus, since the cause of most transverse sinus occlusion is ear disease.

Headache may be so severe as to suggest brain abscess. The incidence of transverse sinus thrombosis in cases of mastoiditis is about 1 per cent. Occlusion of the sigmoid sinus is probable if perisinal suppuration is found at mastoidectomy. The blood culture is positive for infecting organisms in 50 per cent of patients not receiving sulfone compounds or antibiotics, and pyogenic metastases may appear in the joints, subcutaneous tissues and lungs.

Jugular and innominate veins, superior vena cava.—Obstruction of the jugular or innominate veins will cause increased intracranial pressure and stagnant cerebral anoxia if the dominant side is involved acutely. Venous return from the brain is decreased significantly in 25 per cent of patients if the major jugular vein is thrombosed, and inadequacy is extreme in 4–10 per cent (Woodhall). Chronic jugular impedance may be tolerated because of collateral drainage via the posterior vertebral venous system (Fig. 20), which has a potential capacity exceeding that of both jugular channels. Bilateral resection of both internal and external jugular veins has been accomplished with no more than temporary cerebral congestion (Gius and Grier). However, if both sets of vessels are to be removed in radical neck dissection, it is best to do so in two separate operations with an interval between.

Uncompensated superior caval obstruction from thoracic tumors or aneurysms, mediastinitis, thrombophlebitis or constrictive pericarditis results in fulness in the head, headache, vertigo and mental changes. The head, neck, upper chest and arms are cyanotic, regional veins are distended and the eyes bulge. All symptoms and signs are made worse by bending forward. The syndrome subsides as the vertebral venous system becomes adequate. A patient with verified thrombosis of the superior vena cava has survived 25 years with only minimal symptoms from venous obstruction (Rose).

LABORATORY STUDIES

Abnormalities in the hemogram may be those of blood dyscrasia or of inflammatory reaction. An increased "stickiness" of the blood may accompany thromboses in the puerperal, febrile or postoperative states. Urinary findings are nonspecific, and the blood pressure is not necessarily affected unless intracranial pressure is extreme.

X-rays of the skull may show enlargement of the fontanel and widening of cranial sutures in infants or prominence of diploic emissaries from chronic sinus blockage in the adult, but they are usually negative. Special views will reveal mastoid disease with transverse sinus thrombosis. A roentgenogram of the chest for mediastinal tumor may demonstrate the cause of cephalic venous congestion.

The lumbar cerebrospinal fluid pressure is high in all types of phlebothrombotic or phlebitic disease. The cerebrospinal fluid may be clear, xanthochromic or bloody, depending on the degree of transudation or hemorrhage from obstructed vessels. The lymphocyte count may reach

5,000 per cu. mm. and polymorphonuclear cells predominate if the causative process is inflammatory. Protein increase parallels the degree of pathologic activity but is rarely over 100 mg. per 100 ml. in aseptic thrombosis. Gold curves are frequently abnormal.

Queckenstedt's observation of a rise in lumbar cerebrospinal fluid pressure due to engorgement of intracerebral veins when the jugulars are compressed was applied by Tobey and Ayer to the diagnosis of occlusion of the transverse or sigmoid sinuses. With unilateral obstruction, com-

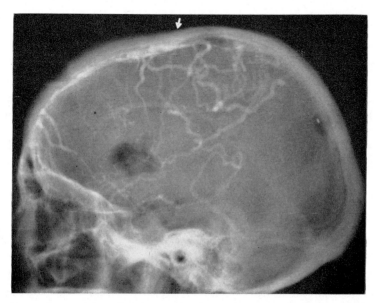

FIG. 100.—Thrombotic occlusion of superior sagittal sinus (arrow); anastomotic veins demonstrated by dural sinus venography. (Courtesy of B. S. Ray *et al.*)

pression of the jugular vein on the involved side will not cause a rise in cerebrospinal fluid pressure, whereas contralateral compression results in a normal rise to 350–400 mm. of water. Anatomic variations in dominance of the lateral sinus will allow small inequalities; no change or very little change in resting cerebrospinal fluid pressure during jugular tamponade must be the criterion of lateral sinus obstruction.

Ventriculography or encephalography in sinus obstruction (pseudotumor cerebri) discloses small ventricles, not displaced, with no or little visualization of subarachnoid spaces. Major cerebral infarction distorts the air patterns.

Arteriography can reveal failure of venous and sinus patterns to appear at appropriate locations and times. The most logical and clearcut method of demonstrating sinus occlusion has been introduced by Ray and associates as dural sinus venography (Chapter 20). Not only is it possible to show exact sites of thrombosis with this method, but the development of collateral flow which will permit sinus resection is also displayed (Fig. 100).

Electroencephalographic changes depend on the degree of cerebral tissue destruction.

DIAGNOSIS

Cerebral venous thrombosis may be diagnosed in the presence of a disease or physical state known to cause spontaneous clotting or embolization, when symptoms and signs are of fairly rapid onset, are multiple in nature and are particularly restricted to abnormalities of the motor system (hemiplegia, aphasia, convulsions). Thrombophlebitis is revealed by accompanying signs of infection, such as fever, leukocytosis and delirium, and more severe changes in the cerebrospinal fluid, expressed as hemorrhage, xanthochromia or frank meningitis.

Venous thrombosis and thrombophlebitis must be distinguished from the more common cerebritis or intracranial abscess. When hemorrhage is a prominent clinical feature, distinction must be made from ruptured aneurysm, cerebral apoplexy, arteriovenous malformation or other cause of subarachnoid bleeding. Multiple tumors may be suggested by a diffusion of neurologic signs.

Superior sagittal sinus thrombosis occurs in the marantic or puerperal state or follows infections of the scalp or skull. Enlargement of superficial veins and edema of the scalp develop, intracranial pressure is increased to high degree, and motor signs appear as the process extends to superior cerebral veins. Cavernous sinus thrombosis, a sequel of inflammatory states in the face, head or throat, is a severe, febrile and toxic condition. The chief local manifestations are orbital and ocular. Transverse or sigmoid sinus occlusion is almost always produced by suppuration of the middle ear and mastoid. It causes local tenderness and regional pain, and the febrile response, headache and evidences of elevated intracranial pressure may simulate symptoms of brain abscess. Diagnosis of transverse sinus thrombosis may be difficult because one tends to think of infections of the ear, bone, meninges or brain first. The Tobey-Ayer test is confirmatory if positive.

Sagittal sinus thrombosis is usually confused with brain tumor in adults, with hydrocephalus in infants and children, and may be mistaken for meningitis at any age. Cavernous sinus thrombosis has to be differentiated from orbital cellulitis, frontal sinusitis, arteriovenous aneurysm, orbital tumor and ophthalmic herpes. Lateral sinus occlusion is hard to distinguish from cervical adenitis, recurrent mastoiditis, meningitis, cerebritis and abscess of the temporal lobe or cerebellar hemisphere.

TREATMENT

Two main courses of medical therapy are mandatory in acute intracranial phlebothrombosis or thrombophlebitis: anti-infective, if there is evidence or suspicion of an inflammatory etiology, and anticoagulant, if hemorrhagic phenomena are not prominent. Antibiotics of appropriate type are to be given in large quantities, as in meningitis, and combinations of antibiotics in high dosage should be used if the infecting organism cannot be identified. Heparin, Dicumarol or other anticoagulant substances are administered to depress the prothrombin time. Intravenous use of trypsin may also be effective (Innersfield *et al.*).

Surgical therapy may be lifesaving. Subtemporal decompressions can accommodate increased intracranial pressure and save vision, if sinus occlusion has caused papilledema, until collateral channels open up sufficiently to drain blood from the brain. Clots have been successfully removed from the superior sagittal sinus, and both sinus thrombectomy and ligation of the jugular vein after transverse sinus thrombosis have long been standard procedures. Complicating brain abscess usually requires appropriate surgical measures. Drainage of a subdural hygroma in a patient of mine with cavernous sinus thrombosis was apparently lifesaving.

PROGNOSIS

It is difficult to appraise the prognosis in intracranial venous and venous sinus disease, now that vigorous use of antibiotics, anticoagulants and early intelligent management of increased pressure in the cranial chamber are becoming standard procedures. Many, if not all, of the foregoing syndromes had a high mortality in the preantibiotic era; cavernous sinus thrombosis, for one, was invariably fatal. There have now been numerous reports of successful treatment of cavernous sinus thrombosis, and the death rate in all varieties of intracranial phlebothrombosis and phlebitis has been reduced to at most one-third the older figures. The incidence of these disorders as complications of common infections, par-

ticularly of the soft tissues and bones of the head, has likewise been
decreased tremendously by early antibacterial therapy.

BIBLIOGRAPHY

Bailey, O. T., and Hass, G. M.: Dural sinus thrombosis in early life: Recovery from acute
thrombosis of the superior longitudinal sinus and its relation to certain acquired lesions
in childhood, Brain 60:293-314, 1937.
Bailey, P.: Peculiarities of the intracranial venous system and their clinical significance,
Arch. Neurol. & Psychiat. 32:1105, 1934.
Bucy, P. C., and Lesemann, F. J.: Idiopathic recurrent thrombophlebitis with cerebral
venous thrombosis and an acute subdural hematoma, J.A.M.A. 119:402-405, 1942.
Gius, J. A., and Grier, D. H.: Venous adaptation following bilateral radical neck dissec-
tion with excision of the jugular veins, Surgery 28:305-321, 1950.
Gurhkelch, A. N.: Subdural effusions in infancy, Brit. M.J. 1:233-239, 1953.
Hyland, H. H.: Intracranial venous thrombosis in the puerperium, J.A.M.A. 142:707-
710, 1950.
Innersfield, J.; Schwarz, A., and Angrist, A.: Intravenous trypsin: Its anticoagulant,
fibrinolytic and thrombolytic effects, J. Clin. Invest. 31:1049-1055, 1952.
Keschner, M., and Davison, C.: Otitic thrombosis of cerebral sinuses and veins simulating
multiple brain tumors, Arch. Neurol. & Psychiat. 47:428-437, 1942.
Mitchell, R. G.: Venous thrombosis in acute infantile hemiplegia, Arch. Dis. Childhood
27:95-104, 1952.
Ray, B. S.; Dunbar, H. S., and Dotter, C. T.: Dural sinus venography as an aid to diag-
nosis in intracranial disease, J. Neurosurg. 8:23-37, 1951.
Rose, L. B.: Obstruction of the superior vena cava of 25 years' duration, J.A.M.A. 150:
1198-1200, 1952.
Smith, J. C.: Primary cerebral thrombophlebitis, J.A.M.A. 148:613-616, 1952.
Tobey, G. L., and Ayer, J. B.: Dynamic studies on the cerebrospinal fluid in the differ-
ential diagnosis of lateral sinus thrombosis, Arch. Otolaryng. 2:50-57, 1925.
Wright, I. S.: Vascular Diseases in Clinical Practice (2d ed.; Chicago: The Year Book
Publishers, Inc., 1952).
Walsh, F. B.: Clinical Neuro-ophthalmology (Baltimore: Williams & Wilkins Com-
pany, 1947).
Woodhall, B.: Variations of the cranial venous sinuses in the region of the torcular
Herophilii, Arch. Surg. 33:287-314, 1936.

CHAPTER 14

Hypertensive Brain Disease

THE MAGNITUDE of the problem of arterial hypertension and associated disease of the brain, heart and kidneys is truly immense; over 4,500,000 persons in the United States alone have high blood pressure, arteriosclerosis or both. Virtually every case of severe and protracted hypertension is complicated by cerebral involvement, and high blood pressure may attack the brain at any age. Although heart and kidney failure account for the majority of deaths from hypertension, approximately 25 per cent of patients die of cerebral hemorrhage or major cerebral infarction, and many more are stricken neurologically before a cardiac or renal death.

ETIOLOGY; PATHOGENESIS

The arterial blood pressure is a product of the cardiac output and peripheral resistance, largely in the arterioles. Hypertensive disease is a pathologic condition in which an unknown pressor mechanism initiates arteriolar vasoconstriction, elevates the blood pressure and produces vascular sequelae.

PSYCHIC FACTORS.—The effect of the stress syndrome in producing hypertension is an elusive factor which has evaded accurate evaluation. Yet it is a matter of common observation that the hypertensive patient is frequently tense, nervous and worrisome and often operates under the same "high pressure" as does his arterial circulation. Stimulation of the frontal lobes and hypothalamus experimentally will raise the blood pressure acutely, and irreversible hydrocephalus in animals will elevate arterial tension chronically. Psychiatrists find traits of obsessive-compulsive makeup in patients with elevated blood pressure.

RENAL DISEASE.—Most attempts to reproduce human hypertensive disease in laboratory animals have concerned the kidney, because of the frequent association of hypertension with renal disease. Goldblatt by

275

partial occlusion of the renal arteries of dogs produced sustained high blood pressure, arteriolar and cardiac lesions in animals which survived for long periods. Modifications of this original technic include the adding or substituting of ureteral ligation, renal encapsulation and systemic injection of tissue extracts. It is probable that none of these studies relates to essential hypertension in man, since experimentally elevated pressure after renal damage does not respond to chemical sympathicolysis and renin is not increased in the outflow of the renal vein. They may apply, however, to the hypertension of clinical kidney disease.

The assumption has been made that renal changes cause essential hypertensive disease by liberation of vasopressor substances from the kidney. Page's investigations of humoral relations in the hypertensive state implicate the interaction of a renal pseudoglobulin, "renin," with a hepatic pseudoglobulin, "preangiotonin," the result being an active vasopressor substance, "angiotonin." The possibility of the elaboration of renin or of like substances after excessive sympathetic nervous discharge is suggested in the finding by Trueta and associates of renal ischemia when the splanchnic nerve is stimulated either directly or reflexly.

ENDOCRINE FACTORS.—Glandular secretions may play an as yet inestimable part in human hypertensive disease by their elaboration in physiologic or pathologic amounts. Cushing became interested in the possible role of the anterior pituitary after his observations of the frequency of hypertension in acromegaly and in pituitary basophilism, one type of Cushing's syndrome. A striking reduction of pathologically elevated blood pressure in a few patients with Cushing's syndrome has followed x-ray therapy directed toward the hypophysis. During ACTH therapy, hypertensive states may be precipitated or aggravated. Although Pitressin, a product of the posterior neurohypophysis, will elevate the blood pressure of animals acutely, its possible contribution to human hypertension has been questioned.

The adrenal directly or as a result of pituitary activation may also be a cause of, or maintain, hypertension by release of hormones from the cortex or medulla. The type of Cushing's syndrome associated with cortical hyperplasia or tumor produces high blood pressure, as does administration of the adrenal steroid, cortisone. Pheochromocytoma causes severe, labile hypertension, and hypertension may be a symptom of thyrotoxicosis. The brain has been found to elaborate a hormone-like vasopressor substance (Taylor et al.).

CLINICAL HYPERTENSIVE DISEASES.—At least 50 pathologic conditions are associated with elevated blood pressure. Most of the patients are included in the diagnostic category of *essential hypertension,* the etiology of which is unknown although a hereditary predisposition is often present. High blood pressure is frequently a manifestation of primary or secondary *kidney disease* other than nephrosis, neoplasm and renal tuberculosis. Additional, fairly common hypertensive states are eclampsia and other toxemias of pregnancy, increased intracranial pressure, coarctation of the aorta, lead poisoning, acute poliomyelitis and paraplegia.

In *eclampsia* the hypertensive and cerebral changes resemble those of acute nephritis or malignant nephrosclerosis. Vasospasm may cause brain softening without thrombosis (Holmberg), and cerebral hemorrhages occur in 15–20 per cent of eclamptic patients who die (Eller). The relationship of *increased intracranial pressure* to hypertension is not obvious. Epidural or subdural hematomas are often accompanied by greatly elevated systolic and diastolic tension, but a massive glioma of equal size may not produce any pressure changes. Compression of the brain stem by herniations through the tentorium and foramen magnum are probably responsible for the appearance of hypertension, which is usually the consequence of only an acute increase in intracranial pressure.

Coarctation of the aorta should always be suspected when high blood pressure is found in a young person. *Lead* in toxic quantities poisons the endothelium of capillaries and arterioles throughout the body and also raises blood pressure by injury to the kidney; thickening of the cerebral leptomeninges and severe brain edema occur in children. The acute high blood pressure of bulbar *poliomyelitis* indicates inflammation of central vasoregulatory nuclei. Paroxysmal hypertension is common in *paraplegia* when distension of the bladder or bowel causes reflex vasoconstriction in the lower half of the body.

PATHOLOGY

The pathologic state of the hypertensive brain varies with the stage of the disease and the degree of accompanying arterial degeneration. Grossly, the brain is a pale, edematous, bloodless sponge in hypertensive encephalopathy. Increased intracranial pressure flattens surface veins, and inexpansibility of the cranium forces the cerebellar tonsils down below the foramen magnum. The arterial input is cut off passively by edema, and the brain on cut section is white in color and drips fluid.

Scheinker attributes hypertensive cerebral edema to paralysis of small vessels following acute vasomotor disturbances. Volhard explained brain swelling in hypertensive crisis as a response to vascular injury, and Pal believed the fundamental reaction was cerebral vasoconstriction. The weight of the brain, especially in children, may increase 20–30 per cent.

Major vasospastic episodes involving chiefly the middle cerebral and internal carotid arteries leave large areas in the cerebrum which are of jelly-like translucency; almost the whole of one hemisphere may be affected. Investigation of the arteries supplying such ischemic zones often discloses narrowing without occlusion. Multiple, tiny, cystic or brown discolored foci on the cut surface of the brain indicate smaller infarctions, old or new; if the latter, red dots are seen.

Microscopically, ball, ring and spot hemorrhages and fields of necrobiosis appear anywhere in the brain. Arterioles are thick and hyalinized,

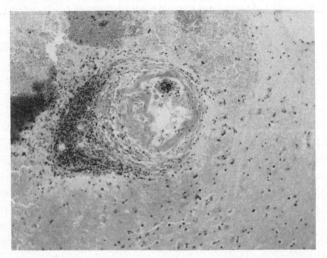

FIG. 101.—Arteriolar necrosis with perivascular hemorrhage. Malignant hypertension.

with reduced lumens (Fig. 101). Small infarcts are numerous. Arteriolar necrosis is unusual but occurs in malignant hypertension; in a very rare case, mitoses of small vascular endothelial cells may be found. Perivascular spaces are widened, owing to edema, and cystic foci are bridged by strands of glia which has proliferated in response to ischemic injury. Spielmeyer considered vasospasm to be the cause of microscopic necrobiotic areas since he could not detect occluded vessels. Rosenberg believed that true arteriolar thrombosis is more frequently responsible for infarction.

SYMPTOMS AND SIGNS

HYPERTENSIVE DISEASE.—Headache is a common complaint. It is usually vertex or occipital in location and comes on in the early morning hours or with excitement. Once started it tends to recur daily and becomes increasingly severe during the progress of the disease. It is of extracranial, not intracranial, origin and resembles histamine cephalalgia. Headache may appear when blood pressure is especially low (early morning) as well as during or preceding a hypertensive crisis. The common factors are relative vascular relaxation followed by acute distention.

Nervousness, irritability and neurasthenic fatigability are common symptoms. A vicious circle exists, increased pressure making the patient more nervous and irritated, which in turn raises arterial tension still higher. Accompanying this reaction is a degree of mental confusion not obvious to the patient or even to others, but recognizable by its absence when hypertension has been controlled. Insomnia may be troublesome, largely owing to the inability to relax. The syndrome of change in the expression of hostility, a new willingness to yield to dependent needs, reduction in perfectionism and anxiety as a response of the organism to brain damage has been said to indicate cerebral decompensation even before the appearance of neurologic signs (Apter and Halstead).

Visual system.—Ocular findings are particularly important prognostically and as an indication for specific therapy. Keith and associates have grouped hypertensive patients into four categories, according to the appearance of the retinal vessels and optic nerves. Group 1 consists of patients in whom mild narrowing and sclerosis of retinal arterioles is present. In group 2, vascular changes are somewhat more advanced with definite arteriovenous "nicking" and increase of the light reflex. Group 3 patients have severe hypertension and diffuse arteriolar changes. Small retinal arteries may be completely obstructed or locally narrowed, and flame-shaped hemorrhages and fluffy exudates are present in the retina. In group 4 or malignant cases, papilledema is added to the pathologic alterations of group 3, and the retina is often edematous as well. Ophthalmoscopic signs correlate closely with the outlook for survival.

Retinal angiospastic changes may be clearly visible during a hypertensive crisis and can cause temporary or permanent blindness, complete or partial. Distinction between the acute papilledema of malignant nephrosclerosis and that of intracranial tumor is often difficult, and bilateral nerve head sclerosis is left as a residuum in both conditions when papilledema subsides. Visual loss may result not only from lesions in the eye but also from temporary constriction of the middle or posterior cerebral arteries.

HYPERTENSIVE CRISIS.—Acute hypertensive edema of the brain is most common in malignant nephrosclerosis but is also seen with glomerulonephritis, eclampsia and lead poisoning. Patients are often under age

40. Prodromes include paroxysmal rise in blood pressure, severe headache, apathy, weakness, paresthesias and extreme anxiety and restlessness. Vomiting, torpor and convulsive seizures appear as the patient passes into a state of coma. The Babinski and Kernig reflexes, stiffness of the neck (cerebellar tonsillar herniation), high cerebrospinal fluid pressure and a slow pulse form a picture suggestive of brain tumor.

Heart failure, Cheyne-Stokes respiration, paroxysmal dyspnea and pulmonary edema may terminate a crisis. Psychosis may result. Osler commented on transient monoplegia and hemiplegia in hypertensive encephalopathy, comparing the attacks to cerebral vasospastic events in Raynaud's disease. Visual phenomena, objective and subjective, are common and papilledema, retinal hemorrhages and vascular spasms can be of very rapid onset.

Hypertensive cerebral attacks without edema (McAlpine) tend to occur in group 3 patients 40–65 years of age. These patients have had hypertension of long standing, and many already reveal chronic neurologic signs. Severe headache is followed by convulsions and coma. The cerebrospinal fluid pressure is normal or nearly so. Recovery is usual, although the process, which is undoubtedly angiospastic in nature, may proceed to infarction or hemorrhage.

LABORATORY STUDIES

Anemia, sometimes of a severe degree, may be revealed. Urinary findings correspond to the stage of nephrosclerosis or nephritic involvement, as do blood chemistry values. The blood pressure is always elevated above normal, sometimes to a level unrecordable on the ordinary mercury or aneroid manometer, during or just at the onset of a vascular crisis.

The cerebrospinal fluid is normal unless a complication such as uremia, heart failure or major stroke exists or the malignant phase of the disease has developed. In malignant hypertension cerebrospinal fluid pressure is elevated, sometimes up to 400 mm. of water, the protein content is often increased, and the colloidal gold curve may be midzone in type.

X-rays of the skull are not altered by hypertension as such. Pituitary tumors should be looked for. Chest films display enlargement of the heart to the left and possibly congestion of the lung fields; coarctation of the aorta may be present in a young patient. Air encephalography or ventriculography discloses small ventricles and sparse subarachnoid spaces in the absence of cerebral infarction or hemorrhage, unless long-standing intrinsic vascular disease has produced brain atrophy similar to that resulting from arteriosclerosis. Arteriography outlines narrowed vessels, often altered by associated atheromatous change. However, angiograms may appear relatively normal.

The electroencephalogram of the hypertensive brain is not diagnostic of the condition and is often unremarkable unless stroke has occurred. Sometimes, however, a combination of slightly but abnormally slow and fast waves may be seen, and voltage increase may produce an irregularly choppy and spiky record (Fig. 102). The principal value of the electroencephalogram in hypertension is to assist in ruling out a complication or

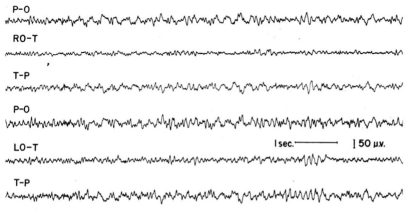

FIG. 102.—Hypertensive cerebrovascular disease. Irregular, spiky record, combination of slow and fast frequencies in the electroencephalogram.

another pathologic process. Electroencephalographic changes in eclampsia are restricted to the period of status eclampticus, during which they resemble epileptic abnormalities.

DIAGNOSIS

Elevation of the blood pressure is the *sine qua non* in making the diagnosis of hypertensive brain disease. The blood pressure is usually but not necessarily sustained at high levels on repeated examinations, and cerebral involvement is ordinarily not present when the systolic and diastolic tensions are not well above the 150/90 limits of normal. A history of kidney disease and evidences of cardiac enlargement or decompensation, renal malfunction and serum chemistry changes support the diagnosis.

There is no uniquely peculiar neurologic syndrome, even in hypertensive encephalopathy, and diagnosis by exclusion must often be relied on in questionable circumstances. Transience of neurologic phenomena such as blindness, hemianopsia, monoplegia, hemiplegia, convulsions and coma suggests a vasospastic etiology. Inspection of the eyegrounds is particularly important. Telltale evidences of severe arteriolar disease, silver-wire vessels, prominent arteriovenous nicking, angiospasm, flame-shaped hemorrhages and exudates, chorioretinopathy, papilledema and edema of the retina may establish the diagnosis of hypertensive encephalopathy as in no other way.

DIFFERENTIAL DIAGNOSIS.—Studies of the urine and blood chemistry indicate or exclude *uremia*. Other metabolic conditions, such as *diabetes,* and drug or metal *poisoning* are detected by a careful history and laboratory analyses. *Coarctation* of the aorta is often visible in a plain x-ray of the chest, when notching of the ribs is also visible. The systolic blood pressure in the legs is usually below 90 mm. of mercury.

Adrenal cortical tumors or hyperplasia results in increased excretion of 17-ketosteroids, and the features of Cushing's syndrome are present in addition to hypertension. *Acromegaly* stigmatizes the patient whose high blood pressure is associated with an acidophil pituitary adenoma, and the sella turcica is enlarged. *Pheochromocytoma* manifests itself in attacks of extremely high arterial pressure, pallor, sweating, angina and "dead" fingers and toes. Histamine or Regitine test results may be positive.

The differentiation of *metastatic* malignancy or *primary* intracranial *tumor* from hypertensive brain disease may be most difficult on clinical grounds alone. Signs of increased intracranial pressure, including papilledema, are often present in equal degree or may be absent in both neoplastic and vascular conditions. Because a person has high blood pressure does not mean that he does not also have a tumor; however, pronounced hypertension results from neoplasm of the brain is only the rarest of instances. The cerebrospinal fluid protein content and gold curve are usually normal in hypertension, unless in the malignant phase, even if the lumbar fluid pressure is high. Electroencephalography is helpful, and serial records aid in observation of the patient. In case of serious doubt, ventriculography or angiography must be undertaken, remembering on the one hand that multiple metastases may not deform the ventricular system and, on the other, that a vasospastic hypertensive patient may not tolerate Diodrast injection. If gross impairment of renal function is evident, the cerebral syndrome is probably due to hypertensive disease and not to brain tumor.

Subdural hematoma is usually eliminated or discovered through cranial trephination, a safe and simple procedure. *Cerebral vasospasm, thrombosis* and *hemorrhage* are discussed at length in other chapters.

TREATMENT

Hypertensive Encephalopathy

Hypertensive encephalopathy is a potentially lethal crisis which demands emergency treatment. Immediate aims are the lowering of the mounting blood pressure, prevention of heart failure, reduction of increased intracranial pressure and control of convulsions. Venesection (400–500 cc.) may not only ease the cardiac strain but can also result in control of seizures.

Hypertonic solutions administered intravenously decrease cerebral edema. Magnesium sulfate is particularly effective as an analeptic and in reducing intracranial pressure. In children it is given as a 25 per cent solution, intramuscularly, in dosage of 0.2–0.4 cc. per kilogram and in adults may be used in 20 cc. amounts of 10 per cent solution, intravenously, every two hours as required (Fishberg). Calcium gluconate is indicated as an antagonist to magnesium if respiratory depression results. Spinal puncture offers only temporary benefit and may be dangerous (cerebellar pressure cone). If no other measure relieves high intracranial tension and papilledema progresses, subtemporal decompression is in order.

The careful and intelligent parenteral use of chemical sympathicolytic drugs such as hexamethonium and Apresoline may well replace the emergency methods of treatment just outlined. The treatment of hypertensive encephalopathy must be individualized.

Medical Management of Hypertension

The fundamental therapy of the underlying disease process is medical control. The low sodium diet is recommended almost universally and has largely replaced the rice-fruit dietary regime. Thiocyanates have had a recurrent vogue; it is difficult to maintain the optimal level of 6–12 mg. per 100 cc. of serum and to avoid toxic effects. Priscoline may succeed in lowering the blood pressure in hypertensive crisis, and Veratrum viride or protoveratrine may be useful in patients with persistent diastolic hypertension. Hydrogenated ergot alkaloids (Hydergine) and rauwolfia prove effective for sympatholysis in selected cases. Psychotherapy is indicated when anxiety-tension states exist.

Hexamethonium, Apresoline.—The most consistently effective sympathicolytic agents which will reduce blood pressure and relieve angiospastic phenomena, cerebral and otherwise, are hexamethonium (C6;

Bistrium) and Apresoline (hydrazinophthalazine). Both drugs act to produce sympathetic blockade, either at the ganglionic or central medullary levels, and have the particular advantage of total effect. Malignant hypertension is especially responsive to chemical sympathicolysis. Cerebral vascular resistance is lowered by Apresoline without reduction of cerebral blood flow; Kleh and Fazekas observed a decided clearing of mental confusion in elderly hypertensive patients treated with this medication. Hexamethonium, on the other hand, seems to have an effect exactly opposite. Whereas vasospasm may be relieved by sympathicolysis, cerebral, coronary or other thrombosis may be precipitated by too sudden or severe a drop of systemic blood pressure. Errors to avoid are giving too large doses of these drugs initially and administration of ineffectually small amounts too late in the course of hypertensive disease. Clinical reactions resembling rheumatoid arthritis and lupus erythematosus may appear when Apresoline is given over long periods (Dustan *et al.*).

Symptomatic therapy.—Hypertensive headache, which usually comes on during the early morning hours, may be relieved by elevating the head of the bed 12 in. Procaine block of the occipital nerves can relieve pain for short periods; occipital neurectomy is rarely of benefit. Ergotamine preparations are contraindicated in the presence of severe organic vascular disease. Intravenous injection of aminophylline, thiocyanate or caffeine sodium benzoate in 0.5 Gm. amounts may afford miraculous, though temporary, benefit.

Anxiety may be alleviated by small doses of phenobarbital or other mild sedatives. Hemorrhagic phenomena are indications for the administration of ascorbic acid and rutin, a flavonol glycoside.

SURGICAL THERAPY

Sympathectomy.—It is difficult to predict the future role of surgical sympathectomy in the treatment of hypertension and hypertensive brain disease in view of the apparent success of chemical sympathicolysis. Before the introduction of hexamethonium and Apresoline, surgical sympathectomy was indicated in patients whose disease did not respond to adequate medical therapy, in malignant hypertension, in chronic refractory hypertensive heart failure and for relief of intractable headache or other incapacitating symptoms. If medical sympathicolysis proves to be effective over a period of years, there will still be occasional cases which will not prove favorable for sympathicolytic treatment and which should be treated surgically.

The most effective type of operation is bilateral removal of the ninth to the twelfth thoracic sympathetic ganglions and the first and second lumbar ganglions, with resection of all splanchnic nerves, major and minor. Two separate procedures are most feasible. Contraindications are patient age above 50–55, cerebrovascular accident or coronary occlusion within the preceding three months and inadequate renal function. Smithwick's long term experience is that the prognosis of patients with hypertensive cardiovascular disease in all stages is significantly improved by thoracolumbar sympathectomy. Fifty of 58 patients treated surgically by Peet and who had had cerebrovascular accidents before operation were free from further intracranial episodes during a five to 10 year follow-up. Cerebrovascular resistance decreases an average of 18 per cent after bilateral thoracolumbar sympathectomy (Shenkin et al.).

Adrenalectomy.—Total or, preferably, subtotal adrenalectomy has been undertaken in many patients with progressive hypertension, usually during removal of the sympathetic ganglions. Near lethal malignant hypertension has been controlled for short periods by this extreme measure, but many patients so treated have lapsed into Addison's disease despite the administration of adrenal hormones postoperatively. Long term results are about the same as those obtained by bilateral thoracolumbar sympathectomy (Jeffers et al.).

Nephrectomy.—Rarely, in a patient with malignant hypertension in childhood or youth, pyelographic studies may reveal a severely diseased kidney. Nephrectomy may be remarkably successful in reducing blood pressure to normal limits, provided the other kidney is not irreparably affected.

PROGNOSIS

Severe hypertension is of more serious import in young patients than in old and is more dangerous in men than in women. Twenty-five per cent of hypertensive individuals die of cerebral hemorrhage or major cerebral infarct. Cerebrovascular accidents tend to be repeated, and the prognosis is grave in hypertensive encephalopathy. The mortality from hypertensive disease during a five to 10 year period varies from 37.6 per cent in group 1 cases (Keith et al.) to 99.5 per cent in group 4 (Smithwick). These prognostic data are improved considerably by chemical sympatholysis or surgical sympathectomy.

BIBLIOGRAPHY

Apter, N. S., and Halstead, W. C.: Psychiatric manifestations of early cerebral damage in essential hypertension, M. Clin. North America 35:133-142, 1951.

Dustan, H. P., et al.: Rheumatic and febrile syndrome during prolonged hydralazine treatment, J.A.M.A. 154:23-29, 1954.

Eller, W. C.: Cerebrovascular complications of pregnancy, Am. J. Obst. & Gynec. 52:488-491, 1946.

Fishberg, A. M.: Hypertension and Nephritis (Philadelphia: Lea & Febiger, 1939).

Goldblatt, H., et al.: Studies on experimental hypertension: I. Production of persistent elevation of systolic blood pressure by means of renal ischemia, J. Exper. Med. 59:347-379, 1934.

Holmberg, G.: Extensive encephalomalacia after toxemia of pregnancy, Acta psychiat. et neurol. 24:175-198, 1949.

Jeffers, W. A., et al.: Evaluation of adrenal resection and sympathectomy in 99 persons with hypertension, J.A.M.A. 153:1502-1505, 1953.

Keith, N. M.; Wagener, H. P., and Barker, N. W.: Some different types of essential hypertension: Their course and prognosis, Am. J. M. Sc. 197:332-343, 1939.

Kleh, J., and Fazekas, J. F.: The use of Apresoline in the hypertensive arteriosclerotic syndrome, Am. J. M. Sc. 227:57-64, 1954.

McAlpine, D.: Hypertensive cerebral attack, Quart. J. Med. 2:463-481, 1933.

Page, I. H.: Disorders of the Circulatory System (New York: The Macmillan Company, 1952).

Peet, M. M.: Hypertension and its surgical treatment by bilateral supradiaphragmatic splanchnicectomy, Am. J. Surg. 75:48-68, 1948.

Rosenberg, E. F.: The brain in malignant hypertension, Arch. Int. Med. 65:545-586, 1940.

Scheinker, I. M.: Hypertensive cerebral swelling: Characteristic clinicopathologic syndrome, Ann. Int. Med. 28:630-641, 1948.

Shenkin, H. A.: Hafkenschiel, J. H., and Kety, S. S.: Effects of sympathectomy on the cerebral circulation of hypertensive patients, Arch. Surg. 61:319-324, 1950.

Smithwick, R. H.: Hypertensive cardiovascular disease: Effect of thoracolumbar splanchnicectomy on mortality and survival rates, J.A.M.A. 147:1611-1615, 1951.

Spielmeyer, W.: Vasomotorisch trophische Veranderunger bei zerebraler arteriosklerose, Monatsschr. Psychiat. u. Neurol. 68:605-620, 1928.

Taylor, R. D.; Page, I. H., and Corcoran, A. C.: Hormonal neurogenic vasopressor mechanism, A.M.A. Arch. Int. Med. 88:1-8, 1951.

Trueta, J., et al.: Studies of the Renal Circulation (Oxford: Blackwell Scientific Publications, 1947).

CHAPTER 15

Cerebral Arteriosclerosis

THE HUMAN BODY is a machine which must wear out, eventually, and susceptibility of the brain to the effects of progressive, degenerative changes in its vessels is a common cause of morbidity and of death in the elderly. The influence of the ravages of cerebral arteriosclerosis on human activity and the course of history is incalculable. On the other hand, brain- and mind-crippling from sclerosis of arteries is not necessarily an inevitable consequence of aging; in many older persons intracranial vessels, although tortuous due to atrophic loss of elastica and muscularis, are open and are patent throughout, and the person remains intelligent and productive to the end. The treasures of wisdom and experience need not always be sacrificed to the deterioration of senility. Studies of cerebral blood flow in aged patients reveal a high percentage of normal values.

The problem of arteriosclerosis is of first-rank prominence in medicine. At least 25,000,000 persons in the United States are over 50 years of age at present; of these, 60 per cent or 15,000,000 will die of cardiovasculorenal disease compared with a predictable 9 per cent mortality from cancer. A large portion of the 60 per cent will succumb to the results of degenerative arterial processes. Over 4,500,000 already suffer from arteriosclerosis or hypertension.

Involvement of the brain in sclerosing changes may be local or general and may be insignificant or dominant compared with implication of other viscera. Seventy-five per cent of brains examined in unselected autopsy series reveal arteriosclerosis to a quantitative degree.

ETIOLOGY; PATHOGENESIS

It is a seeming paradox that the causes of the commonest diseases are the most obscure, and arteriosclerosis is no exception. Two principal theories have been advanced to account for the deposition of atheroma in the walls of vessels and replacement of elastic and muscle tissue by fibrosis, the chief pathologic changes in hardening of arteries.

1. Winternitz' explanation of the pathogenesis of arteriosclerosis is based on a concept of the proliferation of small vessels (vasa vasorum) intramurally as part of an exudative-fibrosing reaction to an exogenous (infectious?) or endogenous (chemical) factor as yet undiscovered. The frequency of subintimal or intramedial hemorrhages in advanced sclerosis supports this contention. Cholesterol plaque formation is explained as a residue of laked erythrocytes. Thrombosis is thought to occur on intimal areas denuded of endothelium by an inflammatory reaction.

2. The dietary theory, long championed by Leary, is of special current interest and debate. According to this hypothesis, the arterial intima is invaded by waves of macrophages carrying crystalline esters of cholesterol, which is present in the plasma in unusually high concentration because of excessive intake of fatty foods or malfunction of endogenous cholesterol-regulating mechanisms. Deposited crystals stimulate the growth of fibrous connective tissue, which thickens the wall of the vessel, strangles its blood supply and narrows the lumen.

Proponents of the dietary explanation of atherosclerosis note that the disease is a common complication of diabetes mellitus, thyroid deficiency and xanthoma tuberosum, conditions in which serum lipid values are elevated. The incidence of arterial involvement is said to decrease in populations subjected to starvation. Tendencies to premature sclerosis are often hereditary. The S_f lipoproteins of the 12–100 class are said to be increased pathologically in patients with coronary artery disease and are reduced in the S_f 35–100 band after weight loss (Gofman and Jones).

Calcific change is considered to be an end stage of saponification of fat deposits no matter how the latter appear. Hormonal influences undoubtedly play a large part in the pathogenesis of arteriosclerosis; susceptibility to the disease is greater in men than in women.

Arteriosclerosis in infancy.—That atherosclerosis is to some extent a "physiologic" change is indicated in the observation that the process which closes off the ductus arteriosus and begins during fetal life is indistinguishable, grossly and microscopically, from sclerosing alterations which characteristically appear in major arteries in later life. Focal calcification and thromboses have been found in the media of coronary vessels in babies, and Altschul discovered cerebral endarteritis obliterans in an infant.

Susceptibility of arteries of the brain.—Development of arteriosclerosis in cerebral arteries is prone to take place at the angles of branching of the vessels, according to Tuthill, because of splitting of elastic and collagen fibers in these areas which predisposes to the absorption of fat. The principal susceptibility of the intracranial arterial system, especially of its small vessels, is to thickening of an already peculiarly well developed internal elastic membrane and further fibroplasia in a constitutionally fibrous media. What would be considered arterial fibrosis elsewhere in the body may be normal in the vessels of the brain.

PATHOLOGY

ARTERIES.—Several types of sclerosing change affect the intracranial arteries. The end stages of atherosclerosis are most familiarly seen grossly in the sinuous, opacified, beaded and pipestem *large* arteries of the circle of Willis and cortex of an aged person. The vessels are stiff and inexpansile and are flecked with yellow; tortuosity and rigidity change their course so that adjacent nerves may be compressed. Small branches are pulled taut from the parent artery on one side and are redundant on the other (Fig. 42). Subintimal deposition of lipids narrows or occludes the arterial lumens, as do intramural hemorrhages and calcific plaques. Destruction of endothelium by pressure atrophy or by exudation results in thrombosis. Degeneration of muscle and elastica leads to fibrous alteration in the media. Vasa vasorum proliferate in the wall. Plaques perforate the media and may open up pathways for arterial rupture. Atherosclerosis is primarily a focal disease, affecting chiefly the angles of branching of the larger vessels at the base of the brain.

Mönckeberg's sclerosis affects *large* and *medium* arteries; the basilar trunk often shows this type of change. Replacement of degenerating media with rings of calcium limits the vessel in expanding, although intimal integrity prevents thrombosis.

Endarteritis obliterans is a fibrosing, hyalinizing, occlusive process, not properly inflammatory, without atheroma or calcium deposition, seen in *small* arteries. It is the vascular substrate of Binswanger's progressive subcortical encephalopathy, a condition in which progressive obstruction of longer subcortical vessels produces slow disintegration of projection fibers, especially in temporal and occipital lobes, with preservation of the cortex.

In diffuse, hyperplastic sclerosis the subintimal tissue of *arterioles* thickens and becomes hyaline, particularly in the hypertensive state, and the altered arteriolar walls are found to be calcific, as an end stage, in arteriosclerotic parkinsonism. *Capillary* sclerosis occurs in Sturge-Weber disease when the cortical and immediately subcortical small vessels are involved to the point of calcification. I have seen similar capillary calcification in the hypothalamus of patients dying suddenly of catatonic schizophrenia.

GROSS PATHOLOGY.—The cerebral consequences of impairment of blood flow resulting from arteriosclerosis in its various forms may be diffuse or focal and may range from multiple microscopic areas of necrobiosis in the cortex to massive hemispheral necrosis. Grossly, the gyri of

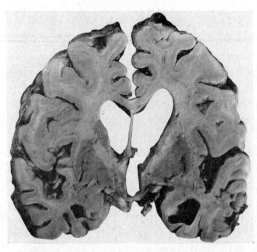

FIG. 103.—Brain atrophy due to arteriosclerosis. (AFIP #AMH 11261A.)

the arteriosclerotic brain are shrunken, alternatingly hardened and softened, and the whole organ appears old (Fig. 103). Widened subarachnoid channels and lakes are covered by a milky arachnoid membrane which partially conceals the cholesterol-studded, rigid, angulated arteries. Here and there yellow-brown areas, palpably soft, are effects of recent minor superficial infarction. On section, the ventricular system is enlarged due to the tissue contraction of gliosis (hydrocephalus ex vacuo) and is full of fluid. Cystic remnants of ancient interior infarcts and tiny round or oval necrotic foci of pea or bean size are prevalent in the basal ganglions, internal capsule, thalamus and brain stem, particularly the pons. Shrinkage of parenchyma from vessels gives the subcortex a spongy feeling on palpation (*état lacunaire*, Fig. 104). Perforating arteries of the brain stem cannot be injected in postmortem specimens obtained from elderly patients.

Significant arteriosclerotic changes afflict the internal carotid arteries most frequently of major vessels, and after the carotids the basilar and the middle cerebral arteries in that order. Vessels may be found occluded by atherosclerosis without cerebral infarction; sudden hypotension or thrombosis must be superadded to cause death of brain tissue. The degree of anastomotic circulation also determines the extent of parenchymal damage.

MICROSCOPIC CHANGES.—In microscopic preparations, ganglion cells

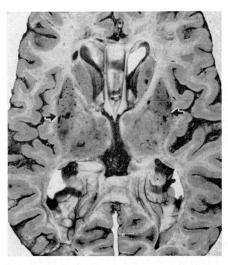

FIG. 104.—*État lacunaire* (arrows) of basal ganglions. (George Washington University Laboratory of Neurology.)

are seen to have undergone lipoid or fatty change or appear dark and contracted with deep-staining nuclei and corkscrew, apical dendrites (chronic cell change). Intraganglionic fibrillary thickening and plaque formation in the ground substance, revealed by silver stains and characteristic of Alzheimer's presenile dementia, are also found not uncommonly in cerebral arteriosclerosis. The cortical ribbon is narrow and depopulated. Relative (condensation) and absolute (growth in response to partial ischemia) increase of all types of glia is seen in the cortex and subcortex. Pale zones of outfall of ganglion cells retaining the ghostlike shadows of necrobiosis are present in any or all cortical areas, and almost always in the Sommer's sector of the cornu Ammonis formation. Spielmeyer considered many of these circumscribed fields of infarction to be the result of vasospasm, since thrombosis was not evident in the feeding vessel, large or small. Simon *et al.* believe that diffuse neuronal degeneration is a senile and not an arteriosclerotic change, and they found this alteration to be predominant in the brains of elderly psychotics. Particularly in the white matter, *état lacunaire* is evident in the enlargement of the perivascular spaces of His and Virchow-Robin, where hematogenous and glial phagocytes are found, many containing the iron from the nuclei of dead neurons. Hyalinized small vessels dot the microscopic fields of basal and brain stem nuclei, especially the former, in which ganglion cell decrease and glial preponderance resemble cortical alterations.

PATHOPHYSIOLOGY.—Studies by Fazekas *et al.* indicate that cerebrovascular resistance is increased and cerebral blood flow reduced in the average elderly person with cerebral arteriosclerosis. These signs of impairment in the efficiency of circulatory channels are more severe in the presence of neurologic involvement, such as hemiplegia. However, evaluations of cerebral metabolic rate suggest that depressed cerebral enzyme activity and impaired oxygen availability also contribute to clinical symptomatology. Coincident hypertension reduces cerebral blood flow still further. In general, cerebral blood flow is depressed to some extent after age 50.

The possibility of intermittent claudication of the arteriosclerotic brain should be mentioned. Local neuronal activity, for example in the pyramidal system, should normally increase cerebral blood flow locally. It is conceivable that the metabolic needs of a cerebral area of functional exaltation may outstrip the blood supply, which is unable to keep up with heightened requirements because of sclerotic changes. The result may be temporary loss of function (hemiparesis) until the balance between neuronal activity and proper circulation is restored. Electroencephalographic studies of an arteriosclerotic man in whom sudden hypotension was induced by the administration of pentamethonium iodide revealed a prolonged delay of recovery of consciousness and normal cortical rhythm even after the blood pressure had been restored to adequate levels. A normal control subject recovered completely and rapidly once the blood pressure rose again above a level of 50 mm. Hg (Bromage).

SYMPTOMS AND SIGNS

Cerebral arteriosclerosis is an entity of inexorable progression. Early symptoms resemble those of neurasthenia. Vertex headache, giddiness, fatigue, somnolence and transient weakness or numbness are complained of. These phenomena are often worse in an upright position and are accentuated by heart block or failure. The patient is "no longer himself," is plagued by failing memory, cannot retain impressions, is subject to uncontrollable mood-swings and manifests poor judgment. Temporal vessels become prominent. A combination of increasing pyramidal and extrapyramidal deficit leads to "arteriosclerotic rigidity" (Foerster). The patient is weak and stiff, and the gait is shuffling. Agnosia, apraxia and dysphasia result from brief apoplectiform attacks. Convulsive seizures occur. Severe mental and physical decline are seen in end stages, with character and conduct changes as the patient slips into a vegetative or childish existence. Early syndromes resemble those of cerebral anoxia, acute or chronic; late in the course, the arteriosclerotic patient is often hard to distinguish clinically from a patient with general paresis.

NEUROLOGIC FINDINGS.—Almost any neurologic sign may be evident, but the physician should recall the normal presence of minor neurologic deficits in the elderly patient. The pupils are usually small and tonic; there may be ptosis of the eyelids. Patches of numbness on the face are found when complaints of tinnitus and vertigo resemble those of Ménière's syndrome. Hearing is often deficient. A nasal type of voice, if present, is associated with a sluggish gag reflex. Gait and station are stiff, uncertain and weak. The Romberg sign is often present. An increase in muscle tonus and rigidity are palpable in manipulation of the extremities, and the cogwheel and clasp knife phenomena are evident on passive flexion of elbow or knee when extrapyramidal disease is prominent.

Increased deep tendon jerks and pathologic reflexes (Hoffmann, Babinski) indicate pyramidal tract involvement. Muscular atrophy, hypotonia, depressed or absent deep reflexes may be the result of accompanying arteriosclerotic disease of the lower brain stem and spinal cord, and fibrillations also bespeak the slow death of anterior horn motor neurons. Gauntlet or glove and stocking hypoalgesia may manifest sclerosing changes in the peripheral nerves. The loss of vibratory and even of position sense in the lower extremities is almost physiologic in age.

MENTAL STATUS.—Confusion and loss of memory, particularly of retention and recall, are frequently apparent in a brief examination of mental status. The patient's inability to speak properly or to understand what is said is evidence of aphasia, and inability to read or write indicates impairment of reception or expression in related spheres of language. One must remember to ask certain questions related to orientation and memory, for successful preservation of ordinary social responses can conceal profound psychic deficiency, when the sclerotic patient resembles "the icing without the cake."

EYE SIGNS.—The fact that the retinal artery is a direct derivative of the internal carotid makes possible the estimation of intracranial arterial change by ophthalmoscopy. Tortuous, irregular and wirelike vessels with increased light reflex and the compression of veins by arteries may be evident and usually indicate parallel cerebral vascular sclerosis. However, Alpers *et al.,* during comparative autopsy examinations, observed that whereas retinal arteriosclerosis indicates the possibility of similar pathologic alteration of the basilar trunk, no conclusions could be drawn concerning the state of the arteries and arterioles of the cerebral cortex or basal ganglions. It is evident from all experience that the correlation between fundic and cerebral arteriosclerotic changes is more significant if positive than if negative. Hickam *et al.* obtained evidences of simultaneous rigidity of retinal and cerebral arteries in arteriosclerosis, finding depressed reactivity of both sets of vessels to physiologic stimuli.

Additional common ocular findings with hardening of the carotid and ophthalmic vessels and compression of the optic nerves or chiasm are optic atrophy and increase in cupping of the papilla due to impairment of the nutrition of the optic nerves, binasal hemianopsia (very rare) due to notching of the chiasm by sclerosed carotids, and altitudinal hemianopsia when the ophthalmic arteries burrow into the overlying optic nerves.

Retinopathy is one of the earliest manifestations of vascular involvement in diabetes. Deep retinal hemorrhages, microaneurysms and yellow exudates lead to a chief complaint of visual impairment.

CRANIAL NERVE PALSIES.—The possibility of compression of other cranial nerves by regional arteries is present in certain vulnerable neurovascular anatomic relations (Sunderland) (Fig. 3). Pressure on the oculomotor nerve may be effected by the carotid, posterior cerebral, posterior communicating and superior cerebellar arteries. The trochlear nerve may be involved by the superior cerebellar artery; the trigeminal nerve, by the superior, middle or inferior cerebellar vessels, the basilar trunk or a persistent carotid-basilar connection. The abducens nerve may be compressed by the cerebellar, basilar or vertebral arteries; the facial and auditory nerves are related intimately to the anterior inferior cerebellar and auditory arteries. The glossopharyngeal, vagus, accessory and hypoglossal nerves are closely neighbored by the cerebellar, basilar and vertebral vessels.

Palsies of the cranial nerves are seen in elderly patients with diabetes and arteriosclerosis; signs usually come on abruptly and eventually subside, leaving residuals. The oculomotor, abducens, optic, auditory, trochlear and trigeminal nerves are usually involved in that order (Grinker and Reich). Dandy believed arteriosclerosis of the anterior inferior cerebellar artery to be a principal cause of tic douloureux; this explanation of the etiology of trigeminal neuralgia is not generally accepted. Arteriosclerosis of the vertebral artery was found to be responsible for paralysis of the palate, vocal cord and tongue in a man, 65, by Anderson and Petch. Buchstein observed elevation of the vagus bundle over a rigid artery in an elderly patient with intractable vomiting.

ARTERIOSCLEROTIC SYNDROMES

Several separate neurologic syndromes of cerebral arteriosclerosis have been described. It should be emphasized that consistency of anatomic changes in these various entities is far from absolute, and distinction among them is largely clinical. In all these conditions there is slow death of nerve cells or fibers surrounding gradually narrowing vessels, and multiple tiny infarcts form the pathologic substrate.

In Binswanger's disease, involvement of long but fine subcortical arteries leads to disintegration of association fibers, particularly in the temporal and occipital lobes. Mental breakdown, uncertain speech and gait and convulsive seizures frequently result. Arteriosclerotic rigidity is the end stage of combined lesions of the internal capsule (pyramidal) and basal ganglion (extrapyramidal) projection systems. Tremors, choreiform movements or other types of uncontrollable motor activity may be prominent reactions. Separation of arteriosclerotic rigidity from Lhermitte and McAlpine's "combined disease" would seem to be largely academic.

ARTERIOSCLEROTIC PARKINSONISM.—Paralysis agitans is a familiar condition appearing in elderly people. It is of gradual or sudden onset and is characterized by rigidity and tremor of the voluntary muscles, often with superadded evidences of pyramidal tract involvement. The face becomes expressionless, the voice low pitched and hurried; the patient is bent forward when erect, often with the head tilted, and is statuesque in immobility. Rigidity flexes the arms slightly and the fingers "roll pills." The gait is uncertain, festinating and propulsive as the patient runs to catch up with his falling-forward center of gravity. The emotional state may resemble that in pseudobulbar disease. Other stigmas of vascular deficiency are present. Behind this hardening façade the mind often remains active and alert.

Distinction between degenerative and arteriosclerotic parkinsonism is made on the basis of earlier onset and greater purity of extrapyramidal signs in the former condition, as well as by a difference of pathologic lesions. The atrophic change in ganglion cells characterizes degeneration, whereas perivascular atrophy and ischemia are present in the arteriosclerotic form. In either case, the brunt of the morbid process in the brain is borne by the globus pallidus of the basal ganglions and the substantia nigra of the mesencephalon, as in other diseases producing Parkinson's syndrome.

These findings do not, however, offer a ready explanation for the clinical picture of paralysis agitans, since experimental investigations thus far have not made very clear the specific functions of the globus pallidus and substantia nigra. Indeed, the closest laboratory approximation of the familiar clinical syndrome has resulted from placing lesions in the mesencephalon and pontile tegmentum of monkeys (Ward *et al.*). Rigidity and tremor may result from release of rhythmic activity from the facilitatory reticular nucleus when supranuclear inhibitory corticobulbar tracts are interrupted. Rigidity may be looked on as tremor "run together," and tremor as rigidity "spread apart." Certain features of Parkinson's disease are being seen in the few patients who recover from the decerebrate state after head injury or evacuation of an intracranial expansile mass.

PSEUDOBULBAR PALSY.—This condition is so named because the causative lesions are not in the cranial nerve nuclei proper but in the divisions of the motor cortical pathways which play upon them, the corticobulbar tracts. Multiple areas of softening involve these tracts bilaterally some place between the cortex and the lower nuclei. The clinical picture in many ways resembles the effect of primary disease of the brain stem in such a process as poliomyelitis.

The voice is nasal, garbled, sparse and is rendered in a hoarse whisper. The jaw hangs partially open and its reflex jerk is increased. The patient drools, and chewing is painfully slow. Swallowing is difficult, the palatal reflex is depressed and death often occurs from aspiration pneumonia. The face is a sad, expressionless mask. Laughing and crying are often uncontrollable and resemble each other in sound and effect. Gait and station are those of parkinsonism with modifications according to the degree of associated pyramidal tract deficit. Hemiplegia is a common complicating disability.

ARTERIOSCLEROTIC PSYCHOSIS.—Factors bearing on the cause of arteriosclerotic and senile psychoses are both organic and psychologic.

Fisher offers the suggestion that some senile psychotic patients suffer from unsuspected occlusion of the cervical carotid arteries. Freyhan *et al.* report increased cerebrovascular resistance and reduced blood flow in patients with arteriosclerotic mental breakdown. Fazekas and co-workers believe that a chronically sluggish state of cerebral enzyme activity adds to impairment of blood flow to reduce cerebral metabolic rate and oxygen uptake still further. From the psychologic point of view, there is little doubt that the ravages of arteriosclerosis, particularly cerebrovascular accident, often precipitate psychosis in older persons already burdened with emotional problems from the inevitable socioeconomic changes in activity and habitat.

The usual time of appearance of arteriosclerotic psychosis is after an apoplectic stroke, major or minor, or other disturbing physical episode. The elderly patient, formerly not noticeably maladjusted, begins to tire easily, becomes dull and loses initiative. Memory fails little by little, at first and largely in the sphere of retention and recall. Emotional instability and clouding of consciousness become apparent. Headaches, dizziness, tinnitus and sleeplessness are frequent complaints; deterioration in personal appearance and tonically small pupils are common signs. Many patients suffer from epileptic and epileptoid syncopal attacks.

LABORATORY STUDIES

The blood count should be checked because anemia, although not necessarily common in elderly people, may be responsible for strokelike episodes in the presence of sclerosed vessels. Urinary findings reflect vascular or nephritic changes in the kidneys. The blood pressure is not elevated by sclerosis; the mean pressure in most patients with clinical signs of cerebral arteriosclerosis is normal although hypertensive disease may be associated.

CEREBROSPINAL FLUID.—Cerebrospinal fluid findings are usually normal unless there is a complication such as stroke, uremia or congestive heart failure. The initial pressure is below 150 mm. and sometimes very low. In only 4 per cent of patients is the cell count above 10 per cu. mm. In 75 per cent of fluid specimens taken from patients without complications the protein content is below 45 mg. per 100 ml. The colloidal gold reaction is usually also normal or only slightly changed.

ROENTGENOLOGY.—X-ray films of the skull may reveal advanced calcification of the intracranial carotid artery (Fig. 105). The pineal gland will sag downward and backward with extreme atrophy of the brain. Calcification in the edge of the tentorium may make the petro-clinoid (Gruber's) ligament visible. Deposition of calcium salts in the walls of basal ganglial arterioles in Parkinson's disease is sufficiently marked on rare occasion to outline the globus pallidus nuclei. Aging of the skull may demineralize the cranial bones and render lacunar vascular channels more easily visible. Atrophy of the sella turcica and clivus of the sphenoid bone due to pulsation of a sclerosed basilar trunk can produce erosion of the posterior clinoids indistinguishable from that caused by

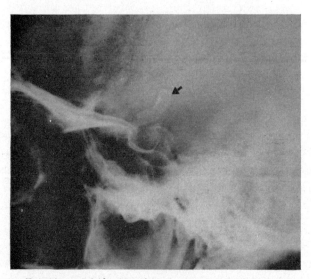

FIG. 105.—Calcification of the intracranial carotid artery.

increased intracranial pressure. Skull vascularity is especially severe in associated Paget's disease. Frontal hyperostosis is sometimes seen with or without diabetes mellitus.

Encephalography or ventriculography typically show widening of intergyral sulci and cortical atrophy (Fig. 106), especially in the frontal and temporal regions, and general symmetrical dilatation of an open ventricular system (hydrocephalus ex vacuo). When arterial stenosis or occlusion is more advanced in one hemisphere than in the other, the respective lateral ventricle will be larger than its mate. Extensive brain atrophy often includes the contents of the posterior fossa, cerebellar degeneration becoming evident in an enlarged cisterna magna and prom-inent cerebellar folia. Encephalographic differentiation of cerebral arterio-sclerosis from Alzheimer's and Pick's diseases may be difficult.

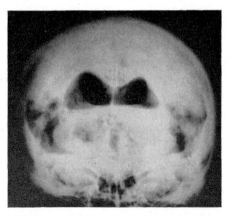

FIG. 106.—Encephalogram, arteriosclerotic brain atrophy.

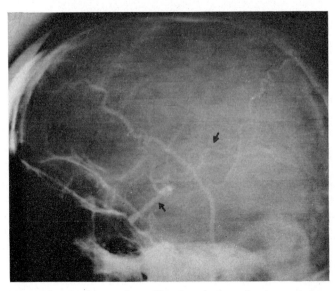

FIG. 107.—Sclerosis of internal carotid and cerebral arteries (arrows) demonstrated by angiography. (Courtesy of J. M. Williams.)

Arteriography reveals arterial alterations directly. Especially in lateral views, vessels are seen to be thicker than normal, irregular and bossed, not undulating but rectilinear in their course (Fig. 107). Fewer arteries are visible than in the angiogram of a young brain, and when thrombosis has occurred in a particular vessel it is absent from view beyond this point. The carotid siphon is uncoiled and straight, and branches of the carotid leave at a high level, are sparse, irregularly thinned and of spoke-like origin. The circulation time of the brain may be prolonged.

ELECTROENCEPHALOGRAPHY.—The electroencephalogram of cerebral arteriosclerosis is far from consistent. It may even be normal in the

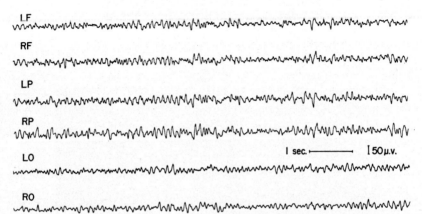

FIG. 108.—Spiky, irregular electroencephalographic record in cerebral arteriosclerosis.

presence of clearcut evidences of brain degeneration, such as arteriosclerotic parkinsonism. However, with cortical involvement, especially if advanced, waves in the bands of slow (5–7 per second) and fast (12–14 per second) frequency appear, the configuration of wave form becomes choppy and irregular, and bursts of pathologic slow activity in the anterior temporal leads may even suggest brain tumor (Fig. 108). Severe alterations of the electroencephalogram are exceptional, however, without major infarction. Compression of the cervical carotid artery may evoke pathologic slow waves in the ipsilateral electroencephalogram (Skillicorn and Aird).

DIAGNOSIS

The diagnosis of cerebral arteriosclerosis may be made in an elderly person with signs of arteriosclerosis elsewhere, particularly in the vessels of the scalp and eye, in whom neurologic disability has progressed slowly and inexorably but with episodes of temporarily more severe deficit. Mental and physical symptoms and signs indicate involvement of the brain generally. There are numerous and widespread neurologic abnormalities of greater and less degree with special reference to the cranial nerves and pyramidal and extrapyramidal projection systems. Physical, laboratory and roentgenographic examinations must eliminate all alternative diagnoses. This last criterion is especially important because all too often a hasty impression of cerebral arteriosclerosis condemns a patient with treatable inflammatory, neoplastic or traumatic brain disease to unnecessary suffering and death.

DIFFERENTIAL DIAGNOSIS.—In older patients *infectious* disease processes anywhere in the body may produce cerebral signs suggestive of intrinsic neurologic involvement which subside as toxicity and the febrile reaction are brought under control. Restoration of a normal cardiopulmonary cycle will distinguish secondary effects of *cardiac failure* from primary sclerotic change. Blood chemistry and urinalysis can reveal *metabolic* disturbances as the cause of signs simulating those of vascular deterioration. Care must be taken to rule out *drug intoxication,* particularly from bromides. Normal serologic reactions eliminate brain *syphilis,* a difficult differentiation to make on purely clinical grounds.

A complete physical check-up with particular reference to chest x-ray and endoscopy as well as inspection of the cerebrospinal fluid sediment for cancer cells is necessary to eliminate *metastatic malignancy* as a source of vague neurologic findings in the elderly. Primary *brain tumor* may not produce headache or pressure signs if infiltrative, and reliance must be placed on objective specialized examinations and observation in differentiation. A history of head injury, particularly in an alcoholic patient, with striking fluctuations in the state of consciousness may lead to the discovery of *subdural hematoma. Cerebral vasospasm, infarction, embolism and hemorrhage* are recognizable as processes additive to the effects of arteriosclerosis in the historical, physical and laboratory findings peculiar to each complication.

TREATMENT

Management of the patient with cerebral arteriosclerosis is largely palliative and regulatory, since no reliable specific therapy is as yet available. A definite program of restricted work and exercise should be outlined, intake of food and fluids in adequate amounts and proportions must be assured and attention directed to regulation of the eliminatory functions of skin, kidney and bowel.

The final decision as to the advisability of withholding all fatty and other cholesterol-containing substances from the diet is still in abeyance as debate continues. It has been observed that the body can manufacture cholesterol and its esters from many foods not considered to be fatty and that total elimination of lipid precursors is almost impossible. A fat-free dietary regime does not satisfy hunger without the addition of excessive bulk. A compromise may be made by forbidding foods of obvious high fat or cholesterol content, while adding vitamin supplements and sustaining an adequate protein intake (1 Gm. per kg. per day). Lipotropic preparations such as Methischol are recommended. Osler called alcohol "the milk of old age," and alcoholic beverages in moderation may be quite helpful.

VASODILATORS.—Use of potentially vasodilating drugs has proved of greater benefit in specific complications of cerebral arteriosclerosis, such as vasospasm or thrombosis, than in diffuse arteriosclerotic disease. One must be particularly sure that a precipitate fall in blood pressure does not occur during use of vasodilators, for cerebral infarction may thus be brought on. With Priscoline orally an aphasic arteriosclerotic patient improved (Smith and Turton), although psychiatric patients have not benefited from this drug (Hall). Hexamethonium and Apresoline are more powerful vasodilators. Cerebrovascular resistance is decreased while cerebral blood flow is maintained, although in the elderly the cerebral blood flow may be reduced by hexamethonium. Improvement in mental status has been seen after injection of Apresoline (Kleh and Fazekas).

The successful use of histamine and nicotinic acid in hemiplegia and organic psychosis (Furmanski et al.) suggests a more vigorous trial of this method in cerebral arteriosclerosis. The value of cervical sympathectomy is yet to be determined, although preliminary studies by Gardner and by Shenkin indicate a reduction in the number of neurologic episodes in sclerotic patients. Scheinberg et al. demonstrated potential reversibility of the increased cerebrovascular resistance of aged patients by administration of carbon dioxide oxygen during cerebral blood flow estimations.

HORMONES.—Administration of male and female sex hormones has not produced anticipated rejuvenation or circulatory benefits, although the pain of osteoporosis may be relieved. Holbrook's experience indicates that small doses of cortisone (25–50 mg. daily) may make the elderly arteriosclerotic patient less forgetful, more alert and happier. Thyroid, also in small doses, has occasionally been found to be beneficial.

SYMPTOMATIC THERAPY.—Aspirin-codeine combinations or mild barbiturates may be given for headache. Potassium chloride, 1 Gm., with

16–32 mg. of phenobarbital, each four times daily may relieve vertiginous sensations. Potassium iodide (10-15 drops three to four times daily) is an old and effective remedy used in cerebral arteriosclerosis. Whether or not lipids are actually removed from the wall of atheromatous vessels by saturation of unsaturated fatty acids, the giving of iodides will often relieve many complaints, including headache.

PARKINSONISM, PSEUDOBULBAR PALSY.—With signs of extrapyramidal disease, one of the many preparations of belladonna, stramonium, scopolamine and related compounds, or newer substances recommended for this symptom complex, is indicated. The latter include Benadryl and other antihistamines, Artane and Panparnit. There is no drug cure for Parkinson's disease, and dramatic, objective control of tremor or rigidity seldom results. However, the patient usually feels better and can be more active on a program of medication optimal for him, possibly because of the extreme suggestibility in this group. Surgical treatment should be limited to patients with unilaterally severe tremor, an uncommon variant of the arteriosclerotic form of the disease.

Small doses of scopolamine hydrobromide are recommended in pseudobulbar palsy. No medication is consistently helpful in this condition, which runs its own course, occasionally with spontaneous remission.

PSYCHOSIS.—Psychiatric treatment measures are discussed in Chapter 19.

PROGNOSIS

There is no cure for cerebral arteriosclerosis, which is a terminal disease, although rapidity of progress may be slowed by measures just outlined. Complicating thromboses and infarctions of the brain or intracranial hemorrhage conclude the deteriorating course of vascular sclerosis, although modern treatment may tide a patient through what might otherwise be a fatal episode. Survival of the patient is limited eventually by his life span, if not by a fatal stroke or heart attack. A total of 60–75 per cent of arteriosclerotic psychotics die in mental hospitals, and only 10–20 per cent are discharged. Death occurs from stroke, arteriosclerotic heart disease, pneumonia or simply old age.

BIBLIOGRAPHY

Alpers, B. J.; Forster, F. M., and Herbut, P. A.: Retinal, cerebral and systemic arteriosclerosis: A histopathologic study, Arch. Neurol. & Psychiat. 60:440-456, 1948.
Altschul, R.: Cerebral endarteritis obliterans in an infant, J. Neuropath. & Exper. Neurol. 8:204-213, 1949.

Anderson, H. J., and Petch, C. P.: Bulbar palsy due to an atheromatous vessel, Lancet 1:665, 1941.

Bromage, P. R.: Some electroencephalographic changes associated with induced vascular hypotension, Proc. Roy. Soc. Med. 46:919-923, 1953.

Buchstein, H.: Personal communication.

Fazekas, J. F.; Alman, R. W., and Bessman, A. N.: Cerebral physiology of the aged, Am. J. M. Sc. 223:245-257, 1952.

Fisher, M.: Senile dementia: New explanation of causation, Canad. M. A. J. 65:1-7, 1951.

Freyhan, F. A.; Woodford, R. B., and Kety, S. S.: Cerebral blood flow and metabolism in psychoses of senility, J. Nerv. & Ment. Dis. 113:449-456, 1951.

Furmanski, A. R., et al.: Histamine therapy in acute ischemia of the brain, A.M.A. Arch. Neurol. & Psychiat. 69:104-117, 1953.

Gardner, W. J.: Personal communication.

Gofman, J. W., and Jones, H. B.: Obesity, fat metabolism and cardiovascular disease, Circulation 5:514-517, 1952.

Grinker, R. R., and Reich, J.: Cranial nerve disturbances due to arteriosclerosis of intracranial arteries, Illinois M. J. 75:453-457, 1949.

Hall, M. N.: Study on effects of Priscoline on patients with psychosis due to cerebral arteriosclerosis, Connecticut M.J. 15:385-389, 1951.

Hickman, J. B.; Schieve, J. F., and Wilson, W. P.: The relation between retinal and cerebral vascular reactivity in normal and arteriosclerotic subjects, Circulation 7:84-87, 1953.

Holbrook, P.: Personal communication.

Kleh, J., and Fazekas, J. F.: The use of Apresoline in the hypertensive arteriosclerotic syndrome, Am. J. M. Sc. 227:57-64, 1954.

Leary, T.: The genesis of coronary sclerosis, New England J. Med. 245:397-402, 1951.

Lhermitte, J., and McAlpine, D.: A clinical and pathological résumé of combined disease of the pyramidal and extrapyramidal systems, with special reference to a new syndrome, Brain 49:157, 1926.

Scheinberg, P.; Blackburn, I.; Rich, M., and Saslaw, M.: Effects of aging on cerebral circulation and metabolism, A.M.A. Arch. Neurol. & Psychiat. 70:77-85, 1953.

Shenkin, H. A.: Personal communication.

Simon, A., et al.: Cerebral arteriosclerosis, Am. J. Psychiat. 108:663-668, 1952.

Skillicorn, S. A., and Aird, R. B.: Electroencephalographic changes resulting from carotid artery compression, A.M.A. Arch. Neurol. & Psychiat. 71:367-376, 1954.

Smith, S., and Turton, E. C.: Restoration of speech in severe aphasia by intravenous and oral priscol, Brit. M. J. 2:891-892, 1951.

Spielmeyer, W.: Vasomotorisch trophische Veränderung bei zerebraler arteriosklerose, Monatsschr. Psychiat. u. Neurol. 68:605-620, 1928.

Sunderland, S,: Neurovascular relations and anomalies at the base of the brain, J. Neurol., Neurosurg. & Psychiat. 11:243-257, 1948.

Tuthill, C. R.: Cerebral arteries in relation to arteriosclerosis, Arch. Path. 16:453-470, 1933.

Ward, A. A.; McCulloch, W. S., and Magoun, H. W.: Production of alternating tremor at rest in monkeys, J. Neurophysiol. 11:317-330, 1948.

Winternitz, M. C.; Thomas, R. M., and Lecompte, P. M.: The Biology of Arteriosclerosis (Springfield, Ill.: Charles C Thomas, Publisher, 1938).

CHAPTER 16

Inflammatory and
Collagenous Diseases

INFLAMMATORY VASCULAR DISEASE

Participation of the cerebral circulation in the pathologic changes attendant on many infectious and inflammatory diseases is commoner than is usually realized. Cerebral vascular reaction may become predominantly important in almost any infectious illness. Many so-called encephalitides are actually the result of extension of systemic inflammatory processes to the intracranial circulation.

BACTERIAL (PYOGENIC) DISEASES.—In almost all of the brains of 300 young subjects dying of various infectious illnesses, including diphtheria, influenza, scarlet fever, pneumonia and typhoid fever, Wiesel found destructive changes in the smooth muscle and elastica of small arteries with accompanying proliferation of the intima, but without evidence of actual bacterial invasion. Mallory was able to demonstrate a bacteria-induced perivascular reaction in the brain in septicemia. Endothelial swelling and proliferation of small cerebral cortical vessels producing microscopic areas of partial or complete softening in the brain were found by Winkelman and Eckel in many toxic conditions.

Hemorrhagic encephalitis.—The intensity of cerebral involvement may reach that of hemorrhagic encephalitis, in which the white matter is studded with yellow or red areas consisting of central dilated and thrombosed blood vessels with surrounding necrosis and hemorrhage. Onset of this syndrome is abrupt, with headache, high temperature, vertigo, convulsions, meningeal signs, focal neurologic findings and rapid passage to coma.

Systemic infections.—Brain petechiae occur in chickenpox. Minute hemorrhages possibly due to air embolism during fits of coughing characterize pertussis "encephalitis." Cerebral thrombosis with hemiplegia has been reported in scarlet fever and typhoid. Multiple small cerebral vascular occlusions have been found at autopsy in fatal pneumonias (Baker and Noran). Naturally, the more septicemic any illness may be, the greater the frequency of vascular lesions in the brain. Bacteria may often be found microscopically with special stains.

Febrile cerebral thrombosis in childhood.—Inflammatory cerebral thrombosis, usually venous but also arterial, is a principal cause of infantile and juvenile hemiplegia. Any severe infection may be responsible; it is possible that normally transient bacteremias in the young, which in combination with trauma will produce osteomyelitis, may also attack intracranial vessels. Most cases occur in children under 10 during convalescence from a systemic infection. Convulsions, paralysis, aphasia and hemianopsia are the usual neurologic signs because of the susceptibility of the middle cerebral veins and artery. Stupor may progress to coma, and the accompanying fever is usually severe. This condition must be differentiated from encephalitis, endocarditis with cerebral embolization, brain abscess and postmeningitic subdural hygroma.

The cerebrospinal fluid is usually not remarkable, but the electroencephalogram may be highly abnormal with a focus of spikes. The ultimate prognosis of these episodes is not good; in many of these young patients hemiplegia does not recede, limbs become spastic and fail to grow. Severe convulsive seizures recur and mental arrest results. Air study may reveal dilatation of a cerebral ventricle or porencephaly.

Meningitis.—In any of the purulent meningitides, the adventitial coats of surface vessels and the pia-glial perivascular membrane internally may be invaded, with resultant angiitis and thrombosis (Fig. 109). This is usually but not exclusively true of veins. Inflammatory vascular invasion is particularly common in pneumococcic, staphylococcic and influenzal infections. Large vessels are surprisingly resistant to tuberculous disease but may be invaded via the vasa vasorum; pan- or periarteritis results, followed by typical tubercle formation with caseation. Endarteritis of the pial vessels is more severe in tuberculous meningitis than in other types of meningeal inflammation. Hemorrhage is rare but infarcts of even large size are not uncommon.

Laboratory findings in all cases of meningitis are typical of the primary disease with modifications due to vascular complications. The cerebrospinal fluid pressure is increased and the fluid is turbid, cloudy or xanthochromic. The increased cellularity is chiefly polymorphonuclear in type with acute, pyogenic illness and is lymphocytic and mononuclear in the chronic granulomatous types. Sugar and chlorides are reduced. Bacteria may be found in stained smears, and in tuberculous meningitis acid-fast bacilli are often present in the protein pellicle which forms after the fluid is allowed to stand. Culture of the cerebrospinal fluid should always be made.

Treatment.—The treatment of bacterial inflammatory angiitis and thrombosis, with or without meningeal reaction, is that to which the responsible micro-organism is most vulnerable. Sulfonamides or antibi-

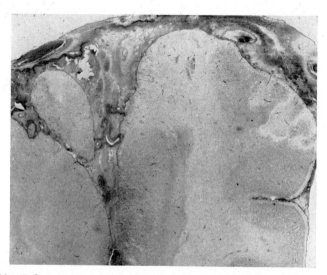

Fig. 109.—Inflammatory pial vasculitis with cortical infarction. Purulent meningitis.

otics are administered parenterally in large dosage; the value of intrathecal medication is questionable. The pathogenic germ should be recovered and cultured and its susceptibility determined by sensitivity titration with antibiotic substances. In tuberculosis of the brain, vessels and meninges, a combination of streptomycin and para-aminosalicylate or the hydrazide of isonicotinic acid is used. Stellate block and anticoagulants are indicated in febrile thrombosis. Subdural membranes should be removed.

RICKETTSIAL INFECTIONS.—*Typhus fever.*—Typhus fever derives its name from the stupor or coma which develops in severe cases. The infection is caused by the rickettsial coccobacillary organism which invades and destroys vascular endothelium throughout the body. Grossly, intense hyperemia of the brain is seen at autopsy, with numerous small hemorrhages visible in meninges and gray matter of cortex and nuclei. Microscopically, minute vessels are occluded by endothelial swelling and are surrounded by nodules of proliferated microglial and adventitial cells. Tiny infarcts are numerous in the gray tissue of the cerebrum. Perivascular round cell accumulations are present in all rickettsial encephalitides. The responsible micro-organisms may be found in the endothelium as inclusion bodies.

Neurologic phenomena often dominate the clinical picture. Febrile delirium, coma and convulsive seizures are common. Inflammatory cerebrospinal fluid changes are present after the tenth day of illness. Diag-

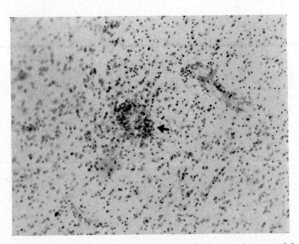

FIG. 110.—Capillary necrosis, glial nodule. Rocky Mountain spotted fever.

nosis is established by a positive Weil-Felix reaction. The mortality is high, and residual hemiplegia, aphasia and other evidences of severe brain damage are present in over one-half the survivors. Chloramphenicol is the specific medication; if depression of the bone marrow is threatened or occurs when this drug is given, aureomycin or terramycin may be substituted.

Rocky Mountain spotted fever.—Rocky Mountain spotted or tick bite fever is a common variant of rickettsial disease in the United States. It is carried by animal ticks, and children are frequently infected. Neurologic symptoms may appear early. Pathologically, inflammatory changes are almost identical with those of typhus, except that lesions are more common in the white matter than in the gray cortex or nuclei (Fig. 110). Mortality rates vary widely, but the disease responds readily to chloramphenicol which should be given early, hematologic studies being constant. However, neurologic residuals are frequently severe. In patients examined one to eight years after spotted fever, the majority showed signs of damage to the central nervous system and electroencephalographic abnormalities (Rosenblum et al.).

SPIROCHETAL DISEASES.—*Syphilis.*—The cardiovascular system is preferentially attacked by the Treponema pallidum, and syphilitic inflammation of cerebral vessels is one of the commonest causes of hemiplegia in young adults. Heubner's arteritis appears during the first year after primary, untreated infection and affects large vessels of the circle of Willis. Vasculitis results in endothelial proliferation, splitting of elastica and medial coats and adventitial degeneration; all layers are infiltrated by chronic inflammatory cells. The plastic process results in great thickening of the wall or in complete occlusion of the involved vessel; aneurysmal dilatation is rare. Thrombosis with or without brain infarction is the usual conclusion. Subintimal fibrosis and medial hyalinization develop as arteritis heals. Arteriosclerosis is particularly common in cerebral syphilis.

Headache, irritability and convulsive seizures result from meningovascular syphilis. General neurologic and psychologic deterioration is the end stage of multiple cystic softenings in the gray and white matter. Clinical syndromes resemble those of arteriosclerosis but differ in the greater rapidity of onset, floridity of signs and frequent spontaneous remission. Argyll Robertson pupils are common and any isolated neurologic sign may be seen. Hemiplegia and convulsions often occur and may rarely be accompanied by aphasia. There is a slow cerebral circulation time in cerebrovascular syphilis. Cerebrospinal fluid reactions other than serologic may be normal or abnormal in the cerebrovascular form of the disease. The Wassermann reaction is positive in the blood in 80 per cent of patients and in the cerebrospinal fluid in 50 per cent.

In treatment, penicillin is the drug of choice, 12,000,000 units of procaine penicillin being administered in an 18 day period. If penicillin is not tolerated or cannot be given for another reason, Terramycin in dosage of 60 mg. per kilogram of body weight per day may be substituted. Herxheimer's reactions are rare. Two years may pass before serologic reversal, although lesions heal rapidly.

Other spirochetal diseases.—Relapsing fever, caused by various species of Borrelia, is endemic in the Middle East and Africa and also occurs sporadically in North, Central and South America. Attacks of prostrating fever and malaise alternate with periods of well-being. Although jaundice, hemorrhages and splenomegaly are the more prominent clinical signs, chronic headache, organic psychosis, meningismus, facial paralysis, hemiplegia, aphasia and convulsive seizures have been reported. Treatment is carried out as in syphilis.

Leptospirosis (Weil's disease, infectious jaundice) results from infection with the Leptospira icterohemorrhagica. The rat is the most common reservoir, and distribution of the disease is almost world wide. Small vessels in the brain are plugged with spirochetes, white blood cells and hyaline thrombi (Kastein and Haex). Hemorrhages of petechial variety result and glial nodules develop. Symptoms of cerebral type are related to toxemia or multiple vascular occlusions. Meningitis may be severe and is evidenced by increase of cerebrospinal fluid pressure, cellularity and protein content. Iridocyclitis is common and ocular hemorrhages may be present.

The diagnosis is established by serum agglutination of the leptospira. The mortality rate is variably high. Convalescent serum, bismuth and neoarsphenamine have had some success therapeutically; the parasites are apparently resistant to penicillin.

MYCOTIC INFECTIONS.—The mycotic diseases, which include actinomycosis, aspergillis, sporothrix infections, etc., produce granulomatous meningitis and abscesses in the brain. The cerebral vessels are involved only secondarily. True mycotic aneurysm of the circle of Willis has been reported. Yeastlike organisms (Torula histolytica, coccidioides, oidiomycetes) cause meningoencephalitis and although they invade the cerebrum along perivascular sheaths do not attack vessels directly or preferentially.

VIRUS DISEASES.—Virus infections of the brain cause generalized nonsuppurative encephalitis. Microscopic or ecchymotic hemorrhages and extreme endothelial swelling may feature the pathologic change in some cases, especially of epidemic encephalitis. Massive intracerebral hemorrhage and occlusion of major brain vessels with thrombotic infarctions of whole lobes of the cerebrum have been found in patients dying of choriomeningitis.

Porphyria, a disease of unknown etiology, causes a diffuse toxic meningopolioencephalomyelitis with pronounced involvement of the blood vessels of the brain stem, cerebellum, diencephalon and cerebral hemispheres.

COLLAGENOUS VASCULAR DISEASE

In those vascular diseases generally classified as collagenous, pathologic alteration of the cerebral vessels, as elsewhere in the body, is featured prominently but not exclusively by mesenchymal reaction. Inflammatory changes may be almost the only changes at certain stages. The etiologies of these loosely related processes are unknown, but the participation of an allergic reaction is at least suspected and the possibility of infection with ultramicroscopic ("l") organisms has been suggested.

RHEUMATIC ARTERITIS.—The etiology of rheumatic fever remains obscure, but its relationship to a preceding beta-hemolytic streptococcic infection is more than casual, and antistreptolysin titers are increased in the blood in acute stages of the disease.

Pathology.—In rheumatic fever, the brain may be involved in one or more of four ways: primary vascular alterations (rheumatic arteritis), focal areas of ischemic softening, embolic infarction and the pathologic changes of Sydenham's chorea. Cerebral vascular lesions are found in small and medium-sized arteries and are characterized by proliferation of intimal and subintimal connective tissue cells. Especially in acute rheumatic fever there is a panarteritis with infiltration of leukocytes and monocytes through the vascularized walls of the vessels. Small round cells lie in the adventitial coats. Endothelial growth can completely occlude the arterial lumen, vasa vasorum growing through to recanalize old thrombi. Denst and Neubuerger described thromboses resembling valvular vegetations in all sizes of intracranial arteries and veins in late rheumatic heart disease. Splitting of the elastica and fibrosis of media and adventitia are similar to the processes in arteriosclerosis. The pathologic change of Sydenham's chorea is primarily encephalitic, although with associated small vessel involvement.

Symptoms and signs.—Neurologic evidences of rheumatic cerebral arteritis correspond to the degree and location of parenchymal ischemia and infarction. Bruetsch declared that 5 per cent of mental hospital patients suffer from rheumatic brain disease, and he found signs of involvement of heart and cerebrum in 9 per cent of autopsies on schizophrenics. He believes that obliterating rheumatic endarteritis, productive of infarcts, scars and glial nodules, may account for many obscure neuropsychiatric syndromes. Laboratory findings in rheumatic cerebral vasculitis correlate with the degree of activity of the underlying process. The sedimentation rate is elevated in acute attacks.

Treatment.—The therapy of rheumatic fever is medical. Prophylactic administration of penicillin, an adequate protein diet and favorable climate seem to prevent recurrences. Antibiotics and corticotropin are helpful in acute attacks. Cerebrovascular complications may call for stellate block and the use of chemical vasodilators or anticoagulants in addition to general medical management.

PERIARTERITIS NODOSA.—Periarteritis nodosa (essential polyarteritis) is a strange and fascinating disease which affects arteries throughout the body. It involves the brain in 8 per cent of cases and the nervous system generally in 20 per cent (Kernohan and Woltman). The cause is obscure. In some patients the illness follows rheumatic fever or hemolytic streptococcic infections. A fundamentally hyperergic etiology is suggested by Rich's relationship of several cases to serum sickness and sulfonamide

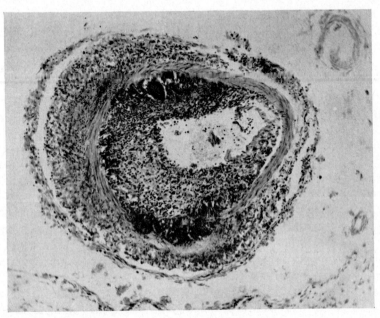

FIG. 111.—Periarteritis nodosa of pial vessel. (Courtesy of N. W. Winkelman and M. T. Moore.)

allergy. Polyarteritis has also developed in patients with thyrotoxicosis who were treated with iodine and with thiouracil.

Pathology.—The arterial process begins as a panarteritis rather than a periarteritis. Mural necrosis is followed quickly by a surrounding and pervasive inflammatory reaction, at first acute and later chronic in cellular constituents. The media and elastica are destroyed, the intima is denuded and the lumen of the vessel is often filled with thrombus (Fig. 111). Aneurysmal dilatation of the weakened wall may cause vascular rupture and intracranial hemorrhage.

Symptoms and signs.—Periarteritis nodosa appears in several clinical syndromes variously featured by fever, pallor, splenomegaly, muscular nodules, skin eruptions, abdominal crises, renal pain and hematuria, asthma and hemoptysis, and evidences of involvement of the central or peripheral nervous system. Neurologic signs indicative of brain injury may include headache, vomiting, vertigo, delirium, convulsions, hemiplegia, cortical blindness, cranial nerve palsies, cerebellar ataxia and mental disturbances. Meningismus and frank subarachnoid hemorrhage may also occur.

Ocular evidences of vascular disease may range from vasospastic retinitis to thrombosis of the central artery, and papilledema has been seen. Eosinophilia, anemia and leukocytosis may be striking. The urinary and blood chemistry changes and hypertension parallel renal arterial destruction. Cerebrospinal fluid abnormalities are noted when vascular lesions approach or perforate the meningeal spaces. The electroencephalogram may indicate focal brain damage secondary to ischemia or hemorrhage.

Treatment.—There is no reliable cure for periarteritis nodosa. Corticotropin or cortisone may be tried, and occasionally the disease will subside spontaneously if the patient is removed from a contributory allergen. The mortality rate is very high.

TEMPORAL (CRANIAL) ARTERITIS.—Since the first description by Horton *et al.* of what has come to be called temporal or cranial arteritis, many cases have been recognized. The youngest patient reported previously was 22 (Meyers and Lord); one of my patients was a 19 year old girl. Most patients are over age 55 at onset. Cranial involvement is sometimes a local manifestation of periarteritis nodosa, but it seems unlikely that this applies to the benign form of the disease which is self-limited or which responds to drug therapy or surgery. Infection in the head or neck seems to result in arterial inflammation occasionally, and in rare instances syphilitic temporal arteritis is encountered.

Pathology.—Temporal arteries, superficial and deep, are always involved. They stand out in bold relief on the temples (Fig. 112) or are obscured by perivascular inflammatory edema and fibrosis, forming tender, prominent masses. Facial, occipital and other external carotid arterial branches may be included in the process. Intracranially, retinal arteritis has caused papilledema, ocular hemorrhages, extraocular palsies or permanent blindness, and inflammation of cerebral or cerebellar vessels has led to related neurologic sequelae. A severe variety of panarteritis is seen in biopsy specimens of the affected vessels; medial necrosis, intimal proliferation and mural hemorrhages are found. The chronic, diffuse, foamy and giant-cellular response extends to the adventitia and resembles tuberculosis, gumma or xanthoma.

Symptoms and signs.—The chief complaint is that of severe, burning headache, beginning in the vicinity of the swollen scalp arteries. The patient often appears really ill, the systemic reaction with fever, malaise, anorexia, weight loss, dizziness and nausea resembling that of a generalized disease. Anemia and an elevated sedimentation rate are often present. The colloidal gold curve of the cerebrospinal fluid may be abnormal.

Treatment.—Only analgesics or periarterial procaine infiltration may be needed to relieve headache. In the absence of general systemic complaints but with persistence of cranial pain and arterial swelling, local excision of the involved vessels will usually afford relief. Cures have been reported with the use of corticotropin and cortisone, and benefit has been said to follow penicillin, histamine and Gantrisin therapy. The mortality

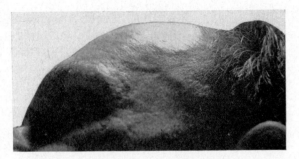

FIG. 112.—Temporal arteritis. Prominent scalp vessels.

rate is 12.5 per cent (Crosby and Wadsworth). In one reported case, death resulted from rupture of the aorta (Broch and Ytrehus) and in another from coronary thrombosis.

LUPUS ERYTHEMATOSUS DISSEMINATUS.—This unusual, disseminated and highly fatal disease is identified clinically by a butterfly type of facial rash involving the cheeks and the bridge of the nose, branny desquamation of the skin elsewhere, lesions of the mucous membranes, fever, arthritis, evidences of renal damage, splenomegaly, pleuritis, pericarditis, weight loss, anorexia and cachexia. The patient is very sensitive to sunlight. The etiology is unknown, although some type of allergy is suspected. There is no apparent relation to discoid lupus and none to tuberculosis. Pathologic changes are distributed throughout the connective tissue of the body, in association with small blood vessels, in the kidney and in the endocardium.

Pathology.—Endothelial proliferation, medial necrosis and fibrosis and infiltration of the adventitia with serum, blood and chronic inflammatory cells are evident. "Wire-loop" hyaline thickenings are seen in the renal glomeruli, and verrucous endocarditis is often present (Libman-Sacks disease). Recent and old infarcts, large and small, are found in the brain. In most of 15 autopsied cases (Dubois *et al.*), death was due to cerebral angiitis as a local effect of systemic lupus erythematosus.

Symptoms and signs.—Cerebral complications are evidenced by vascular spasm, exudates and hemorrhages in the eyegrounds, appearance of the organic mental syndrome, focal neurologic signs, electroencephalographic changes (Fig. 113) and convulsive seizures. L.E. cells are present in the bone marrow and peripheral blood. Anemia, leukocytosis and an

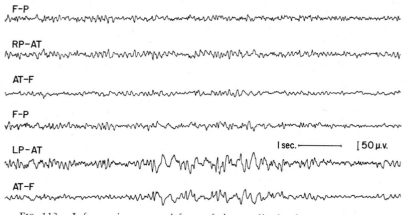

FIG. 113.—Left anterior temporal focus of abnormality in electroencephalogram of patient with lupus erythematosus disseminatus.

increase in sedimentation rate are also found, as are urinary abnormalities. Hypertension accompanies severe renal injury.

Treatment.—Present therapy includes the use of corticotropin and cortisone in large doses (Dubois *et al.*; Soffer and Bader). There have been spontaneous remissions of variable duration in 20 per cent of reported cases; the disease is ultimately uniformly fatal.

ANGIONEUROTIC EDEMA; SERUM SICKNESS.—Convulsive seizures, transient or permanent hemiplegia, aphasia, hemianopsia, papilledema and retinal edema have been observed by Kennedy and by Park and Richardson in the course of allergic angioneurotic edema and generalized serum disease. The cerebrospinal fluid pressure was very high in these patients. Kennedy interpreted these episodes as being due to localized meningeal hydrops. However, in view of the evidences of cerebral parenchymal involvement, it seems reasonable to assume that the reactions in the brain were vascular in nature although autopsy examination was not reported.

THROMBOANGIITIS OBLITERANS.—Thromboangiitis obliterans (Winiwarter-Buerger disease) is considered to be either of inflammatory origin or a collagen disease of blood vessels. The pathologic process attacks the extremities primarily, the incidence of cerebrovascular complications being less than 0.5 per cent (Lippmann).

The one etiologic relationship on which all agree is that of tobacco allergy, and diagnosis of Buerger's disease in a nonsmoker is suspect. It is almost exclusively encountered in men; the rare instances of thromboangiitis obliterans among women appear in those of mannish disposition who are heavy smokers. Originally thought to occur only in people of the Jewish race, it has been recognized in individuals of all racial derivations and nationalities. Sulzberger's studies disclosed hypersensitivity to tobacco proteins (not nicotine) in 78 per cent of patients with thromboangiitis, twice the incidence of allergy in healthy smokers. Scheinker compared the appearance of vascular changes to those seen in ergotism and periarteritis nodosa. Functional, reversible phenomena such as migrating phlebitis often precede anatomic alterations.

Pathology.—The extremities are particularly disabled, the legs more than the arms, and the heart is often involved, but any vessel in the body may be attacked, veins as well as arteries. In a few cases, only the brain is involved. Krayenbühl reported several instances of cervical Buerger's disease leading to carotid thrombosis (Fig. 31).

On the surface of the brain, thickened leptomeninges cover white, pulseless and cordlike arteries (Davis and Perret). The middle cerebral arterial vessels are primarily diseased. Occasionally cortical veins are thrombosed. The cortex proper appears yellow, granular and atrophic. On coronal sections of the cerebrum, minute areas of softening are present in the white matter. Microscopically, foci of fat granule cells, tissue rarefaction and glial scars represent tiny ischemic infarcts; major infarction may be present as well. The arteries and veins are damaged by panvasculitis and true necrosis with polymorphonuclear and small round cell invasion. The intima and lumen are replaced by masses of granulation tissue and organizing thrombi. Intramural hemorrhages may occlude the ostium of the vessel from without. In chronic phases of the disease, an artery and its accompanying vein are bound together in fibrous scar which includes the perivascular nerves. Recanalization takes place to a limited degree.

Symptoms and signs.—The general systemic syndrome begins with pains in the legs, limitation of walking, migrating phlebitis and absence of pulsations in the extremities. Later, peripheral gangrene and coronary thromboses occur. Any type of neurologic symptom or sign can be produced by cerebral thromboangiitis obliterans. Fleeting paralyses, transient visual disorders and convulsions are common. Segmentation of arteries and veins, papillary changes and retinal extravasations may be found on ophthalmoscopy.

Treatment.—Therapy of the intracranial form of thromboangiitis obliterans has been unsatisfactory. Arterial resections, the use of spasmolytics and cervical sympathectomy have not been effective. The only known measure of benefit is the absolute cessation of tobacco smoking. Adrenalectomy has been reported to be helpful in selected cases.

BIBLIOGRAPHY

Baker, A. B., and Noran, H. H.: Changes in the central nervous system associated with encephalitis complicating pneumonia, Arch. Int. Med. 76:146-153, 1945.

Broch, O. J., and Ytrehus, O.: Three new cases of arteritis temporalis, Nord. med. 34:1111-1113, 1947.

Crosby, R. C., and Wadsworth, R. C.: Temporal arteritis: Review of the literature and report of 5 additional cases, Arch. Int. Med. 81:431-464, 1948.

Davis, L., and Perret, G.: Cerebral thromboangiitis obliterans, Brit. J. Surg. 34:307-313, 1947.

Denst, J., and Neubuerger, K. T.: Intracranial vascular lesions in late rheumatic heart disease, Arch. Path. 46:191-201, 1948.

Dubois, E. L., *et al.:* Corticotropin and cortisone treatment for systemic lupus erythematosus, J.A.M.A. 149:995-1001, 1952.

Horton, B. T.; Magath, T. B., and Brown, G. E.: An undescribed form of arteritis of the temporal vessels, Proc. Staff Meet., Mayo Clin. 7:700-701, 1932.

Kastein, G. W., and Haex, A. J. Ch.: Histopathologic investigations in icterohemorrhagic spirochetosis, with special consideration of vascular disturbances, Acta. med. scandinav. 101:256-288, 1939.

Kennedy, F.: Cerebral symptoms induced by angioneurotic edema, Arch. Neurol. & Psychiat. 15:28-33, 1926.

Kennedy, F.: Certain nervous complications following use of therapeutic and prophylactic sera, Am. J. M. Sc. 177:555-559, 1929.

Kernohan, J. W., and Woltman, H. W.: Periarteritis nodosa, Arch. Neurol. & Psychiat. 39:655-686, 1938.

Krayenbühl, H.: Zur Diagnostik und chirurgischen Therapie der zerebralen Erscheinungen bei der Endangiitis obliterans v. Winiwarter-Buerger, Schweiz. med. Wchnschr. 75:1025-1029, 1945.

Lippmann, H. I.: Cerebrovascular thrombosis in patients with Buerger's disease, Circulation 5:680-692, 1952.

Mallory, F. B.: Infectious lesions of blood vessels, Boston City Hosp. Rep., 148, 1913.

Meyers, L., and Lord, J. W., Jr.: Cranial arteritis, J.A.M.A. 136:169-171, 1948.

Park, A. M., and Richardson, J. C.: Cerebral complications of serum sickness, Neurology 3:277-283, 1953.

Rich, A. R.: The role of hypersensitivity in periarteritis nodosa, as indicated by seven cases developing during serum sickness and sulfonamide therapy, Bull. Johns Hopkins Hosp. 71:123-140, 1942.

Rosenblum, M. J.; Masland, R. L., and Harrell, G. T.: Residual effects of rickettsial disease on the central nervous system, A.M.A. Arch. Int. Med. 90:444-455, 1952.

Scheinker, I. M.: Cerebral thromboangiitis obliterans and its relation to periarteritis nodosa, J. Neuropath. & Exper. Neurol. 4:77-87, 1945.

Soffer, L. J., and Bader, R.: Corticotropin and cortisone in acute disseminated lupus erythematosus, J.A.M.A. 149:1002-1008, 1952.

Sulzberger, M.: Recent immunologic experiments in tobacco hypersensitivity, Bull. New York Acad. Med. 9:294-317, 1933.

Wiesel, J.: Der Erkrankungen Arterieller Gefasse im Verlaufe akuter Infektionen, Ztschr. Heilk. Abt. path. Anat. 27:69, 1907.

Winkelman, N. W., and Eckel, J. L.: Endarteritis of the small cortical vessels in severe infections and toxemias, Arch. Neurol. & Psychiat. 21:863-875, 1929.

CHAPTER 17

Blood Dyscrasias;
Vitamin Deficiencies; Poisons

BLOOD DYSCRASIAS

IN MOST IF not all the blood dyscrasias, physiologic or anatomic cerebrovascular complications often occur and may be responsible for neurologic disability or death. The anoxic syndrome, acute or chronic, results if the erythrocyte concentration in the blood is inadequate. When blood viscosity is reduced in severe anemia, the body's compensatory attempt to supply more oxygen to the brain results in lowered cerebrovascular resistance and increased cerebral blood flow. Conversely, thickening of the blood by an excess of cellular elements, as in polycythemia, will slow the rate of cerebral circulation. The majority of frank intracranial episodes in the hematologic diseases are hemorrhagic in nature, but thromboses may develop also. Blood dyscrasia should always be suspected when bleeding, intracranial or otherwise, occurs without evident cause.

THE ANEMIAS.—*Acute anemia.*—Rapid and prolonged hemorrhage may cause permanent blindness. Retinal hemorrhages and even papilledema have been observed by Walsh in patients with severe secondary anemia. In a patient I saw, severe intellectual deterioration, aphasia and parietal lobe dysfunction were the long term consequences of severance of the jugular vein. The necessity of rapid replacement of blood by transfusion is obvious.

Pernicious anemia.—Paranoid psychosis and other impairment of mental function in pernicious anemia has been correlated by Scheinberg with reduced cerebral oxygen consumption. Endarteritic and perivascular hemorrhagic changes develop in the hypothalamus and brain stem, as they do in Wernicke's polioencephalitis hemorrhagica superior. Small vessel alterations may be associated with patches of demyelination in the brain. Retinal extravasations, pallor of the optic disks and, rarely, papilledema are seen in severe pernicious anemia.

Scheinberg found the cerebral blood flow to be increased and cerebrovascular resistance to be reduced in patients with a hemoglobin level of less than 7 Gm. per 100 ml., but the reverse was true when the hemoglobin concentration was above this value. Diagnosis of pernicious anemia is made by the findings of achlorhydria in gastric analysis, macrocytosis and reticulocyte increase in the peripheral blood smear and megaloblastic activity in bone marrow specimens. Degeneration of the pyramidal tracts, posterior columns of the spinal cord and cauda equina (com-

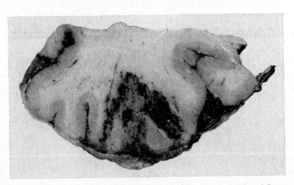

FIG. 114.—Confluent cortical hemorrhages. Sickle cell anemia. (Courtesy of R. K. Thompson *et al.*)

bined system disease) is common in advanced cases. Treatment includes transfusion, liver extracts and vitamin B_{12}.

Sickle cell anemia.—The brain is affected in approximately one third of all cases of sicklemia, a disease which is fairly common among American Negroes and also affects white persons of Mediterranean stock. The disease is hereditary, carried by a mendelian dominant. The etiology is unknown; red blood cells become slipper or sickle shaped when exposed to a low oxygen tension and agglutinate in clumps.

The lumens of meningeal and intracerebral vessels, large and small, are plugged with clumps of pathologic erythrocytes, and thromboses follow. Lobar or less extensive infarctions of the brain are visible grossly, and necrobiotic foci are numerous in microscopic preparations (Fig. 114). The meninges are thickened and rust stained. Petechial and massive intracranial hemorrhages are not uncommon; a capsular hemorrhage indistinguishable from that of hypertension caused death in a 12 year old boy with sickle cell anemia.

Neurologic symptoms include headache, dizziness, convulsions, hemiplegia and coma. Systemic complaints are referable to the skin (leg ulcers), joints, abdomen and the cardiovascular system generally. Tortuosity of fundic vessels, engorgement of veins, retinal edema and pallor of the optic disks are seen. The finding of sickled erythrocytes in plain blood smears or in anoxic preparations establishes the diagnosis. Anemia is often severe. The lumbar fluid pressure may be high, and the cerebrospinal fluid is xanthochromic or bloody and has a high protein content and many cells. The skull is osteoporotic due to decalcification associated with increased blood flow. Electroencephalographic abnormalities are present in many children who may not otherwise show neurologic involvement (Patterson *et al.*).There is no effective treatment for sicklemia other than transfusion.

DEFECTS IN THE CLOTTING MECHANISM.—*Hemophilia.*—The hemophilic disorder is hereditary and affects males almost exclusively. Severe hemorrhages follow trauma or occur spontaneously. The clotting time of the blood is greatly prolonged, apparently owing to failure of platelet disintegration. Subdural, subarachnoid or intracerebral hemorrhages occur frequently and may be extensive and even lethal. Retinal extravasations are rare. Mortality is high; one-half the patients die before age 7 (Ford). Transfusions are the only effective therapy, although histamine may shorten the clotting time temporarily (Sanford *et al.*).

Thrombocytopenic purpura.—Diminution in platelet concentration and prolonged bleeding but normal clotting time characterize thrombocytopenic purpura. The disease appears in childhood and is featured clinically by repeated and multiple spontaneous hemorrhages in the skin, mucous membranes, serous cavities and viscera. Thrombocytopenia may be secondary to toxic bone marrow depression or to replacement of marrow by neoplasm, but it is often idiopathic in etiology. Symptomatic purpura may result from drug reactions or senility or may be of the Schoenlein-Henoch type. Although platelet counts may be normal, intracranial bleeding can occur.

Meningeal and intracerebral hemorrhages are either pinpoint and diffuse or massive and localized and are the usual cause of death. Cranial nerve palsies, convulsions, aphasia and hemiplegia have all been reported. All types of ocular hemorrhage are seen. Engel *et al.* and Ladwig found widespread occlusions of capillaries, arterioles and venules in thrombotic thrombocytopenic purpura. Neurologic symptoms are particularly varied and manifold in this type of purpura, which is thought to be associated with periarteritis nodosa.

Splenectomy often cures idiopathic cases. Transfusions are always indicated and corticotropin and cortisone are said to be of benefit. Other more rare hemorrhagic diseases which are complicated by intracranial episodes are hereditary pseudohemophilia (thrombasthenic purpura), idio-

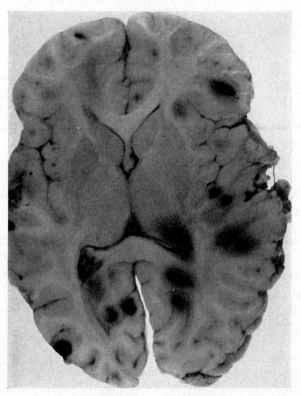

FIG. 115.—Multiple cerebral hemorrhages. Acute lymphatic leukemia. (George Washington University Laboratory of Neurology.)

pathic (familial) hypothrombinemia and afibrinogenemia. Cerebral hemorrhage has been reported in all.

NEOPLASTIC BLOOD DYSCRASIAS.—The designation neoplastic is applied here to the leukemias and to polycythemia vera. Invasion of the bone marrow and liver by carcinoma and sarcoma may also cause hemorrhagic phenomena in the brain by replacement of megakaryocytes or by interference with prothrombin formation.

Leukemia.—Cerebral and meningeal hemorrhages, small and large, are not uncommon in both myelogenous and lymphatic leukemia, more often in the acute than in the chronic stages of the disease (Fig. 115). Major intracerebral hemorrhage may cause death. Histologic study of the brain often reveals perivascular extravasations and distended small vessels which may be thrombosed with plugs of leukemic cells. The latter are also identifiable distally in the cerebral tissue or sheaths of cranial nerves. Transverse sinus thrombosis has occurred.

General evidences of leukemia include fever, weight loss, adenopathy, splenomegaly, hepatomegaly, jaundice, anemia and purpura. Retinal hem-

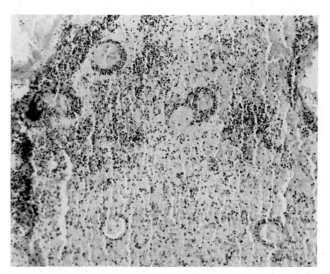

FIG. 116.—Perivascular extravasations of nucleated erythrocytes in cerebral infarct. Polycythemia vera.

orrhages appear in the fiber layer but may be subhyaloid. Diagnosis is established by finding immature myeloid or lymphoid elements in the peripheral blood, bone marrow or lymph nodes. The etiology of leukemia is unknown but in certain occupational groups such as roentgenologists the disease incidence is far greater than that in the general population. Most cases speed to fatal termination, but x-ray therapy to spleen, liver and the body generally and the use of corticotropin, cortisone or antifolic drugs may retard the progress appreciably, particularly of the lymphatic type. Radioactive phosphorus is also said to be somewhat successful. Transfusions are indicated when there is severe secondary anemia. A new chemical agent, 6-mercaptopurine has been found to have an antileukemic effect which may be promising.

Polycythemia vera.—Symptoms referable to the head outnumber those of any other body system in polycythemia vera. Cerebrovascular lesions include subdural, subarachnoid or intracerebral hemorrhage and arterial or venous thromboses (Fig. 116). The most sluggish cerebral circulation time ever recorded was in a patient with polycythemia (Kety). Etiology is obscure; the disease appears to be related to leukemia, in which it may terminate. Occasionally, removal of a cerebellar hemangioblastoma has resulted in disappearance of polycythemia. The usual symptoms and signs are hypertension, red-blue cyanosis and enlargement of spleen and liver. Headache, convulsions, aphasia and hemiplegia are related to brain involvement. The retinal veins are engorged, the arteries purple and the optic disks edematous. Hemorrhages are frequently seen in the fundus, either the central retinal artery or vein may be occluded.

Hematologic findings of erythrocytosis (up to 10,000,000–12,000,000 per cu. mm.) and rapidity of coagulation establish the diagnosis. Cerebrospinal fluid pressure may be extreme and the fluid is often bloody. Many patients die of heart failure or cerebral accident; others become leukemic. Venesection is an excellent emergency treatment and may restore the comatose patient to normal, indicating the role which simple intracranial plethora due to increased blood volume and viscosity may play in producing cerebral signs and increase in intracranial pressure. Oral administration of radioactive phosphorus is a simple and effective method of keeping polycythemia vera under control (Duffy and Howland). Every patient should be surveyed for hemangioblastoma of the cerebellum. Very high red blood cell counts are also found in patients with congenital heart disease and pulmonary emphysema, arteriosclerosis or fibrosis. Thrombosis of cerebral arteries has been encountered in patients with congenital cardiac disorders.

VITAMIN DEFICIENCIES

AVITAMINOSIS C.—Intracranial hemorrhages, subdural and subarachnoid but intracerebral as well, occasionally complicate severe scurvy. Subdural hematoma usually implies trauma in addition. Thrombosis of the basilar artery has also been reported. Avitaminosis C is most common today in neglected infants. Subperiosteal hemorrhages, ecchymoses in the skin and mucous membranes and changes in the bones and teeth are general signs. The diet must really be deficient in all forms of fresh vegetables, meat and fish to produce scurvy, which takes about six months to develop. Treatment depends on giving vitamin C, as orange juice, other fruit and vegetable extracts or ascorbic acid. Vitamin P is also usually lacking.

AVITAMINOSIS K.—Deficiency in vitamin K causes bleeding because of an impaired formation of prothrombin by the liver. This takes place in adults with severe hepatic disease but is much more common in infants. Hemorrhagic disease of the newborn may result from an accentuation of normally low prothrombin production just after birth or from sepsis, syphilitic hepatitis, icterus gravis or erythroblastosis fetalis (Fig. 117). It appears three to four days to two to three weeks after birth.

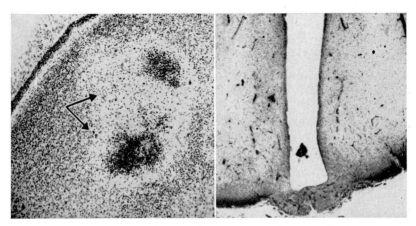

FIG. 117 *(left)*.—Ring hemorrhages (arrows) in cerebellum. Erythroblastosis fetalis.
FIG. 118 *(right)*.—Minute hypothalamic hemorrhages. Wernicke's disease (thiamine deficiency).

Petechiae and ecchymoses are multiple in the body. Intracranial hemorrhage, the commonest cause of death, develops in 10–20 per cent of these infants and is manifested in convulsions, stupor, coma, a bulging fontanel and bloody or xanthochromic cerebrospinal fluid. The newborn infant is severely anemic, and the clotting time may be prolonged to 10 minutes or more.

Total blood replacement is the treatment for erythroblastosis due to Rh incompatibility in the parents. Other infants with hemorrhagic disease should receive 25 mg. of vitamin K twice a day for three days, in addition to transfusion of 5–8 cc. matched parent's blood per pound of body weight. Mortality from cerebral hemorrhage is over 50 per cent. Heparin or Dicumarol given to the mother ante partum may be responsible for deficiency of vitamin K and intracranial vascular accident in the infant.

AVITAMINOSIS B.—Severe deficiency of vitamin B intake of sudden appearance will result in Wernicke's polioencephalitis hemorrhagica superior. This syndrome is usually attributed to alcoholism, but of the cases originally reported by Wernicke (1881), one was associated with esophageal cicatrix after a suicidal attempt and another with severe gastric pathologic change. The single common factor is lack of absorption of vitamin B_1 (thiamine). Varicose deformities of blood vessels, vascular proliferations, fresh and old hemorrhages and ganglion cell necrosis are found in the gray matter lining the third and fourth ventricles and intervening cerebral aqueduct (Fig. 118). The hypothalamic, cranial neural and cerebellar nuclei are particularly involved.

Clinically, delirium tremens passes into a state of chronic psychosis featured by retrograde amnesia filled in with confabulation—the Korsakoff syndrome. Ophthalmoplegias, alterations of the state of consciousness, nausea, vertigo, ataxia and other vestibulocerebellar signs are common. Beriberi polyneuropathy and cardiac failure are often present. Administration of remarkably small amounts of vitamin B_1 have cleared symptoms and signs of Wernicke's disease, but large doses of thiamine (50 mg. one to three times daily) are in order for safety's sake. Other dietary factors should also be supplied in large quantity.

CEREBROVASCULAR POISONS

CARBON MONOXIDE.—Carbon monoxide inhalation produces lesions in the brain not only by a direct or anoxic effect on neurons but also through damage of cerebral vessels. Carbon monoxide unites with hemoglobin more readily than does oxygen, and a stable compound is formed. Carboxyhemoglobin is detectable in spectroscopic analysis of the blood and imparts to the tissues of the monoxide victim a cherry red color. In fatal cases, the brain is congested, edematous and bright pink. Petechial hemorrhages are seen on section; the globus pallidus nuclei and substantia nigra may be visibly necrotic if life has been sufficiently prolonged. Softened areas are present elsewhere in the cortex and interior of the cerebrum and cerebellum, particularly where end-arteries exist (internal capsule, Ammon's horn). Vasodilatation, paralysis and thromboses are seen histologically; the medial coats of larger vessels may be destroyed and even calcified chronically. Endothelial proliferation and swelling further tend to occlude vascular lumens. Perivascular hemorrhages, infarction and demyelination are often present; necrobiotic foci and laminar destruction in the cortex are of purely anoxic origin.

If 10–20 per cent monoxide saturation is present in inspired air, symptoms are minor; with 30–50 per cent saturation, complaints are severe, and with 50–60 per cent, unconsciousness and convulsions ensue. Above this level, paralysis of respiration and of heart beat result (Ford). The usual subjective sensations are headache, flushing of the face and vertigo. More extensive toxicity produces nausea and vomiting, ataxia, weakness, tremor and collapse. On recovery from severe exposure, chronic parkinsonian states, focal neurologic deficit, spasticity, convulsions, psychosis or a vegetative existence may be serious residuals. In milder cases, the only defect may be one of retrograde amnesia. Peripheral neuropathy can result as well and may mimic poliomyelitis. Diagnosis depends on the recognition of carbon monoxide hemoglobin (spectroscope) or on experienced observation. Treatment includes inhalation of 5–7 per cent carbon dioxide with oxygen in concentration below 80 per cent and circulatory support, particularly with transfusions.

LEAD.—Lead is a diffuse vascular poison. It affects the child much more often than the adult not only because of the infant's frequent ingestion of lead paint but because of some immature susceptibility. Anemia may be severe and is accompanied by colic, neuritis and encephalopathy. Cerebral symptoms may be the first evidence of lead poisoning, especially in children. Convulsive seizures, hypertension and signs of greatly increased intracranial pressure with or without focal neurologic deficit form the picture of lead encephalopathy. In autopsy specimens, the brain is swollen, pale and edematous, with a well marked cerebellar pressure cone. The leptomeninges are thickened and fibrous. Petechial hemorrhages are visible in microscopic sections in which proliferation of capillaries and the endothelium of larger vessels has occurred almost to a granulomatous degree. In chronic disease, there is hyalinization of the arterial media. One form of "hemorrhagic encephalopathy" is caused by inhalation of lead tetraethyl gasoline.

Diagnosis is established by the finding of stippled erythrocytes in blood smears and the detection of excessive amounts of lead in the serum and urine. In children, increased density is visible on x-rays of the metaphyseal, growing ends of the long bones. With lead encephalopathy in infants the cerebrospinal fluid pressure may be as high as 1,000 mm. of water; the fluid is yellow, the protein content may be increased to above 100 mg. per 100 ml., and the cell count may attain several thousand per cu. mm. Increased convolutional atrophy is evident in skull films.

BAL (2, 3-dimercaptopropanol) is used in treatment. Dosage is 3 mg. per kilogram of body weight six times a day for two days, four times during the third day, and twice daily for 10 days. Calcium versenate seems to be particularly effective in mobilizing lead for urinary excretion while keeping it in an inactive form. The prognosis in lead encephalopathy is not very favorable. Convulsions must be controlled. Subtemporal or suboccipital cranial decompressions can be undertaken to save vision and life while the process of "de-leading" is carried out (Haverfield et al.).

ARSENIC.—Arsenic is also toxic to the cerebral vascular endothelium. Small vessel damage and perivascular extravasations in the meninges and cerebrum produce the picture of "hemorrhagic encephalopathy" in severe cases. Capillary thromboses and rhexes with acute neuronal change are visible microscopically.

Hemorrhagic encephalopathy can appear one or two days after the first intravenous injection of an arsenical compound. Headache, fever, irritability, stupor, vomiting and convulsions progress to coma and death in a high percentage of these patients. The diagnosis of arsenic poisoning is made by examination of gastric contents, hair, nails and urine. The cerebrospinal fluid pressure may be elevated, and specimens are bloody or show slight pleocytosis and hyperproteinism. Injections of epinephrine, atropine, sodium thiosulfate and calcium gluconate are useful in arsenical encephalopathy, and BAL is also recommended.

OTHER TOXIC AGENTS.—Mercurialism may cause vascular changes similar to those of lead and arsenic, and perivascular ring hemorrhages appear in the brain. Basal ganglial degeneration results in a form of parkinsonism. Manganese (industrial) poisoning thickens and occludes small cerebral vessels as well as attacking the striate bodies.

Carbon disulfide inhaled in toxic amounts causes widespread degenerative changes in the ganglion cells of basal ganglions and substantia nigra and also produces endothelial proliferation and thickening and hyalinization of arterioles. Hemiplegia from cerebral hemorrhage has been reported.

The vasoconstricting drug ergot and its compounds affect brain arteries and arterioles. Weakness, headache and dysesthesias are followed by convulsions, jerkings, hallucinatory and delusional psychosis and coma. Ischemia and infarction are evident grossly in the brain in fatal cases; thromboses and hyaline degeneration are seen microscopically. The therapeutic use of vasodilating substances (sympathicolytics, histamine) is mandatory.

Larger vessels are stated to be unaffected by major therapeutic doses of roentgen rays (Wachowski and Chenault). In a series of microscopic sections from brains that were heavily irradiated during the treatment of glioma I have seen significant endothelial proliferation and medial hyalinization and thickening of arterioles and venules.

BIBLIOGRAPHY

Duffy, B. J., and Howland, J. W.: Clinical uses of radiophosphorus, New York J. Med. 52:551-554, 1952.

Engel, G. L.; Scheinker, I. M., and Humphrey, D. C.: Acute febrile anemia and thrombocytopenic purpura with vasothrombosis, Ann. Int. Med. 26:919-933, 1947.

Ford, F. R.: *Diseases of the Nervous System in Infancy, Childhood and Adolescence* (Springfield, Ill.: Charles C Thomas, Publisher, 1937).

Haverfield, W. T.; Bucy, P. C., and Elonen, A. S.: The surgical treatment of lead encephalopathy, J.A.M.A. 114:2432-2437, 1940.

Kety, S. S.: The physiology of the human cerebral circulation, Anesthesiology 10:610-614, 1949.

Ladwig, H. A.: The central nervous system in thrombotic thrombocytopenic purpura, Neurology 3:267-276, 1953.

Patterson, R. H.; Wilson, H., and Diggs, L. W.: Sickle cell anemia: A surgical problem, Surgery 28:393-403, 1950.

Sanford, H. N.; Hall, F. R., and Butler, S.: Further studies on the influence of histamine on platelet activity, with especial reference to its action on the blood of the hemophiliac patient, Pediatrics 9:212-219, 1952.

Scheinberg, P.: Cerebral blood flow and metabolism in pernicious anemia, Blood 6:213-227, 1951.

Wachowski, T. J., and Chenault, H.: Degenerative effects of large doses of roentgen rays on the human brain, Radiology 45:227-246, 1945.

Walker, D. W., and Murphy, J. P.: Sickle cell anemia complicated by acute rheumatic fever and massive cerebral hemorrhage, J. Pediat. 19:28-37, 1941.

Walsh, F. B.: *Clinical Neuro-ophthalmology* (Baltimore: Williams & Wilkins Company, 1947).

CHAPTER 18

Headache

HEADACHE IS a common presenting complaint of patients seeking medical assistance. The incidence of various types of headache among adults of all ages and occupations is almost 65 per cent. Rare in childhood and infrequent in old age, headache afflicts 75 per cent of persons aged 21–30, sporadically or chronically. Women are more subject to headache than are men. Single persons suffer from headache more than do the married. Eighty per cent of college students but only 40 per cent of young adults with little or no education have headaches. Among those whose work involves tension, worry and responsibility, headache is of frequent occurrence; laborers are relatively free from headache.

PHYSIOLOGY OF HEADACHE

Vasosensory, vasomotor innervation.—Within the cranium the large vascular channels, arterial and venous, are pain sensitive; those above and in front of the tentorium cerebelli are supplied by the trigeminal nerve and those in the posterior fossa by the glossopharyngeal, vagus and hypoglossal cranial nerves and the upper three cervical posterior sensory roots. Extracranially, all soft tissues are sensitive, particularly the arteries.

One function of the greater superficial petrosal division of the facial nerve is presumably that of vasodilation of the intracranial circulation. Gardner *et al.* and others have reported relief from paroxysmal unilateral cephalalgia in some patients after removal of the parasympathetic innervation of the facial complexes. Vasodilator fibers in the trigeminal nerve are believed to account for true headache and other vasomotor phenomena accompanying tic douloureux. The possible participation of the sympathetic nerves in painful phenomena of the head and neck is obscure; Leriche and Fontaine declared that the cervical sympathetic chain conducts pain impulses from the craniocervical region, and attempts to relieve headache by interruption of sympathetic pathways have been successful on rare occasion (Campbell and Evans).

Mechanisms of headache.—There are six fundamental processes which can produce headache of intracranial origin (Wolff): (1) displacement of the great venous sinuses and traction on entering veins; (2) traction on the middle meningeal arteries; (3) torsion or displacement of the large arterial members of the circle of Willis and their immediate branches; (4) distention and dilatation of intracranial arteries; (5) inflammation in or about pain sensitive structures within the head, and (6) direct pressure by tumors on cranial and cervical nerves conducting pain afferent fibers from the head to the brain.

Headache of extracranial origin may be caused by (1) dilatation of arteries of the scalp; (2) trauma to scalp arteries and nerves; (3) contraction of and inflammatory changes in the muscles inserting on the skull; (4) inflammation of other soft tissues of the head, including the blood vessels; (5) errors of refraction, injury or inflammation of the eye; (6) pathologic changes in the nose and paranasal sinuses, and (7) neuralgias of the trigeminal and occipital nerves. Arterial dilatation is the single most common factor in all headaches, particularly if "throbbing" in character, when each systolic impulse gives an excessive stretch-stimulus to painful, distended vessels.

Associated phenomena.—The concomitance of dizziness, nausea and vomiting, irritability and vasomotor phenomena with headache is more than coincidental. It appears that these symptoms are in some way the direct result of head pain, since the giving of pure analgesics or periarterial infiltration of procaine in tender areas of the scalp will often relieve vertigo and nausea as headache disappears. Trigeminal reflexes activating autonomic nuclei in the hypothalamus and brain stem may be responsible for these features of the headache syndrome.

Differential Diagnosis

The diagnostic features of headache of various etiologies are summarized in Table 2.

Migraine (Hemicrania)

Migraine is one of the most painful, obstinate and widespread of functional diseases. It was known to Aretaeus of Cappadocia in the first century A.D., so it cannot be considered entirely a legacy of the frenetic modern age although paroxysmal headache has been called the com-

TABLE 2.—Differential Diagnosis of Headache

Type or Cause of Headache	Etiology	Pathogenesis	Location	Onset	Frequency	Neurol. Signs	Neuro-radiology	EEG	CSF
Migraine	?, psychogenic, allergic, hereditary	Vasoconstriction, dilatation, edema	Hemicranium, elsewhere	Gradual, A.M.	Cyclic	±	−	±	−
Histamine headache	?, psychogenic, allergic	Vasodilatation, edema	Hemicranium, face, neck	Sudden, early A.M.	Series with intervals	−	−	−	−
Cerebrovascular accident	Hemorrhage, thrombosis, embolism	Vascular torsion, occlusion	Head generally, locally	Sudden or gradual	Persistent after CVA	+	+	+	+
Subarachnoid hemorrhage	Aneurysm, vascular anomaly, other	Vascular rupture, nerve irritation	Head generally, locally, neck	Sudden, severe	Constant until subsidence	±	±	±	+
Cerebral arteriosclerosis	Arterial hardening	Vascular rigidity	Head generally, vertex	Gradual	Constant, remissions	±	±	±	±
Intracranial mass	Neoplasm, hematoma, abscess	Vascular torsion, dural tension	Head generally, locally	Gradual, early A.M.	Intermittent, becoming constant	+	+	+	+
Hypertension	"Essential," other	Vascular rigidity, dilatation	Vertex, occipital	Gradual or sudden	Daily	±	±	±	±
Post-traumatic	Head injury	Vasodilatation, scalp contusion, neck sprain	Vicinity of trauma, neck	After trauma or later	Constant until subsidence	±	±	±	−
Tension, anxiety	Psychogenic	Vasodilatation, muscle spasm	Vertex, band, neck	Gradual, sudden, P.M.	Daily or constant	−	−	−	−
Menopausal	Hormonal, psychogenic	Vasodilatation, muscle spasm	Vertex, neck	Gradual, A.M.	Intermittent or constant	−	−	−	−
Ocular	Astigmatism, inflammation	Ocular muscle pain, referred	Frontal, suboccipital	Gradual, P.M.	Regular	−	−	−	−
Nasal, sinal, dental	Inflammation, allergy, neoplasm	Trigeminal nerve irritation	Frontal, face	Gradual, sudden, early A.M.	Intermittent or constant	−	−	−	−
Cervical spine	Arthritis, spondylitis, discogenic	Cervical radiculitis	Cervico-occipital, frontal	Gradual, sudden	Intermittent or constant	±	+	−	−
Myositis, fibrositis	Inflammation, psychogenic	Muscle spasm, painful nodules	Cervico-occipital	Gradual	Constant until subsidence	−	−	−	−

monest complaint of civilized peoples. The condition is particularly rife among professional "brain" workers; many vivid descriptions of personal attacks of headache have been given by physicians.

Etiology.—Heredity plays a definite role; in the family of a migraine patient, one in 10 is also afflicted and one in 55 is epileptic. The disease is sex-linked to the extent that it occurs in women in the ratio of 2:1. Personality characteristics include perfectionism, rigidity and pronounced aggressive drives. Migraine patients are meticulous and obsessive and have a fear of failure and criticism. Psychogenic precipitation of an attack is often obvious in an individual to whom every problem, major or minor, is a "real headache;" Wolff calls the migraine patient "stress-addicted."

Elevation of the serum sodium level and hydration of the blood accompanies edema of the body in the premigraine phase of the disease. Onset of headaches at puberty, their cessation during pregnancy and at the menopause in women implicate a hormonal influence, possibly operating through regulation of body water. The urinary excretion of 17-ketosteroids is increased in an attack. More than a few patients are allergic to certain foods, particularly chocolate, milk, wheat, pork and inhalants, intake of which will set off a typical headache.

Intracranial aneurysm must always be thought of in ophthalmoplegic migraine when ocular palsies develop in an otherwise typically migrainous situation. Typical migraine headache is rarely symptomatic of cerebral arteriovenous malformation.

Pathogenesis.—The excruciating headache in migraine has been proved to be the result of paroxysmal dilatation of branches of the external carotid artery, particularly the superficial temporal, deep temporal, middle meningeal and occipital vessels, with accompanying enlargement and swelling of major arteries of the circle of Willis to a variable degree. Neurologic phenomena which precede the headache and may represent an attack in entirety are undoubtedly of cerebral angiospastic origin. Objective studies of the pulse waves of cranial arteries during migrainous vascular headache confirm the progression of change from vasoconstriction through vasodilatation to vasoedema (Tunis and Wolff) (Fig. 119). Temporal pulse changes may precede the onset of headache by several days.

External vasodilatation may compensate for intracranial vasoconstriction. Hemicranial pain can be precipitated or reproduced in the susceptible by injection of histamine, administration of nitroglycerin sublingually or induction of the partially anoxic state by simulated high altitude. Headache is relieved at least temporarily by compressing the superficial temporal or external carotid arteries but not by increasing intracranial pressure experimentally. This indicates a lesser participation of intracranial arteries in migraine than in histamine headache.

Symptoms and signs.—Onset is usually in adolescence but may take place in childhood; cyclic vomiting is often a precursor of later headache. There is almost always a history of similar attacks in the immediate family. Headaches are recurrent, begin in the frontotemporal region, are throbbing and unilateral (hemicrania) and at onset appear against a

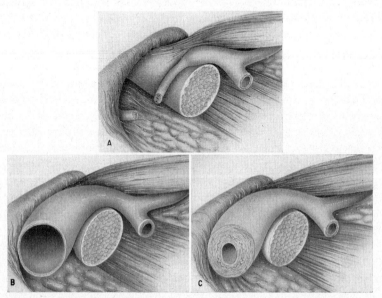

FIG. 119.—Vascular changes in migraine. *A*, vasoconstriction; *B*, vasodilatation; *C*, arterial edema. (Courtesy of Sandoz Pharmaceuticals Co.)

background of relative well-being. Vasospastic visual disorders often precede pain. These may take the form of scintillating scotomas, photophobia, blurred vision or hemianopsia. There may be severe neurologic deficits such as aphasia, hemiparesis, paresthesias or mood change of an organic character. Nausea, vomiting, other autonomic phenomena and irritability occur at the height of an attack. The superficial temporal arteries become rigid, pipelike and exquisitely sensitive as headache becomes agonizing. Each seizure usually lasts from "sunup to sundown" but can be longer or shorter in duration. The victim often passes large quantities of pale urine at or near the termination of an attack and the next day is unusually bright and clear, as a morning after a rain.

Variations of the classic hemicranial pattern and "migraine equivalents" are several. When intracranial vessels are participating in an attack, dilatation of the anterior circle of Willis causes pain in the eye or forehead, and postauricular or occipital headache results from swelling of the basilar or vertebral arteries. Painful sensation may be experienced only in the face or jaw. "Equivalent" states include attacks of pain in the chest (precordial migraine), abdomen (abdominal migraine or epilepsy) or extremities, gastrointestinal upsets, mental depression, diffuse edema and otherwise unexplained fever. In some patients vasospasm of the vessels of the brain with resultant temporary loss of vision, speech, orientation, sensation or motor power constitutes the entire attack and headache is minimal or absent. Hemiplegic migraine may be familial.

Organic complications.—The ocular palsies of ophthalmoplegic migraine are usually but not invariably reversible. In two patients Alpers and Yaskin did not find an anticipated berry aneurysm and attributed the syndrome to vasomotor changes in cranial nuclei or to recurrent pressure on extraocular nerves by enlargement and edema of the circle of Willis. Permanent occlusion of the central artery of the retina has been observed and is considered to be the result of spasm of a vessel already sclerosed. Dunning described verified instances of both cerebral infarction and cerebral hemorrhage in migraine, without discoverable thrombosis or evident vascular rupture at autopsy.

Electroencephalography.—In 1,000 cases of nonorganic headache, Ulett and associates found abnormal electroencephalograms in 9.7 per cent of males and 20.5 per cent of females. Sugar called attention to the frequency of asymmetry of amplitude in the electroencephalograms of patients with migraine, relating this finding to diminished cerebral blood supply. Low potential is ipsilateral with brain involvement, as indicated by hemianopsia, but is not necessarily present on the same side as headache. Abnormal electroencephalograms were found in 60 per cent of a group of migraine patients with predictable neurologic phenomena (Dow and Whitty).

The relation between migraine and epilepsy is strengthened by such observations; 26.5 per cent of patients with migraine examined by Cohn had moderate to maximal electroencephalographic irregularities, indistinguishable from the patterns of certain convulsive disorders or of arterial hypertension. A common finding in epileptic migraine is a choppy, irrregular resting electroencephalogram with breakdown into sustained, high-voltage slow waves of paroxysmal appearance during and after hyperventilation.

Diagnosis and therapy.—The diagnosis of migraine must be restricted to the typical syndrome and not applied loosely to any type of periodic headache. Of essential character are a hereditary or familial history, rigid and perfectionistic personality traits, prodromes usually of a visual type, recurrence of unilateral cephalalgia, association of nausea and vomiting and relief by the usual remedies. The general physical and neurologic examinations are usually negative, as are x-rays of the skull and cervical spine and results of spinal puncture. Electroencephalograms are normal except in the epileptic type of the disease. Typical vasodilating headache may be induced in most migraine patients by the sublingual administration of 1.3 mg. (1/50 gr.) of nitroglycerin.

Medical treatment in migraine is the treatment of choice, and surgery is to be used only occasionally and as a last resort. In the management of migraine or of any other headache, it should be emphasized that analgesia without further investigation may lead to disability or death.

Psychotherapy is helpful prophylactically in one half to two thirds of the patients. The migraine patient should be advised to seek more relaxation, avoid worry over minor problems, make his ambitions commensurate with his capabilities and develop tolerance of himself and others.

During an actual attack, few patients are interested in the elaboration of psychodynamisms and all demand relief from pain. In headache of low intensity, aspirin or compounds of aspirin, phenacetin and caffeine orally in doses of 0.3–0.6 Gm., with possible addition of 32–65 mg. of codeine, may be sufficient. When pain is of high intensity, specific therapy is in order, and it must be used during the spastic or dilatory vascular stages before the development of vessel edema (nausea and vomiting).

Ergotamine tartrate may be injected intramuscularly in 0.25–0.5 mg. doses or used sublingually as 4–5 mg. tablets which may be repeated once or twice at 30 minute intervals. Not more than 0.5 mg. intramuscularly or 11 mg. orally should be given per week, and the drug is contraindicated in infectious conditions, hypertension, impaired hepatic or renal function, pregnancy and general vascular diseases, spastic or sclerotic. Disagreeable side effects include numbness and tingling of the extremities, muscle cramps and stiffness, and nausea and vomiting.

Dihydroergotamine (DHE-45) is better tolerated and may be used during pregnancy. It is given subcutaneously or intravenously in 0.5–1 mg. amount. Approximately 80-85 per cent of patients will be relieved with either ergotamine or dihydroergotamine, provided the drugs are used early enough in an attack. Oral combinations of ergotamine with belladonna, phenobarbital or caffeine (Cafergot) may be quite effective in aborting attacks of migraine or other head pain. One mg. of ergotamine tartrate may be administered with 100 mg. of caffeine citrate by mouth, or 2 mg. of ergotamine combined with 100–200 mg. of caffeine, 0.4 mg. of atropine sulfate or 0.25 mg. of Bellafoline may be used as a rectal suppository in patients unable to retain oral medication. Octin (methylisooctenylamine) is also useful as a vasoconstrictor to relieve dilating headaches, but it raises the blood pressure considerably.

Restriction of salt for two weeks before onset of the menses and diuretics are recommended for dehydration in menstrual migraine. Foods to which the patient is allergic should be forbidden. Hormonal therapy is reported to be valuable in women (Blumenthal and Fuchs). Progesterone in the latter half of the menstrual cycle may prevent edema, or testosterone can be used to suppress ovulation. Histamine desensitization is sometimes successful, as it is in histamine cephalalgia. Nicotinic acid in 100 mg. amounts intravenously or orally may rarely and paradoxically be helpful. Inhalation of carbon dioxide-oxygen mixtures may stop an incipient migraine episode if used in the vasoconstrictive phase. If the electroencephalogram is abnormal, anticonvulsant drugs are indicated and may quite effectively control headache.

Surgery may rarely be in order if a patient cannot take ergot derivatives because of vascular disease or is dominated by unalterable habits and life situations. When external pressure on painful scalp vessels or the periarterial infiltration of procaine will eliminate headache temporarily, resection of portions of the temporal or occipital arteries will relieve pain ipsilaterally for a time. If cephalalgia is diminished by temporal compression and is stopped by common carotid occlusion, ligation of the middle meningeal artery may be effective. Alcohol injection of the gasserian ganglion or retrogasserian neurotomy will prevent anterior headache at the cost of anesthesia of the face, including the cornea.

HISTAMINE HEADACHE

The concept of histamine headache was introduced into clinical medicine by Horton of the Mayo Clinic. True histamine cephalalgia is relatively rare, occurring most often in men of middle age. The severe unilateral headache comes on suddenly, lasts for one to two hours or more, involves the orbit, nose, teeth, temple and neck and is associated with stuffiness of the homolateral naris and tearing of the eye. Discomfort is often so intense as to make the victim contemplate suicide. Pain distribution corresponds to the branching of the external carotid artery, which is tender. Associated dilatation of the internal carotid is indicated by the relief from head-ache during jugular compression, experimental elevation of cerebrospinal fluid pressure or increase in positive g by centrifugal force which drains blood from the cerebral arteries. Conversely, jolting the cranium makes headache worse.

The fundamental cause is unknown, but excess production of hista-mine or an "H-substance" in the body in some reactive manner is believed to be pathogenetic of cranial vasodilatation. Psychogenic factors are re-sponsible at least to a degree comparable to that in migraine. Gastric acidity increases during a bout of headache and a relationship exists between peptic ulcer and histamine cephalalgia.

Diagnosis and therapy.—Diagnosis is made by reproduction of an attack when 0.35 mg. of histamine base is injected subcutaneously. Not only does an immediate, generalized headache appear, but the full blown syndrome comes on 30–50 minutes after injection. Adrenalin (1:400,000) given intravenously will stop the headache but must be used with caution.

An acute attack may be aborted by intravenous injection of 1 mg. of dihydroergotamine, the breathing of pure oxygen or use of a rectal sup-pository containing 2 mg. of ergotamine tartrate and 100–200 mg. of caffeine. A program of desensitization is often effective prophylactically. Histamine base (0.275 mg. in 1 cc.) is used, beginning with 0.05 cc. injected subcutaneously and repeated in six to eight hours. Two injections are then given daily, increasing the amount 0.05 cc. each time until 0.5–1 cc. is reached (Horton). Milk or aluminum gel tablets should be given with each injection to prevent activation of peptic ulcer. Treatments may then be carried on twice a week or more often, as necessary. Precipitation of symptoms by histamine desensitization calls for no or minimal increase in dosage. Daily or twice weekly intravenous infusions of 0.275 mg. of histamine in 500 cc. saline solution may be used instead. The success of these programs is attributed to the psychologic effect of ritualism by critics of the organic interpretation of the syndrome. Benadryl and other antihistamines may be of diagnostic or temporary therapeutic value. Apres-oline in small doses (5–10 mg. four times daily) has been reported to prevent attacks of histamine headache.

Dandy reported cure in two patients who had what must have been histamine cephalalgia by extirpation of the ipsilateral inferior cervical and first thoracic sympathetic ganglions; this experience has not been confirmed by others. Resection of the greater superficial petrosal nerve has relieved attacks in about one third of patients, but regeneration of the nerve prevents permanent relief (Gardner *et al.*).

Atypical Facial Neuralgia

This common complaint, baffling in etiology and therapy, is closely related to migraine and histamine headache. Indeed, the condition often represents a topographic variant of either. Atypical facial neuralgia was described and so named by Glaser. There is no reason to believe that buccal neuralgia, Sluder's (sphenopalatine) neuralgia, vidian neuralgia and carotid pain are essentially different conditions.

The etiology is ill defined, although atypical facial neuralgia appears to be a truly psychosomatic disease (Engel). Facial pain often seems to be only one of many neurotic elaborations; a history of nervous breakdown, alcoholism or peptic ulcer is common in this group of patients. Fay, Hilger and others regard dilatation of the carotid artery and external branches to be responsible for disagreeable sensations. Hardly a patient is ever relieved by surgical therapy directed to the nose or paranasal sinuses. Watts believes that hypothyroidism often causes atypical facial pain and advises thyroid medication if the basal metabolic rate is low. Diseases of the cervical spine, such as ruptured disk or arthritis, may occasionally be accompanied by head and face pains resembling atypical neuralgia. Intracranial aneurysm is also a cause of facial dysesthesias.

The disease chiefly affects white adults, women more often than men, and the general personal background is psychoneurotic. Pain often comes on at night (4 A.M.) and begins in the interior or at the base of the nose, upper jaw or just below the rim of the orbit in the vicinity of the infraorbital foramen. It is unilateral and is described as "boring," "grinding" or "drawing." Pain is steady and not lancinating, as is true trigeminal neuralgia, and lasts for hours or days. Tearing and nasal congestion develop, as in histamine headache, and spread of the pain often includes the whole half of the head, neck, shoulder, arm and sometimes radiates to the heel. Painful areas on the head and the carotid artery are tender. The carotid bifurcation may be thought to be a "swollen gland." Discretely sensitive and edematous areas often correspond to the distribution of a specific arterial division. The patient becomes depressed, hopeless and often suicidal if relief is not obtained.

Atypical facial neuralgia must be distinguished from true trigeminal neuralgia, because alcohol or surgical destruction of branches or roots of the fifth cranial nerve, which is so effective in tic douloureux, not only does not usually relieve the atypical neuralgic patient, but may make him worse as anesthesia and paresthesias are added to the original complaint. In contrast to trigeminal neuralgia, the pain spreads beyond the confines of the fifth and ninth nerves and is not relieved by local anesthesia of branches of these nerves; the pain is steady, not paroxysmal, and there are no trigger zones. The age group is younger in atypical than in trigeminal or glossopharyngeal neuralgia. Finally, vasodilators make pain worse, whereas vasoconstrictors may relieve, the reverse being true in tic douloureux.

Therapy.—Treatment is largely medical and psychotherapeutic. If psychodynamic factors are predominant, the patient should be made to realize this. On the other hand, the antimigrainous or the histamine desensitization program may prove to be rewarding. An oral preparation of ergotamine, belladonna and phenobarbital (Bellergal) is often effective during acute attacks. Caution must be used in ordering opiates because of a strong tendency to addiction. If thyroid deficiency or a pathologic change in the cervical spine is present, it should be corrected.

Procaine derivatives should be used if nerve blocks are to be done. Alcohol is not to be used except as a last resort. In almost all cases, no relief is obtained by coagulation, neurectomy or neurotomy of the trigeminal nerve or its branches. Greater superficial neurectomy has been of benefit occasionally. Application of cocaine or Pontocaine to the sphenopalatine ganglion is sometimes effective; however, cocaine dependency may develop. Reichert observed that resection of peripheral arteries in the face and head may benefit an occasional patient. Perhaps superior cervical ganglionectomy should be given a further trial, since the nerve supply of the external carotid tree comes from the superior cervical ganglion. In particularly refractory and potentially suicidal cases, prefrontal lobotomy is in order when all other measures have failed and the situation is desperate.

POST-TRAUMATIC HEADACHE

In the absence of intracranial hematoma, post-traumatic cephalalgia is of three kinds and origins. Local pain or tenderness at the fresh site of impact or in a scar is due to bruising or fibrosis of nerve endings in the scalp. Caplike or vertex pressure discomfort is caused by sustained contraction of skeletal muscles and is accentuated by tension and anxiety. Attacks of throbbing pain, resembling migraine or histamine headache, result from paroxysmal dilatation of arteries (Wolff).

The pathogenesis of many sustained postinjury states involves all etiologic factors—scalp contusion, anxiety and vasodilatation. In any head trauma, the striking force is usually sufficient to produce soft tissue damage, which is particularly painful if branches of the trigeminal or cervical plexuses are involved. Loss of self-confidence and fear are induced by the patient's belief that following injury to the all-important cranium he cannot now "use his head" or "keep his head above water" (Wolff). This psychologic pattern is perpetuated if insurance compensation offers a soft bed meanwhile. If the pretraumatic makeup of the patient is potentially migrainous, an otherwise insignificant blow may be sufficient to initiate a cycle of recurrent spontaneous headaches. Many post-traumatic headache syndromes result from wrenching and spraining of cervical ligaments and direct contusion or indirect pinching of the upper cervical nerves in a whiplash snapping of the head and neck.

Post-traumatic head pains resemble other vascular headache syndromes. An icecap, bed rest, simple analgesics, reassurance and the passage of time are usually sufficient for relief. Ergotamine in 0.5 mg. amounts intramuscularly often controls severe attacks, and ergot preparations may be given orally. Histamine desensitization may occasionally be effective. If pain persists in one particular area of the head, procaine should be infiltrated into tender muscles or around scalp arteries, which may also be resected. Head traction and physiotherapy to the neck is helpful in whiplash injuries. Avulsion of the occipital nerves or intraspinal rhizotomy of the second or third cervical nerves may relieve intractable post-traumatic occipital neuralgia associated with nausea and dizziness.

OTHER VASODILATORY HEADACHE

Hypertensive headache comes on in the early morning hours when vessels of the cranium have been relaxed and are therefore subject to expansion by pressure thrust. The patient may obtain relief by assuming the upright or semi-sitting position, by caffeine, aminophylline, thiocyanates or ergotamine and by pressure on the carotid, temporal or occipital arteries. Paraplegics are subject to similar headache when distention of the bladder or rectum causes reflex vasoconstriction in the lower half of the body, which results in temporary elevation of blood pressure. *Menopausal* cephalalgia is of paroxysmal vasodilatory character and is accentuated by cervical muscle spasm. The headache of *fever* and sepsis is due to enlargement of cranial vessels by toxic substances.

Anoxia and *anoxemia* likewise produce vasodilatation in the head, and *polycythemia* distends intracranial vessels with blood. *Postconvulsive* headache is vasodilatory. The head-crushing agony of alcoholic *hangover* resembles histamine cephalalgia in most regards and may be the result of failure of detoxification of "H-substance" by the temporarily malfunc-

tioning liver or of the loss of sodium or potassium. It is not due to alterations of cerebrospinal fluid pressure. The headache of *constipation* is
probably of vasodilatory nature.

SPINAL PUNCTURE HEADACHE.—In the upright position, drainage of
as little as 20 cc. of cerebrospinal fluid (less than 1 per cent of the total
volume) will bring on severe head pain, generalized in location but most
severe in the back of the neck, owing to traction on all intracranial vessels
by the sagging brain. Pain is made worse by distention of the cerebral
veins, as in bilateral jugular compression, and is relieved by lying flat or
by simply flexing or extending the head. Postpuncture headache, coming
on hours or days after a lumbar tap, is caused by the same drainage-
traction mechanism following slow leakage of fluid from a persistent hole
in the spinal arachnoid and dura. Avulsing injuries of the spinal nerve
roots, caused by shoulder-girdle trauma or by hyperextension of the leg to
relieve sciatica, may also be accompanied by head pain of the same type.

The use of a small bore needle for puncture is supposed to avoid this
annoying but innocuous complication, but a certain number of postpuncture headaches will occur anyway. Fear of the procedure increases the
likelihood of disability. Bed rest, the forcing of fluids, an icecap, analgesics and the passage of time are rewarding. Intravenous administration
of 0.5 Gm. of caffeine sodium benzoate will stop headache like magic,
but the pain soon recurs. Replacement of the fluid withdrawn by sterile
saline is said to be a good preventive at the time of lumbar tap; few patients will permit a repuncture for restoration of intraspinal fluid balance.
Desoxycorticosterone is said to relieve spinal puncture headache.

REFERRED HEADACHE

Pain from *brain tumor* is referred to the superficial distribution of the
trigeminal, glossopharyngeal, vagus or upper cervical nerves which supply
the dura over or near the neoplasm and adjacent vessels. Tumor headache
is not due to increasing intracranial pressure per se but rather to brain
shift which distorts arteries and veins, as does direct compression by the
neoplasm. *Cerebrovascular accidents* cause pain according to the location
of the vessel involved and its proximity to the circle of Willis. Reference
is made to the corresponding external innervation of the scalp, often as
a "spot" of pain.

The *eye* is only rarely the source of headache despite the many types
of cephalalgia which begin in and around the orbit. Severe errors of refraction (astigmatism) and ocular inflammatory processes can cause pain

which arises in the domain of the ophthalmic division of the trigeminal nerve and extends generally. *Nasal* and *sinus* pain is referred chiefly to the maxillary and ophthalmic trigeminal fields. Tearing of the eye and cervical muscle spasm develop. Sphenoid sinus blockage produces excruciating pain immediately below the occiput. Sinus pain is made worse by reclining and is often brought on during sleep.

Strong stimulation of the *teeth* causes headache by spread of central excitation to the soft tissues in the corresponding trigeminal domain and by sustained muscle contractions of face, jaw and neck. Head pain from inflammation or a destructive process in the *ear* is carried by numerous filaments of the multiple innervation of this organ (trigeminal, facial, glossopharyngeal, vagus and cervical nerves). If headache is not relieved by aural or mastoid surgery, intracranial complication is usually present. Pathologic changes in the *cervical vertebrae* or *disks* will refer pain not only to the distribution of the cervical, brachial and occipital nerves but also to the eye and forehead.

TENSION HEADACHE; HEADACHE OF MUSCULAR ORIGIN

Sustained contraction of the skeletal muscles of the head and neck which insert on the skull will cause headache by traction on pain endings in the periosteum and in the muscular insertions proper. Extracranial muscle spasm and vasodilatation are the chief causes of head pain associated with emotional *tension* and *anxiety,* a common source of cranial discomfort. For good reasons we describe a difficult or disagreeable situation or person as "a real headache . . . . a pain in the neck." Psychotherapy relieves 60 per cent of headaches due to nervous tension. Many headaches in children also are of emotional origin (Krupp and Friedman).

A favorable therapeutic response to psychotherapy, placebo or sedative medication serves to distinguish the tension headache from similar syndromes. *Myositis* and *fibrositis* of inflammatory or traumatic origin are also accompanied by cephalalgia, principally occipital, which is relieved by procainization of tender nodules in the neck or back of the head. Muscular spasm and stiffness, largely cervical, add to the discomfort of headache from disturbances of eye, ear, nose, sinuses and upper spine and increase the vascular pain accompanying hypertension.

BIBLIOGRAPHY

Alpers, B. J., and Yaskin, J. E.: Pathogenesis of ophthalmoplegic migraine, A.M.A. Arch. Ophth. 45:555-566, 1951.

Blumenthal, L. S., and Fuchs, M.: Headache clinics: Endocrine therapy in migraine, Am. Pract. & Digest Treat. 2:755-757, 1951.

Campbell, J., and Evans, J. P.: Carotidynia, Neurology 3:391-392, 1953.

Cohn, R.: *Clinical Electroencephalography* (New York: McGraw-Hill Book Company, Inc., 1949).

Dandy, W. E.: Treatment of hemicrania (migraine) by removal of inferior cervical and first thoracic sympathetic ganglion, Bull. Johns Hopkins Hosp. 48:357-361, 1931.

Dow, D. J., and Whitty, C. W. M.: Electroencephalographic changes in migraine, Lancet 2:52-53, 1947.

Dunning, H. S.: Intracranial and extracranial vascular accidents in migraine, Arch. Neurol. & Psychiat. 48:396-406, 1942.

Engel, G. L.: Primary atypical facial neuralgia, Psychosom. Med. 13:375-396, 1951.

Fay, T.: Atypical facial neuralgia, a syndrome of vascular pain, Ann. Otol., Rhin. & Laryng. 41:1030-1062, 1932.

Gardner, W. J.; Stowell, A., and Dutlinger, R.: Resection of greater superficial petrosal nerve in treatment of unilateral headache, J. Neurosurg. 4:105-114, 1947.

Glaser, M. A.: Atypical neuralgia, so-called: A critical analysis of 143 cases, Arch. Neurol. & Psychiat. 20:537-558, 1928.

Hilger, J. A.: Carotid pain, Laryngoscope 59:829-928, 1949.

Horton, B. T.: The clinical use of histamine, Postgrad. Med. 9:1-23, 1951.

Krupp, G. R., and Friedman, A. P.: Recurrent headache in children: Study of 100 clinic cases, New York J. Med. 53:43-46, 1953.

Leriche, R., and Fontaine, R.: Sur la sensibilité de la chaine sympathique cervicale et des rameux communicants chez l'homme, Rev. neurol. 1:483-487, 1925.

Reichert, F. L.: Buccal neuralgia: A form of atypical facial neuralgia of sympathetic origin, Arch. Surg. 41:473-486, 1940.

Sugar, O.: Asymmetry in occipital electroencephalograms, Dis. Nerv. System 8:3-12, 1947.

Tunis, M. M., and Wolff, H. G.: Analysis of cranial artery pulse waves in patients with vascular headache of migraine type, Am. J. M. Sc. 224:565-568, 1952.

Ulett, G. A.; Evans, D., and O'Leary, J. L.: Survey of EEG findings in 1,000 patients with chief complaint of headache, Electroencephalog. & Clin. Neurophysiol. 4:463-470, 1952.

Watts, F. B.: Atypical facial neuralgia in the hypothyroid state, Ann. Int. Med. 35:186, 1951.

Wolff, H. G.: *Headache and Other Head Pain* (New York: Oxford University Press, 1948).

CHAPTER 19

General Management
of the Patient

THE ROUTINE of general care of the patient with a cerebrovascular accident is similar to that employed in the management of severe head injuries. There are special problems referable to increased intracranial pressure, the heart and circulation, the lungs and respiratory cycle, regulation of temperature, the urinary and gastrointestinal tracts, the skin, nutrition, sedation and analgesia. In most acute, many subacute and some chronic cases of cerebrovascular accident the chief therapeutic difficulties are those of coping with and sustaining an unconscious patient. Important in treatment of the subacute and chronic phases of stroke are physiotherapy and re-education designed to compensate for or to regain lost or crippled functions.

HOME OR HOSPITAL?

Many elderly patients flatly refuse to enter a hospital. Few carry hospitalization insurance, which was not available when they were in the subscription time of life. Moreover, to remove some elderly persons from their personally familiar environment and usual pattern of activity is to condemn them to a reactive mental depression. Delirium may be precipitated by a sudden transfer to the unfamiliar surroundings of a hospital. For these and other reasons, an older patient with mild cerebral infarction may remain at home under the care of relatives or a nurse. This is especially true if consciousness is not lost and biologic functions can be carried on without much assistance, if diagnosis is obvious, making complicated diagnostic procedures unnecessary, and if surgery is not contemplated. Adequate physiotherapy can often be carried out at home.

Younger people, in whom differential diagnosis is usually less obvious and the probability of active treatment, medical or surgical, is greater, should always be hospitalized. Whenever a potentially fatal outcome seems likely, the patient should be admitted to the hospital, if only to relieve the family of anxiety and give them assurance.

INCREASED INTRACRANIAL PRESSURE

Increased intracranial pressure is present in two thirds of the patients with cerebral hemorrhage, one-third with cerebral infarction, and may be present in various other types of cerebrovascular disease. This state demands preferential control.

It is not the increase of tension inside the skull in itself which is important; brief experimental elevations of cerebrospinal fluid pressure to 1,400 mm. of water are tolerated by healthy young adults with no loss of consciousness (Evans *et al.*). The secondary effects of high intracranial pressure on cerebral blood flow, the flattening of veins and capillaries and the compression of midbrain and lower medulla by herniations of adjacent brain tissue through the tentorial incisura and foramen magnum are the dangers. These impair cerebral nutrition, produce coma by distortion of the upper brain stem and hypothalamus and finally cause death when hemorrhages are induced in the mesencephalon and pons.

The brain becomes edematous after anoxic injury of its small vasculature. Rapid intravenous administration of water as 5–10 per cent glucose solution aggravates edema and raises intracranial pressure still further. "Water intoxication" can in itself cause convulsions, and it is doubtful that normal saline solution has any greater edema-increasing effect. A tap-water enema can kill in the presence of high intracranial pressure, as that with cerebellar tumor. Yet the patient must have fluids for general body needs.

MANAGEMENT

The proper procedure is to attempt to reduce the high intracranial pressure first, before proceeding further with treatment. When the initial pressure is not above 300 mm. of water, spinal puncture may be used therapeutically by removing more than the usual amount of fluid. If it is higher than this, fluid removal must be cautious and to no more than a diagnostic amount, or the appearance of intracranial herniations will be accelerated. By and large, spinal puncture even when repeated is not a maneuver that successfully controls increased intracranial pressure.

Definitive surgical drainage or removal of an intracerebral hematoma and subtemporal decompression are excellent methods for reducing brain swelling or preventing its lethal effect but are restricted to special circumstances. Ventricular taps may be undertaken in the course of investigation for hematoma or as a measure of last resort when death from increased intracranial pressure threatens. In a rare case, ventricular drainage has carried a patient though a critical period.

INTRAVENOUS HYPERTONIC SOLUTIONS.—The most effective way to handle heightened intracranial pressure is by the use of hypertonic solutions. As demonstrated by Shenkin and associates in patients with brain tumor, general brain dehydration induced osmotically will increase cerebral blood flow, whereas intracranial circulation does not necessarily improve after removal of fluid from the cerebral ventricles.

When substances having a volume of distribution approaching that of sodium are injected intravenously in greater than isotonic concentrations, there results a prolonged fall in cerebrospinal fluid pressure and reduction in the volume of uninjured brain. Substances having a volume of distribution approaching that of total body water, for example, urea, when infused hypertonically produce an initial fall in cerebrospinal fluid tension which is followed shortly by a secondary rise to a new high. Hypertonic sucrose, lactate and magnesium sulfate are solutions of the first, sodium-like type used in clinical practice for dehydration of the brain, and concentrated glucose is a dehydrant frequently employed which diffuses throughout the body (Moyer).

The choice of substance is not this simple, since both types of solution may injure the renal epithelium. However, sucrose is more destructive to the kidney than is glucose. A hypertonic sucrose solution may therefore be used only if renal function is assumed to be adequate; if there is renal damage as well as high intracranial pressure, glucose should be employed despite an anticipated secondary rise of pressure. Each sugar is administered intravenously in amounts of 50 cc. of 50 per cent solution through a No. 19 or 20 caliber needle, in order to assure a relatively slow injection. One 50 cc. ampule may be given at four hour intervals for not more than four to six doses. These hypertonic substances sclerose veins.

MAGNESIUM SULFATE PROCTOCLYSIS.—Magnesium sulfate may be administered intravenously, giving 4 cc. of 15 per cent solution every three to four hours, but is usually given orally or rectally in the form of a dehydrating proctoclysis. There is a direct and immediate relation between tonicity of fluid in the lower bowel and intracranial pressure.

The magnesium sulfate proctoclysis is made up by mixing 100 cc. of a saturated solution with 200 cc. of tap water (for adults). The solution is run into a rectal tube through a Murphy drip. The nurse must understand that this clysis is not to be absorbed but will be retained and expelled.

The components and total volume are used in one-fourth to one-third amounts in children. This is an excellent and effective method of withdrawing fluid from the brain. Magnesium-potassium antagonism should be kept in mind; too much magnesium may itself produce coma and respiratory paralysis, in which case potassium must be given to restore respiratory activity.

SERUM ALBUMIN.—Human serum albumin is one of the most effective dehydrants, also the most expensive. It can reduce intracranial pressure when all other means fail. From 60 to 80 cc. of serum albumin is administered in eight to 10 minutes and all fluids are withheld during the next eight hours.

DIURETICS.—Mercurial and other diuretics may occasionally lower intracranial pressure in the course of delivering fluid via well functioning kidneys. The dosage is that ordinarily recommended for diuresis.

HEART AND CIRCULATION

Coronary thrombosis is often associated with cerebral infarction. Cardiac failure may be responsible for brain softening, and the heart is almost always the source of cerebral embolism. The myocardium may be in a precarious state due to hypertension and is easily overwhelmed when blood pressure rises still further as intracranial pressure increases. The cardiac status must always be evaluated carefully in a patient with cerebrovascular accident.

An electrocardiogram should be taken and the patient should be digitalized if there is evidence of cardiac involvement or failure. The placing of tourniquets around extremities, venesection (250–500 cc.) and use of diuretics may also help to restore the failing heart. Aminophylline, while increasing the tonus of intracranial vessels, speeds coronary flow and exerts a direct effect on the respiratory center which may stop Cheyne-Stokes respiration. The sitting position improves cardiac function and is a means of lowering cerebral venous pressure.

If anemia or hypotension is present, a blood transfusion is indicated and this may have to be given intra-arterially if shock is severe. Hypertensive crisis that is responsible for cerebrovascular accident or is a secondary result of rising intracranial pressure may end in heart failure. Sympathetic blocking agents can prevent such a terminus.

LUNGS AND RESPIRATION

So important are the pulmonary aspects of cerebrovascular accidents that it may be said that "if the brain does not kill, the chest will." Frank aspiration pneumonia is becoming a pathologic rarity thanks to an increasing interest in the pathophysiology of the lungs during comatose states and the use of the suction machine. Mortality statistics in cases of stroke, head injury and in neurologic patients in general have been lowered accordingly.

OXYGEN THERAPY.—Oxygen inhalation is in order when cerebral blood flow is decreased, pulmonary interchange is inadequate or heart failure is present or impending. It is easiest to keep a patient oxygenated in a properly functioning oxygen tent. However, engineering supervision is necessary to keep moisture and carbon dioxide accumulation within physiologic limits, otherwise the tent does more harm than good. Failure of refrigeration will accentuate a tendency to hyperthermia in the patient with a stroke. A mask is excellent if tolerated, but it frightens many patients. Nasal catheters are easy to pull out, and necrosis of the posterior pharyngeal wall has occurred when a steady jet of oxygen has been allowed to play on one particular spot for more than 12 hours. If the catheter is inserted too far down into the esophagus, the abdomen becomes distended as the stomach inflates. The method of administration of oxygen should be suited to the individual patient.

Addition of 5–7 per cent carbon dioxide to the oxygen is of value because of its cerebral vasodilating properties. However, carbon dioxide should not be inhaled for long periods by the emphysematous patient because of a vasodilatation-induced critical rise in intracranial pressure (Mithoefer). Oxygen concentrations of greater than 75–80 per cent may depress the arteriosclerotic and elderly patient and even cause delirium or coma ("oxygen poisoning"), apparently because of the weak cerebral vasoconstricting effect of almost pure oxygen and the retention of carbon dioxide. The recommended rate of flow of oxygen is 4–6 L. per minute by nasal catheter and 8–10 L. per minute in a tent. Oxygen concentrations are thus kept around 45 per cent.

POSITION IN BED.—The orthopneic cardiac should and must sit up, other circumstances notwithstanding. Intracranial pressure is also lowest in this position. Elevated intracranial pressure, by causing bradycardia, will increase pulmonary venous tension. When the systemic arterial pressure rises because of medullary stimulation and heart failure supervenes, the circulation of the lungs is hampered still more.

On the other hand, if choking, gagging, aspiration of vomitus or simple failure to cough out nasopharyngeal drippings from the tracheobronchial tubes interferes with respiratory interchange and will soon end in pneumonia, the patient should lie flat, on the side or face. Spontaneous coughing is easier in this position and gravity does not spread foreign material farther into pulmonary parenchyma. Suctioning of the pharynx is also facilitated.

When hemiplegia impairs movements of the diaphragm and inter-costal muscles, the head-down position may permit better diaphragmatic excursion. Any position of the body should be changed every three or four hours to prevent unequal pressure on the skin and passive congestion of one part of the lungs.

MAINTENANCE OF AIRWAY.—An oral airway may aid respiratory exchange by holding the tongue and jaw forward. Suction-aspiration of the pharynx must be faithfully and intelligently carried out. Many nurses are fearful of introducing a suction tube too far down the throat and assiduously but ineffectually clean out the mouth only with a metal tonsil suction tip. This does little good. A lubricated soft rubber catheter (14 F.) should be introduced through the nose and the end pushed down far enough so that the epiglottis or vocal cords are brushed. The catheter is moved in and out rapidly and for short distances, the vacuum bottle of the attached suction apparatus being turned on and off meanwhile. In this way the tube is not obstructed by clenching of the teeth, and holes in the tip of the catheter do not become plugged with mucus. Also, the patient coughs vigorously and raises material from below the larynx. The nose may bleed and the patient cough up blood; the nurse should be re-assured in advance that this does not mean that the lung is being injured.

A ureteral catheter may be used in place of the rubber one, and with practice can actually be introduced into the trachea and major bronchi without preceding anesthesia of the vocal cords. Bronchial plugs may be thus removed. One disadvantage is that the ostia of these catheters are tiny and easily occluded.

If major pulmonary atelectasis develops despite these simple meas-ures or in their absence, bronchoscopy should be undertaken without hesitation no matter what the intracranial status, for otherwise the patient will surely die.

Tracheotomy has been advocated in the management of acute head injuries and it also has a place in the treatment of the patient with a stroke. By furnishing an open and accessible artificial airway, tracheotomy allows easy ingress of air and oxygen and ready and effectual removal of mucus, blood and vomitus. It also relieves the edema-producing negative pull on the interior of the lung when snoring respiration is present. Im-pressive mucus and clotted bronchial casts have been withdrawn through a tracheotomy opening after pharyngeal suctioning had supposedly cleansed the trachea. Endotracheal tubes which are left in place for pro-longed periods cause extreme swelling of the vocal cords; thus, if the general situation seems critical enough to call for an intratracheal airway, tracheotomy is preferable.

PULMONARY EDEMA.—Edema of the lungs is dangerous because froth in the alveoli blocks the respiratory interface and will not move in or out, causing the patient to become asphyxiated. Pulmonary edema may result from acute left ventricular heart failure, as blood pressure rises in crisis or in response to intracranial pressure, but often it is an expression of injury of the vagus nuclei in the medulla. Methods of treatment include the intravenous administration of aminophylline in hypertonic glucose solution, subcutaneous injection of atropine, vigorous suctioning of the tracheobronchial tree, procaine blockade of the *right* stellate ganglion and inhalation of alcohol vapor produced by the bubbling of oxygen through alcohol (Luisada). Alcohol vapor breaks up pulmonary edema by decreasing the surface tension of the foam. Its use has been noted to be associated with emergence of patients from coma but it should be remembered that alcohol-oxygen is a highly explosive mixture. Addition of an inhalant detergent may be preferable.

PNEUMONIA.—Atelectasis accompanied by fever is therefore also pneumonia and should be treated with sulfonamides or antibiotics. The bacterial flora is usually mixed in these cases and broad-spectrum therapy is indicated. Reliance should not be placed on antibiotic therapy alone to the neglect of the suction machine.

URINARY TRACT

A full and tense bladder can account for the restlessness of an unconscious patient. Involuntary urination macerates the skin and hastens the appearance of bedsores. Therefore, an indwelling catheter should be used in the comatose patient. Open drainage is satisfactory for a day or two. However, if constant artificial withdrawal of urine is necessary for longer periods, the catheter should be clamped off and released every six to eight hours to prevent contraction of the bladder, or Munro's tidal apparatus should be attached. A nontoxic sulfonamide such as Gantrisin should be given by mouth or stomach tube since penicillin will not control gram-negative organisms. The appearance of renal and cystic calculi, as in all cases of prolonged recumbency, should be watched for in patients with chronic hemiplegia who are bedfast.

GASTROINTESTINAL TRACT

VOMITING.—Persistent vomiting may feature the early clinical course of cerebrovascular accident. It is a manifestation of increased intracranial pressure or of neurologic involvement of the brain stem, in which instance it is often accompanied by hiccough. Not only is there the possibility of the patient aspirating vomitus, but straining and retching increase the pressure in cerebral veins and repeated vomiting depletes the body of fluid and electrolytes.

If persistent, vomiting must be approached as a problem in itself. Sedatives such as Luminal sodium (65 mg.) or scopolamine (0.2 mg.) may be effective, or Dramamine may be used orally or rectally. All intake by mouth is withheld. The volume of fluid lost must be replaced parenterally. If pharmacologic control is not effective, Wangensteen suction should be instituted to stop vomiting by keeping the stomach empty.

HICCOUGH.—Hiccough is a particularly annoying symptom, often seen with lesions of the brain stem, and is capable of causing death by interfering with rest, respiration and nutrition and because of associated vomiting. Rebreathing into a bag, inhalations of 10 per cent carbon dioxide, peppermint water by mouth, atropine or Dramamine may be tried. In intractable hiccough, certain local anesthetic methods may give relief. These include ethyl chloride spray applied over the anterior triangle of the neck or along the insertion of the diaphragm and procaine infiltration of the phrenic nerve. Simple finger massage of the phrenic nerve just above the clavicle may be effective. Rarely, phrenicophraxis must be performed.

GASTROMALACIA.—If the vomitus is hemorrhagic or contains changed blood, or if the stools are tarry, acute gastric or esophageal ulceration should be suspected. Acute neurogenic ulcers, first described by Rokitansky and brought to attention by Cushing, are common preterminal events in severe cerebrovascular accident. They result from hemorrhages in the brain stem and hypothalamus due to downward herniation of the temporal lobe through the incisura. Lesions may consist of lysis of the wall of stomach or cardiac esophagus or may be entirely hemorrhagic.

If the wall of the stomach or esophagus has "blown out" and gastric contents pour from an ever-widening hole into the abdominal and thoracic cavities through a digested diaphragm, nothing can be done. But if bleeding is the problem, Wangensteen drainage of the upper gastrointestinal tract and blood transfusions are mandatory, and several patients have been saved by this regime. Atropine or Banthine should be administered and a Sippy diet given by stomach tube.

BOWEL EVACUATION.—Enema or cathartic evacuation of the bowel should be effected at least twice a week. Tap-water enemas are forbidden in the presence of increased intracranial pressure. Dehydrating oral purgatives or, better, a magnesium sulfate proctoclysis will accomplish elimination and reduce intracranial pressure simultaneously. If desired, a less vigorous "1-2-3 enema" (one part glycerin, two parts saturated magnesium sulfate solution, three parts water) may be substituted. Enemas are preferred to drastic cathartics because evacuation is better controlled and the patient is less likely to soil himself.

SKIN: DECUBITUS ULCERS

Bedsores are usually thought of as plaguing paraplegic patients, but neglected hemiplegic patients are prone to have them as well. Nutrition is a prominent factor in their development. Experience with spinal cord injuries demonstrates that keeping the hemoglobin level at 14 Gm. and the serum protein concentration at least at 6.5 Gm. by use of transfusions and a high vitamin, high protein diet are excellent precautionary measures which also tend to prevent the formation of urinary calculi.

Other factors predisposing to the formation of bedsores are the slowing or arrest of capillary circulation that results from compression of blood vessels between bony prominences and the mattress; a lack of cushioning by subcutaneous tissues; circulating toxins and bacterial infection; the increased metabolic needs of tissues due to fever, local inflammation and trauma, and mechanical or chemical irritation from urine and perspiration.

PREVENTION AND TREATMENT.—Constant turning of the patient from one physiologic and comfortable position to another helps to distribute the weight of the body, and special beds with alternating-pressure mattresses are ideal in this regard. "Sandwich beds" (Stryker frame) allow a severely paralyzed person to be turned completely over with very little trouble and with no sheet burns in transit. Keeping the patient and the sheets dry also tends to minimize chafing and local irritation. Sawdust-filled boxes are occasionally of practical assistance when the individual is uncontrollably incontinent of urine and feces. Antipyretic and antibiotic therapy gives the tissues a chance for recovery by reducing the metabolic rate and eliminating bacterial activity. The anabolic effect of testosterone may also be of benefit.

Once a decubitus ulcer has developed, half the battle is lost. The list of pastes, liquids, unguents and other preparations advocated for the cure of bedsores is almost endless. Most materials in use come under one of four headings: protectives and astringents, of which tannic acid and tincture of benzoin are examples; solutes of dead tissue, such as allantoin, streptokinase and streptodornase; bacteriostatic and bactericidal mixtures, and stimulators of healthy granulations, vitamin A and D cream being particularly good. Each preparation is recommended at the appropriate stage of treatment. Heat lamps aid by keeping the skin dry. In advanced and chronic decubiti, plastic surgery is indicated, although spontaneous healing of enormous bedsores has occurred.

FEVER

Neurogenic hyperthermia is a bane of the existence of the neurosurgeon. Really fantastic temperatures have been recorded in various kinds of acute brain lesions, particularly in the immediate postoperative period following exploration of the region of the third ventricle and posterior fossa. Patients with cerebral hemorrhage are prone to develop high temperatures; hypothalamic nuclear or tract injury seems to be the anatomic basis. If uncontrolled, hyperthermia of itself will kill, by accelerating cerebral metabolism beyond the range of compensatory cerebral blood flow and by finally and literally "cooking the brain." Greatly elevated internal temperature and icy-cold, dry skin is prognostically the worst form of central fever, indicating that the thermostat (hypothalamus) has lost control. The necessity of following the rectal temperature is indicated; oral temperature readings are inaccurate in a patient breathing through his mouth, and axillary records are valueless.

TREATMENT.—The room should be cooled by air-conditioning or a fan and the bedcovers removed. Icebags may be applied to axillae and groins, if they are warm. Sponging of the hot skin with ice water or alcohol should be kept up assiduously until the temperature is below 102.2 F. (39 C.). In severe cases the patient may be packed in ice. Tepid or even hot water sponging is indicated before the use of external cold if the skin is not warm. Blood must be brought to the surface if superficial cooling is to do any good.

Aspirin (acetylsalicylic acid), an excellent antipyretic, is given in large doses by stomach tube or rectally in amounts of 1–2 Gm. every three to four hours while the rectal temperature remains above 39 C. One-third this dose may be used in children. Repeated injections of minute quantities of morphine (1–2 mg.) may be beneficial. Luminal sodium (0.65–0.1 Gm.) is helpful in controlling restlessness and is also hypothermic to a degree.

Blood transfusion is indicated if a shocklike vascular state results and should be given early. This may be lifesaving. Salt retention increases hyperpyrexia. When the intracranial condition is known to be febrile in reaction, vigorous antipyretic measures should begin when the rectal temperature reaches 39 C. and should be continued as long as it is above this level.

NUTRITION

FLUIDS.—Loss of consciousness places the patient's fluid balance completely in the hands of the physician. Usually 2–3 L. of fluid daily should be given subcutaneously or intravenously to the average adult stroke victim. One liter should contain sodium chloride and other inorganic solutes, such as potassium, and the rest should consist of 5–10 per cent glucose solution. Investigations of the problems of fluid balance in brain disease show that whereas this plan may be satisfactory in many patients, in others careful observance of serum and urinary sodium and chloride levels is necessary and demands an individualized program. Experimental investigations indicate that intracranial pressure is increased to a greater extent by salt-free solutions (glucose in water) given intravenously than by isotonic saline solution despite popular medical belief to the contrary (Fishman and Halla).

SALT RETENTION.—In some patients, alteration of the pituitary-renal relationship resembles diabetes insipidus; water is excreted by the kidney without salt, the osmolar concentration of body fluids is increased and the temperature rises. In patients with head injury analogous to cerebral hemorrhage studied by Higgins et al., hyperchloremia with depression of urinary chloride excretion was present before death. In all patients lesions were present near the basal diencephalon. Complete tubular resorption of chloride ion was thought to be responsible for salt retention.

Serum sodium determinations are indicated if an accurate method is available. Sodium chloride solutions, isotonic or otherwise, should not be administered until the serum chloride level approaches normal or the urinary output becomes greater than 1 Gm. of salt per liter. Depression of serum potassium may require correction.

Increased loss of water by the kidney may be due to interference with neurogenic control of the posterior hypophysis in the brain-injured patient. The antidiuretic hormone (vasopressin) is not the only intracranial influence on renal physiology, since lesions in the upper fourth ventricle cause loss of both salt and water by the kidneys, which reaction is not rectified by pituitary extract (Welt et al.). The use of hypertonic solutions intravenously to decrease high intracranial pressure can coincidently concentrate serum sodium, chloride and urea.

A less complex but equally important factor leading to dehydration is the decrease of natural water intake by the comatose or confused patient who does not recognize his thirst, cannot pick up and drink from a glass or cannot swallow because of an accumulation of mucus or paralysis of the throat muscles. An extrarenal loss of water in excess of salt is also seen in the perspiration which often bathes the individual who has recently had a cerebrovascular accident.

Peters and associates have described a salt-wasting syndrome that is exactly the opposite of salt retention in patients with vascular or other lesions of the brain. In this state, the primary defect is an inability to reabsorb salt on the part of the proximal kidney tubules. Respiratory influences may contribute. The salt-wasting stroke patient needs more than the standard recommendation of 1 L. of saline solution per day, if he depends on fluids alone.

POTASSIUM DEFICIENCY.—The necessity for intake of potassium must be remembered, particularly if magnesium sulfate is being used as a dehydrant (magnesium-potassium antagonism), if vomiting has been or is severe or if gastrointestinal suction has been prolonged. Weakness, aphonia, abdominal distention and electrocardiographic changes signalize potassium deficiency. An oral solution of 1 Gm. each of potassium citrate, potassium acetate and potassium bicarbonate dissolved in 8 cc. of water may be given therapeutically in such a state, or 2.23 Gm. of potassium chloride, an adequate daily maintenance dose, is given in 1 L. of infusion fluid. Administration of potassium has revived several patients in otherwise reversible metabolic coma (Stark and Barrera).

FOOD.—The unconscious or confused patient must have food supplied parenterally. The daily metabolic need for 1 Gm. of protein per kilogram of body weight and approximately 3,000 calories for an ill adult must be acquired artificially if intake of food is not resumed at least by the end of one week. Although protein hydrolysate solutions can meet caloric, protein and salt requirements, Levin tube-feeding is better. The mixtures supplied by trained dietitians supply an almost normal diet, all factors included. Two disadvantages of tube-feeding are the tendency to increased nasopharyngeal secretion, causing atelectasis, and diarrhea. Use of suctioning will clear the pharynx, and the addition of paregoric and bismuth will combat looseness of stools. Large amounts of vitamins should be given if premorbid dietary habits were poor.

RESTRAINTS

Some patients who have had cerebrovascular accidents persist in attempts to get out of bed, risking head injury and fractures of other parts of the body. Some tear and burn themselves up despite sedation or may be wildly psychotic and even dangerous. Under such circumstances and in the face of an increasing shortage of nurses and hospital orderlies, it is only intelligent to restrain a patient judiciously in order to prevent further injury, reduce metabolism and permit nursing care to proceed. The situation should be explained to the family and their written permission obtained if this is felt necessary. All concerned should realize that physical restraint is much safer than constant sedation to the point of anesthesia, when pneumonia will surely develop.

There are many types of restraining methods, some of which are relatively inconspicuous, others bizarre. A simple effective maneuver is to place cuffs on one arm and the opposite leg, tying each to the bedframe; a certain amount of activity is permitted, the extremities and body are accessible for therapy, yet the patient cannot get out of bed or into a dangerously awkward position. If this restraint is not enough all four limbs may be strapped, although when this is done there is much more straining against the bands by the confused patient. Cuffs should be well padded to avoid chafing. Camisole jackets confine the chest and arms and hold the patient firmly and usually immovably to the bed, but such immobilization may predispose to the development of pneumonia. Nettings of steel wire or rope over the bed will keep the patient within bounds and prevent him from climbing over the siderails.

CONTROL OF PAIN AND CONVULSIVE SEIZURES

HEADACHE.—Headache of any type should not go unattended because of the traditional avoidance of depressant drugs in the presence of stroke. Aspirin in 0.05–1 Gm. doses by mouth or an oral preparation of aspirin, phenacetin and caffeine often affords much welcome relief. There should be no hesitancy in adding 32 mg. of codeine if necessary; codeine sulfate may also be injected subcutaneously in 65 mg. doses every four hours without fear, even in the presence of high intracranial pressure. If codeine sensitivity exists, 100 mg. of Demerol can be substituted. Demerol is not a significant respiratory depressant in this amount, but it does not relieve pain as does codeine.

Morphine sulfate (10 mg.) is used in only one type of cerebrovascular accident, subarachnoid hemorrhage, and then not unless other analgesics fail to relieve the particularly severe headache. The problem of controlling a patient who is writhing in agony and may sustain a second arterial rupture is paramount. If morphine toxicity develops, N-allylnormorphine will combat depression. The routine use of morphine in all strokes and head injuries is deplorable and has accounted for many deaths.

RESTLESSNESS.—Sedation is necessary if there is restlessness or overactivity. Safe medications include Luminal sodium in doses of 65–130 mg. subcutaneously every four to six hours, chloral hydrate, 1.3–1.95 Gm. by mouth or rectum, and paraldehyde, 4–5 cc. orally or rectally. In the recovery period, capsules of barbiturates, 0.1 Gm., may be given for sleep, which is often elusive due to inactivity.

THALAMIC PAIN.—Thalamic pain, a burning, constant dysesthesia in the paretic and anesthetic side of the body affected by hemiplegia, is a not infrequent chronic sequel of cerebral thrombosis or hemorrhage especially when the thalamogeniculate artery is occluded and an irritative focus remains in the sensory thalamus. The syndrome may be full blown or partial, involves at least the shoulder and arm, is often associated with mental phenomena and may be permanent.

Benadryl in large amounts has been reported to give relief. Cortisone is also recommended. Stellate block, on the painful or on the opposite side, may produce dramatic symptomatic cure, especially of shoulder-hand pain. Ankylosis of joints must be combated by physiotherapy. In patients with intractable thalamic hyperpathia complicated by an obsessive mental state, prefrontal lobotomy of a minimal type has relieved suffering when all else has failed.

CONVULSIVE SEIZURES.—Convulsive seizures may complicate the acute phase of any type of cerebrovascular accident, can occur at any time in the chronic state and are common in such diffuse varieties of cerebrovascular disease as arteriosclerosis and syphilis. About 15 per cent of all vascular hemiplegic patients sustain epileptiform attacks after the acute phase of illness is over.

A combination of Dilantin and phenobarbital is most effective therapeutically. Dilantin, 0.1 Gm., is given four times daily with the addition of 32 mg. of phenobarbital to each dose or 65 mg. at night only. Double the dose of Dilantin may be given by rectum to the patient who is unconscious or unable to swallow, the capsules being perforated with a pin before insertion. Phenobarbital may be injected as the sodium salt. Both medications should be reduced in amount when seizures are relieved.

Other anticonvulsant drugs may be substituted if Dilantin is ineffective in controlling chronic seizures.

More vigorous therapy is usually necessary in status epilepticus. Oral or rectal use of paraldehyde is particularly good. Barbiturates such as Amytal or Pentothal sodium may be given intravenously to break up the run of seizures, but their effect is not as persistent as that of paraldehyde and attacks may soon start again.

The electroencephalogram is abnormal in 75 per cent of patients with chronic vascular hemiplegia but may be normal even in the presence of obvious epilepsy. Treatment should not be withheld if the diagnosis is apparent but the electroencephalogram is not corroborative. Many supposedly vasospastic or further thrombotic episodes following a major cerebrovascular accident are really of a convulsive nature and should be handled accordingly.

PHYSICAL THERAPY

It is a tribute to the specialists in physical medicine that an increasing number of patients with chronic hemiplegia are being salvaged and rehabilitated to a degree enabling them to leave bed and hospital and even to return to gainful employment. Current statistics show that 60–90 per cent of all hemiplegics can be taught ambulation, self-care and control of fecal and urinary incontinence and that 30 per cent or more can learn to work again.

The earlier that physiotherapy and other rehabilitation procedures are begun, the better, but chronicity and advanced age do not necessarily mean hopelessness. Rusk and collaborators, working with a group of 134 patients whose average age was 63 and some of whom had hemiplegia for a decade, were able to teach 93 per cent to walk and carry on the activities of daily care; 33 per cent eventually became employed. Of course, in many patients with the syndrome of anosognosia (denial of disease), psychosis, malignant hypertension, inoperable brain tumor or senility it is foolish to try obviously ineffectual retraining. Anosognosia is particularly common in patients with left hemiplegia. Rigidity of personality, limited interpersonal resources and lack of a desire to improve all hamper a rehabilitation program.

IN THE ACUTE STAGE.—Instead of caring for the bodily needs of the hemiplegic and assisting him in every regard for an indefinite time, modern practice is to initiate physiotherapy as soon as the cerebral lesion is thought to be stabilized and the patient's mental status is one capable of co-operation. Bed activities may often begin 24 hours after thrombosis,* and active physical treatment can be instituted seven to 10 days later. It is wiser to wait longer following hemorrhagic episodes for fear of recurrence of bleeding. Since psychologic factors are so important, it is helpful to assure the patient that if he can move his arm or raise the affected leg 1 in. from the bed he will be able to walk again and thus regain the activity he most desires.

Several simple procedures will help prevent deformities in the acute stage of hemiplegia (Fig. 120). Use of a footboard or posterior leg splint will avoid footdrop, and sandbags placed along the length of the lower extremity will keep the leg from rotating outward. A pillow placed in the axilla prevents adduction of the shoulder. Quadriceps setting maintains muscle strength about the knee, and a cock-up splint on the forearm wards off flexion contractures. The insertion of a bedboard under the mattress will prevent sagging of the inactive body.

When the patient is ready for more active exercise, he is allowed to sit up. This will facilitate his retaining a sense of balance; recumbency for four to six weeks means that balance will have to be learned all over again. The patient should manipulate the paralyzed arm through the shoulder joint by hand or indirectly with the use of a rope-pulling attachment. Frozen shoulder may thus be prevented. A loop fastened around the instep permits self-administration of passive or active assisted motion through the ankle joint. A knotted rope attached to the foot of the bed can be grasped by the patient to assume the sitting position.

Meanwhile, the physiotherapist or home nurse can apply heat to stiff joints, always remembering that loss of sensation may result in burns. Work is begun on the affected side with passive motion in sessions of 15 minutes, three times a day. Rhythmic volitional movements against progressively increased resistance are particularly effective. Electrical stimulation is impressive but is of less value in maintaining the tonus of paralyzed or paretic muscles than actual motion, passive or active.

The use of Tolserol or other mephenesin preparation may help to relieve spasticity. The usual adult oral dosage is 1–3 Gm. three to five times a day. Neostigmine is not as effective. Cortisone may facilitate recovery from hemiplegia, and curare may be indicated.

Setting up of a definite plan of rehabilitation as early as possible gives the patient hope and insures the regular performance of remedial activities which may at first seem unavailing and must be repeated to be successful. With the day fully occupied, vegetation and rumination are kept at a minimum.

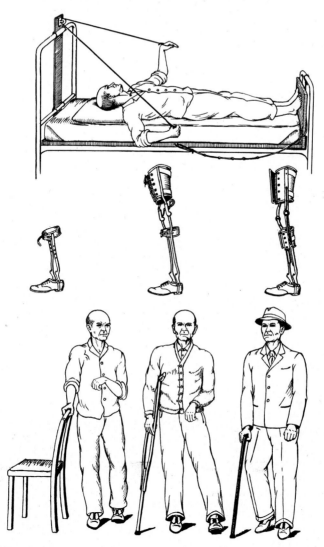

FIG. 120.—Rehabilitation of the hemiplegic patient. (Courtesy of L. N. Rudin.)

IN THE CHRONIC STAGE.—As soon as possible, the hemiplegic patient—now hemiparetic as strength is being regained in the leg at least—is allowed to stand beside the bed and to start relearning to walk. The deteriorating effects of bedrest on the general vascular system will now begin to be reversed. The effect on morale of standing erect is tremendous, especially in a patient who secretly believed that he never again would be able to do so. In initial sessions, the patient should often be reminded that "every hemiplegic can walk again."

He starts out on a smooth floor with either hand on the back of a chair. First with assistance and later by himself, the patient learns to advance the left foot with the right chair, the right foot with the left chair. Walking may also be begun with the patient holding on only one chair with the good hand, which is laced to the back if necessary. He supports himself on the single chair and the strong leg as the weak leg is swung forward. Transition from the chair to a crutch under the unaffected arm is easy; later the crutch is replaced with a cane. At least 50 per cent of patients need support for the paretic leg, either in the form of a short leg brace with footdrop attachment or in the form of a long leg brace with footdrop correction and kneelock or mechanical quadriceps (Rudin and Cronin). A forearm splint which cocks up the wrist may have elastic bands attached for finger exercise.

Rehabilitatory activities are most effective if practiced in a group, but members of the family may encourage and advise the patient in his quest for the regaining of balance and motion. Exercise periods should be kept at 20 minutes once a day in the beginning and repeated and extended as strength improves. There is a remarkable tolerance for what would appear to be agonizingly difficult activity by the elderly, arteriosclerotic or hypertensive stroke victim. The use of special facilities of a department of physical medicine speeds recovery, as does competition with others afflicted similarly, under the sympathetic guidance of trained therapists and physicians. In these circumstances the patient is best taught personal care, to dress himself, carry out toilet activities and to get in and out of bed.

Most attention is concentrated on the leg, because walking is more valuable than the use of even the right arm and because the affected hand is always slowest to regain function. The patient and family should know that the activity of the fingers may never return. If there is absolutely no motor recovery after four to six months of intensive physiotherapy, the program may be abandoned. Individualized treatment should continue for six to 18 months if any gains have been made. Little further improvement may be expected thereafter.

TREATMENT OF APHASIA.—Speech therapy holds out hope in aphasia, even in older persons. Re-education of this type should also commence as soon as feasible, and initial garbled verbalizations should be encouraged. Even the mute or those in whom pharyngeal and laryngeal muscles are affected can benefit from a speech training program. The first sequences taught should be those most useful, and the aphasic, like the child, learns to speak better in sentences than in words. Children's books may be helpful in this stage. The goal is to re-establish speech corresponding to the life situation to be entered.

Mental confusion or deterioration prevents correction of aphasia, as of hemiplegia, and the euphoric aphasic patient who has chosen to ignore or to enjoy his disability, so to speak, may be particularly refractory to assistance. Complete lack of recognition of spoken words, pictures or symbols precludes any recovery of ability to communicate.

THE BASIS OF RECOVERY

How the hemiplegic and aphasic patient regains strength and function even partially after a cerebrovascular accident, in view of the known incapacity of the central nervous system to regenerate, is an intriguing and unsettled question. Much speculation has been undertaken along the line of "takeover" or reorganization of function, which assumes transfer of neuronal connections of face and arm cortical areas to those of the leg, for example, and even implies that sensory ganglion cells can become motor neurons. Another point of view contends that ipsilateral representation, particularly of speech and leg function in the cortex, is responsible for the regaining of activity.

In a critical review of pertinent experimental and clinical observations, Sperry concluded that there was no real evidence for reorganization or takeover of function in the neuraxis at any level, even in such plastic forms as amphibians. In man, ipsilateral movements of the extremities have never been obtained by cortical stimulation.

There are other more reasonable explanations for improvement of hemiplegia. The usual stroke involves the distribution of the middle cerebral artery, which supplies the cortex controlling the face, arm and speech, and does not include the anterior cerebral artery which runs to most of the leg cortex. Therefore, the leg may recover more than the arm.

Moreover, the effective motor area of the cortical gray mantle is probably not confined to a mosaic of neatly arranged and small tiles lying only in the precentral gyrus and adjacent part of the postcentral convolution, as is usually shown in a typical functional map. It consists rather of broad regions of neuronal representation, extending over at least one third of the lateral aspect of the cerebral hemisphere, with wide overlap of face with arm and arm with leg. The reserve of potentially effective motor tissue is great (Murphy and Gellhorn).

When the whole of the potential motor cortex (in the monkey) is extirpated, contralateral hemiplegia results. After the passage of time, recovery of leg function is almost complete and the arm improves to a certain extent. If now the opposite hemisphere is treated exactly the same, hemiplegia is produced on the other side, but the initially paralyzed and largely recovered leg does not become immobile again (Murphy and Arana). This indicates that ipsilateral cortical representation has nothing to do with improvement in strength of the leg after central paralysis, in the monkey at least, and strongly suggests the importance of motor function of subcortical nuclei, particularly in the basal forebrain. Direct stimulation of these internal centers results in just the tonic postural type of movement characteristic of the hemiplegic gait.

It is probable that speech *is* a function bilaterally represented, at least in some persons. In children, stuttering and stammering often follow the changing from left- to right-handedness. Speech therapists note improvement in communication parallel with development of vigor of the left side of the body when aphasia is associated with right hemiplegia.

PSYCHIATRIC TREATMENT

Although any vascular syndrome producing cerebral injury may result in psychiatric illness, the effects of arteriosclerotic and senile changes account for most psychoses following cerebrovascular disease. The mounting incidence of breakdowns in the elderly is proportionate to the increase in longevity of the population as a whole, and the admission rate of aged persons to mental hospitals has doubled in the past 20 years.

Concerning acute cerebrovascular episodes, it is a matter of common observation that emotional stress or crisis may precipitate a stroke. Psychiatric analysis of many patients who have sustained hemiplegic or other intracranial attacks reveals a premorbid life pattern of hostility, chronic anger and aggression often unfulfilled. The paramount necessity of psychologic readjustment and the relaxation of rigidity in a concerted effort to avoid further cerebral vascular insults is obvious.

HOSPITALIZATION.—In any mentally deranged but presumably harmless individual a paranoid streak may erupt into savage and even murderous behavior. It is always the wiser plan to place arteriosclerotic or senile psychotic patients in a custodial institution if there is any suggestion of suicidal or aggressive trends. Moreover, association with others similarly afflicted or even more seriously deranged sometimes seems to be helpful in "shocking" the individual back to prepsychotic sanity, contrary to the family's usual belief that such association will make him worse. The hospital or sanatorium also has the advantages of an established routine and the aid of trained and understanding attendants, two factors important in recovery and often lacking in even the best-ordered household.

GENERAL HYGIENE, SEDATION.—Nutrition must be rectified and maintained, often under trying circumstances. Special attention is given to the intake of fluids, proteins and vitamins, components which the patient tends to leave out of a self-administered diet. Sleep is often difficult to achieve; although the elderly tend to spend fewer hours a night in sleep than do the young, a restless and fretful person needs rest and may exhaust himself without it.

Chloral hydrate (1–2 Gm.) or paraldehyde (4–8 cc.) are better than barbiturates for sedation. One combination of barbiturate and amphetamine, Dexamyl (32 mg. amobarbital, 5 mg. of dextro-amphetamine sulfate), is particularly effective in relieving the mood of depression, with which sleeplessness is associated. Bromides are often employed injudiciously; the treatment and not the disease may become responsible for many symptoms.

OCCUPATIONAL THERAPY.—Too much bed rest, on the other hand, is bad for elderly patients. The services of physical and occupational therapists may be utilized in creating an atmosphere of interested employment, if only in the usual hobby crafts. However, it may be rather late in life to train an elderly artisan in rug weaving, an activity he may regard as silly, and it is better to encourage the patient to resume his usual trade or occupation if and when he is able. Many aged persons have salvageable skills, as war-time emergency situations demonstrated. Occupational therapy is particularly attractive in a group.

ELECTRIC SHOCK.—The older, arteriosclerotic patient with intractable mental depression or in a paranoid episode often responds surprisingly well to shock therapy (Kalinowsky and Hoch). The usual precautions against deleterious side effects should be carefully observed in the elderly and fragile; in addition to orthopedic and cardiac complications, cerebral thrombosis has been precipitated. If vascular contraindications to electric shock are present and a severe psychiatric syndrome of depression, pain or extreme agitation can be controlled in no other way, prefrontal lobotomy can be performed with benefit.

INCREASE OF CEREBRAL BLOOD FLOW.—A direct approach to the problem of increasing the cerebral circulation when major ischemia of the brain is responsible for deterioration and mental symptomatology may some day be made. Euphoria and transient relief from morbid preoccupation and psychomotor retardation have been observed after bilateral stellate ganglion block (Karnosh and Gardner). However, long term effects in a large series of senile depressions have not been reported. A similar study of beneficial results (if any) from cervical sympathectomy has not been undertaken, but this therapeutic approach would seem to have merit. Another less radical method of trying to increase cerebral blood flow is by intravenous administration of histamine and nicotinic acid. Large doses of nicotinic acid (300 mg. orally and three times daily and 100 mg. daily by injection) are said to benefit patients with psychoses of senility (Gregory). Metrazol orally alone or in combination with nicotinic acid may increase mentation in the senile and forgetful.

BIBLIOGRAPHY

Evans, J. P., et al.: Acute head injury, U.S. Armed Forces M. J. 2:1001-1020, 1951.

Fishman, R. A., and Halla, R. J.: Effects of isotonic intravenous solutions on normal and increased intracranial pressure, A.M.A. Arch. Neurol. & Psychiat. 70:350-360, 1953.

Gregory, I.:Nicotinic acid therapy in psychoses of senility, Am. J. Psychiat. 108:888-895, 1952.

Higgins, G., et al.: Metabolic disorders in head injury: Hyperchloremia and hypochloruria, Lancet 1:1295-1300, 1951.

Kalinowsky, L. B., and Hoch, P. H.: Shock Treatments, Psychosurgery and Other Somatic Treatments in Psychiatry (New York: Grune & Stratton, Inc. 1952).

Karnosh, L. J., and Gardner, W. J.: Effects of bilateral stellate ganglion block on mental depression: Report of three cases, Cleveland Clin. Quart. 14:133-138, 1947.

Luisada, A. A.: The mechanism and treatment of pulmonary edema, Illinois M. J. 100:254-257, 1951.

Mithoefer, J. C.: Increased intracranial pressure in emphysema caused by oxygen inhalation, J.A.M.A. 149:1116-1120, 1952.

Moyer, C. A.: Fluid Balance: A Clinical Manual (Chicago: The Year Book Publishers, Inc., 1952).

Murphy, J. P., and Arana, R.: Extirpation of the cortical arm area as defined by stimulation under conditions of primary facilitation, J. Neuropath. & Exper. Neurol. 6:194-200, 1947.

Murphy, J. P., and Gellhorn, E.: Multiplicity of representation versus punctate localization in motor cortex, Arch. Neurol. & Psychiat. 54:256-273, 1945.

Peters, J. P., *et al.*: A salt-wasting syndrome associated with cerebral disease, Tr. A. Am. Physicians 63:57, 1950.

Rudin, L. N., and Cronin, D. J.: A mechanical quadriceps, Arch. Phys. Med. 33:15-19, 1952.

Rusk, H. A.: *Hemiplegia and Rehabilitation* (West Point, Pa.: Sharp & Dohme, 1952).

Shenkin, H. A., *et al.*: The acute effects on the cerebral circulation of the reduction of increased intracranial pressure by means of intravenous glucose or ventricular drainage, J. Neurosurg. 5:466-470, 1948.

Sperry, R. W.: The problem of central nervous reorganization after nerve regeneration and muscle transposition, Neurosurgery report no. 59, Committee on Medical Research of the OSRD, October, 1944.

Stark, W., and Barrera, S. E.: Use of potassium in protracted insulin coma, Arch. Neurol. & Psychiat. 62: 280-286, 1949.

Welt, L. G., *et al.*: Role of the central nervous system in metabolism of electrolytes and water, A.M.A. Arch. Int. Med. 90:355-378, 1952.

CHAPTER 20

Diagnostic Technics

LUMBAR SPINAL PUNCTURE

PROCEDURE.—Spinal tap should always be performed with the patient in the lateral recumbent position, in order to obtain a valid measurement of intracranial pressure. Knees are drawn as far as possible toward the chest and the legs flexed, so that the spine is curved forward. An interspace below the third lumbar vertebra is selected and creased with the thumbnail. The skin is prepared and procaine is infiltrated between two spines down to the interspinous ligament. Reassuring the patient that lumbar puncture is simple, painless and not dangerous will facilitate the procedure.

A long, sharp spinal puncture needle, 19 or 20 gauge, fitted with a stilet, is inserted exactly in the midline. This maneuver is assured by grasping the spinous process just above between the thumb and index finger of the left hand and pushing the needle point through the skin and into the thick interspinous ligament at a point half way between the thumb and index finger at exact right angles to the flat surface of the back. Further advancement of the needle is made along a path of moderate resistance. Too easy progress often means that the needle is entering the muscle and will strike bone, with resultant pain and withdrawal of blood. Usually one aims toward the umbilicus, but if the patient's body is not flexed, the needle goes straight in and sometimes even runs caudally. Perforation of the dura and arachnoid often produces a palpable "click." Progress is made with care to prevent nerve injury and to avoid a traumatic tap. The depth of the subarachnoid space from the surface is variable in thin or thick individuals. When the subarachnoid space is entered by the tip of the needle, cerebrospinal fluid appears as the stilet is withdrawn.

Pressure measurements.—Before measurement of pressure, the patient should be entirely relaxed, with the head in midposition or slightly extended to avoid compression of the jugular veins and with the thighs and knees also extended to relieve flattening of the abdomen. Deep breathing is encouraged to insure further relaxation. After the stilet is withdrawn from the needle, a three-way stopcock connected with an Ayer water manometer is attached quickly to prevent loss of fluid. Readings of pressure should be taken only if pulsations are free and the patient is relaxed. It is erroneous to believe that intraspinal tension can be estimated without use of a manometer.

The upper limit of normal spinal and intracranial pressure determined under these circumstances is 150 mm. of water. With the manometer in place, a sample of fluid is drawn off, 1–2 cc. if the pressure is above 300, 10–20 cc. if pressure is normal. A rapid drop of high intraspinal tension indicates an expansile intracranial mass. There is no need for determining intraspinal hydrodynamics in a patient with cerebrovascular disease except to ascertain whether or not a lateral sinus or jugular vein is occluded. If so, the lumbar cerebrospinal fluid pressure will rise to great heights when the noninvolved jugular is compressed unilaterally in the neck and not at all when the obstructed vein is squeezed (Tobey-Ayer test). This observation is of interest only if the response from the pathologic side is zero or nearly so. Owing to normal inequality in distribution of the intracranial sinuses, increases in lumbar pressure when each vein is tested separately are almost always different to a degree.

Intracranial hemorrhage vs. "bloody tap."—Important information to be obtained from a spinal puncture in cerebrovascular disease concerns the presence or absence of intracranial hemorrhage. One must be certain that blood, if present, is of pathologic and not traumatic origin. Careful attention to the details of puncture will assure an atraumatic lumbar tap. Fluid pressure is often low with a "bloody tap" and is usually high in subarachnoid hemorrhage. Pathologic subarachnoid blood remains in the same concentration as fluid flows from the needle, whereas in a traumatic puncture the last sample obtained is clearer or clear compared with the first bloody drops. A clot forms in cerebrospinal fluid obtained traumatically. Crenated erythrocytes and xanthochromia of a visible degree appear four to seven hours after spontaneous hemorrhage; therefore, the specimen should be centrifuged and inspected immediately. In very fresh intracranial hemorrhages, the uniformity of sanguineous appearance of cerebrospinal fluid must be depended on, since the lapse of time may not be sufficient for crenation of red cells and xanthochromia to become evident.

PNEUMOENCEPHALOGRAPHY

If signs of increased intracranial pressure are absent, cautious encephalography may help to differentiate intracerebral hematoma from cerebral infarct, cerebral arteriosclerosis from brain tumor and ruptured aneurysm from bleeding vascular malformation. In the standard procedure, 90–150 cc. of cerebrospinal fluid is withdrawn by lumbar puncture from the adult patient, sitting upright and under anesthesia. This fluid is replaced with an equivalent amount of air or oxygen.

A "small encephalogram" (Monrad-Krohn) is preferable and may be informative in critical cases and in debilitated and elderly patients or those who have bled recently. Spinal puncture is performed in bed with the patient sitting or leaning sideways on pillows. After 20–30 cc. of fluid is withdrawn, a like amount of air is injected. General anesthesia is unnecessary. Films are made of the skull with the head erect or with the subject lying flat. In a surprising number of cases excellent ventricular filling is obtained and lesions may be visualized. The examination can be combined with arteriography, if indicated.

VENTRICULOGRAPHY

This diagnostic study is ordinarily undertaken before planned, definitive intracranial surgery and is a major operative procedure in itself. The ventricular system is punctured at the junction of the posterior horns and bodies of the lateral ventricles through bur holes placed 5 cm. above the external occipital protuberance and 3 cm. from the midline. Special blunt needles are directed toward the pupil of the eye; the ventricles are ordinarily encountered at a depth of 5–6 cm. from the skin surface. Openings over the anterior horns may be made in the skull 10–11 cm. from the glabella and 3 cm. lateral to the interparietal suture. Fluid is aspirated or is drained by gravity and is replaced with air to the usual amount of 10–30 cc. By placing the head in four standard positions, the ventricular system is visualized roentgenographically in all parts. The third and fourth ventricles are particularly difficult to see clearly. Indentation, collapse of a part of the system or its displacement indicate a mass lesion.

ANGIOGRAPHY

The differential diagnosis and treatment of cerebrovascular disease have been revolutionized by the introduction of intracranial angiography as a diagnostic method. First suggested and described by Moniz in 1927, the procedure has been adopted enthusiastically and has been applied widely by neurologists and neurosurgeons. Angiography is peculiarly suited to the problems of cerebrovascular disease. In this neuroroentgeno-graphic technic, arteries and veins of the brain may be seen directly and clearly. The size, branching, filling and position of intracranial vessels can be compared with the normal, and aneurysms, the vascular supply of tumors and arteriovenous communications and malformations can be filled with radiopaque material and visualized accurately instead of indirectly as in air studies.

Angiography is indicated when surgical treatment is under consideration and a precise diagnosis is required; it is not done when differential distinction is of academic interest only. Contraindications to the procedure include extreme age, advanced arteriosclerosis, severe hypertension, cardiac decompensation, recent cerebral embolism or thrombosis and nitrogen retention. Under these circumstances, the risk of angiography is great and only absolute necessity permits the examination. Active bleeding from an intracranial aneurysm need not preclude arteriography, for it has been demonstrated that injection of 10 cc. fluid into the common carotid artery does not increase the pressure in the internal carotid above (Sweet *et al.*).

MATERIALS

The needle for cannulation of the carotid artery should be sharp, preferably new, and of 17 or 18 gauge. It may be specially curved, tapered to a point or have a steplike bayonet shaft. The Huber needle, which has the opening on the side of the end rather than at a beveled tip, is especially useful. An 18 gauge spinal needle is advocated for puncture of the vertebral artery. The hub of any needle should fit the adapter of a rubber connecting tube or stopcock which is attached after successful insertion has been made in the artery or is continuous with the needle during its entrance into the vessel under direct vision. It is helpful to have a three-way stopcock between tube and syringe, to the side-arm of which an intravenous drip of 5 per cent glucose solution may be connected for measurement of intracarotid pressure and to keep the needle and artery open between injections. The stilet may be replaced in the needle after injection is finished, to prevent clotting.

Syringes should be of 10 or 20 cc. size, must fit the end of the connecting tube or needle hub snugly and should have pistons which are not loose but which slide easily. This last is necessary in order that increased resistance to injection will mean that the tip of the needle is out of the lumen of the artery.

Contrast mediums.—Thorotrast (colloidal thorium dioxide) was first employed by Moniz and was used exclusively in intracranial angiography before the introduction of Diodrast by Gross. Disadvantages of Thorotrast are the production of minor cerebral thromboses and the development of chronic, cicatrizing and strangling granulomas in the neck when the contrast material leaks out of an artery into which it is injected percutaneously. Sarcogenesis has also been reported, since Thorotrast is radioactive.

Today, its use in intracranial angiography is restricted to patients with severe iodine sensitivity and older patients in whom degenerative or inflammatory cerebrovascular disease is suspected.

Diodrast (iodopyracet, perabrodil, umbradil, Diodone) is much superior in all-round usage. Although Thorotrast gives sharper x-ray pictures of vessels, Diodrast may leak into the neck with impunity, leaves no significant scar and only temporary soreness and is an adequate contrast medium. However, Diodrast is a vascular irritant, causing vasospasm and change in permeability of capillaries (Broman and Olsson) and has a direct, toxic action on nerve cells apparently through alteration of the blood-brain barrier (Foltz et al.).

A solution no stronger than 35 per cent should be used for intra-arterial injection. The total volume of dye injected in one day should not be over 40 cc. Warming Diodrast is believed to reduce its vasospastic properties. Prolonged application of this contrast medium to the interior of vessels through which flow is pathologically slow is apt to injure the endothelium; therefore, it is recommended that intervals between repeated introductions be at least 15 minutes long. Before administration of Diodrast by any route, the patient must be examined for iodine sensitivity by an eye or skin test.

CAROTID ANGIOGRAPHY

Anesthesia.—Local infiltration of procaine into the neck and deeper tissues with special blockage of the carotid sinus may be used. By and large, general anesthesia is preferable, since it allays pain and anxiety, insures constant position of the head and freedom from motion, permits a lengthy session if this should be necessary, and prevents convulsions due to cerebral irritation. Pentothal is the anesthetic agent of choice with use of an endotracheal tube and the addition of gas if necessary. If local anesthesia is used, preliminary injection of phenobarbital or Nembutal is indicated, because experimental study has shown that barbiturates exert a protective effect against Diodrast toxicity (Ziperman et al.).

Carotid puncture methods.—In the open method (Fig. 121), the common carotid artery is exposed (Chapter 21) and is brought to the surface of the skin with a rubber drain or loop of umbilical tape. The needle is then inserted under direct vision.

The percutaneous method is preferred in most instances if Diodrast is to be used. When the two-plate x-ray technic is employed, the patient's head is slightly extended and rests with the occiput on a sand bag, face upward, with a pillow placed under the shoulders. The cassette is held against the side of the head and the roentgen tube is directed laterally

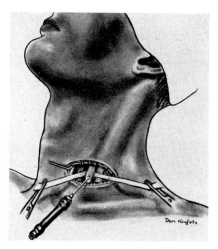

FIG. 121.—Direct (open) carotid angiography. (Courtesy of S. W. Gross.)

toward the opposite side. Or the head may be turned laterally, parallel to the table top, with the rays directed down from above as in a lateral skull film. If a multiple exposure seriograph is to be used, the shoulders slope off the edge of the cassette holder and the head is applied against the flat upper surface of the film compartments, with the noninjected side down. The x-ray tube is superior and the rays directed downward (Fig. 122).

The carotid pulsation is palpated medial to the sternocleidomastoid muscle just below the cricoid cartilage, and the artery is held in place by moderate pressure. The needle is introduced through the skin and toward the artery. The vessel will slip and slide around, especially in a loose neck, and often must be pinioned against the vertebral transverse processes. Directing the needle tip laterally rather than toward the midline is helpful, and the wall of the vessel is encountered superficially rather than deep. A sense of resistance may or may not be felt as the cannula enters the artery: the only valid test of correct placement is a vigorous spurting stream of arterial blood when the stilet is withdrawn. One must be sure that the needle tip is entirely within the lumen and not half in, half out. In the latter event, the force of injection will blow the needle point out of the interior of the carotid and dye will be injected into the carotid sheath. A trial injection of glucose solution is of value to prove proper introduction. The needle may have to be held in place manually or the shaft rested against a folded towel on the chest. The tube system is connected, the glucose drip started, if desired, and the examination then pro-

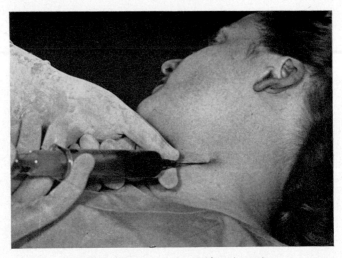

FIG. 122.—Percutaneous carotid angiography.

ceeds. The operator may prefer to attach the syringe directly to the needle or stopcock without using an intervening tube.

Injection, taking of films.—Injection of 35 per cent Diodrast into the carotid artery is made in amounts of 8–15 cc. and as rapidly as possible to keep the dye together on the arterial side. If severe resistance is felt injection should be stopped, since contrast medium is going into the neck or is blocked by a thrombosed artery. Close co-operation of operator and x-ray technician is essential. If a two-plate technic is used, the first film, of the arterial phase, is called for when 8 cc. of Diodrast has entered the artery. The second, venous stage is taken four seconds later on a cassette protected from the first exposure by a lead shield.

Both lateral and anteroposterior projections should be taken in carotid angiography. If a choice must be made between the two, the lateral film is more informative in the greater number of cases. Hence, lateral films are usually made first, since technical difficulties may develop later. While the anteroposterior view is being made, compression of the opposite carotid during injection will result in bilateral visualization of intracranial derivatives of the carotid trunks (Fig. 22).

Multiple exposure methods involve the rapid and serial changing of x-ray plates or recording on a moving roll of film (Fairchild camera). Advantages of multiple exposure methods are freedom from the need for replacing cassettes by hand and, particularly, the visualization of many vessels and lesions not seen when only two exposures are made.

Arteries begin to appear above the floor of the skull when 5–6 cc.

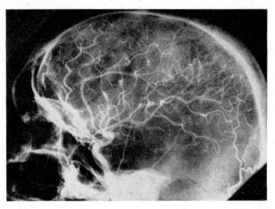

FIG. 123.—Normal arteriogram, internal and external carotid arterial circulations.

of Diodrast has been injected; at 8 cc. the full pattern of the carotid artery and its branches is shown in detail (Figs. 6, 10 and 123). Superficial cerebral veins appear two seconds later, large veins and venous sinuses fill four seconds after the arteriogram (Fig. 18) and all dye has left the skull after two more seconds. Between arterial and venous stages there is a capillary phase.

False interpretation of artefactual "abnormalities" of both arteries and veins due to technical difficulties must be guarded against in the analysis of angiograms. A single vessel cannot be said to be absent without repeated attempts to visualize it.

VERTEBRAL ANGIOGRAPHY

For vertebral puncture by the open method, a transverse incision is made parallel to and just above the clavicle. The vertebral artery (first branch of the subclavian) is isolated directly, after retraction of the phrenic nerve and cutting of the anterior scalene muscular insertion. Or the subclavian artery is exposed by dissection lateral to the scalene, is occluded still further laterally, as is the thyrocervical trunk, and the vertebral artery is injected indirectly against the flow of blood in the subclavian.

In the percutaneous method (Sugar *et al.*), the head is slightly extended, as in carotid puncture. The left hand pulls the carotid sheath laterally from the trachea at the level of the cricoid, and the transverse process of the fifth cervical vertebra is palpated. The 18 gauge spinal needle is advanced, bevel down, through the skin upward, dorsally and laterally. It is helpful to seek the tip of the transverse process and then to move 1 cm. medially to find the vertebral foramen transversarium. The needle tip slides off the body of the lower vertebra into a funnel shaped by the inferior surface of the transverse process of the upper vertebra, and so into the vertebral artery. Tubing or a syringe is connected when an arterial spurt appears. The rest of the procedure progresses as in carotid angiography. The vertebrae hold the needle fairly firmly in place.

Arterial patterns appear in the posterior circulation after 20 cc. of 35 per cent Diodrast has been injected into the cervical vertebral artery (Fig. 11). Veins are seen after an interval of time comparable to the delay after carotid angiography (four seconds).

Two projections are important in vertebral angiography; a lateral view, with care taken to be sure that the suboccipital part of the head is on the film, and a submentovertical (axial) view, replacing the usual anteroposterior view taken in carotid visualization. Oblique x-rays may also be helpful in both carotid and vertebral arteriograms.

COMBINED CAROTID-VERTEBRAL EXAMINATION (Ecker).—The carotid artery is cannulated as low in the neck as possible, and angiography is performed. Compression of the opposite carotid during injection will result in bilateral filling of the intracranial carotid systems. A blood pressure cuff is then wrapped around the ipsilateral arm high in the axilla and is inflated to a pressure above that in the brachial artery. The common carotid artery is compressed manually above the point of needle insertion, and 20 cc. of Diodrast is injected. Films are taken at the end of the injection. Thus, the vertebral artery and its intracranial branches are visualized via the carotid, a method particularly advantageous in children in whom the cervical vertebral vessel is small.

COMPLICATIONS

Untoward effects of angiography range from persistent soreness in the neck to death as a result of the procedure. Local consequences of manipulation or perforation of arteries include needle bruises in the larynx and pharynx, massive hematoma in the neck, occlusion of a vessel by the injection of dye into its sheath, carotid sinus syncope, injury to the cervical sympathetic nerves and thrombosis of the cervical carotid or vertebral arteries. Major reflex cerebral arterial vasospasm, due to trauma to the parent vessel in the neck or to passage of Diodrast through intracranial vessels, has caused cerebral infarction without thrombosis, postarteriographic hemiplegia or other neurologic deficit of transient character and blindness due to retinal angiospasm or hemorrhages. Direct irritation of peripheral vessels may result in convulsive seizures, multiple tiny cerebral infarcts or petechial hemorrhages in the eye and face. Air and blood-clot embolisms have occurred. The blood-brain barrier may be disturbed. Severe reactions in iodine-sensitive patients have terminated in death. Instances of radicular pain, the Brown-Séquard syndrome and "peduncular hallucinosis" have followed vertebral angiography.

The toxic effect of Diodrast is partially suppressed by preinjection administration of a barbiturate or the use of Pentothal anesthesia. Vasospasm is minimized by performing stellate block and by giving 65–130 mg. of papaverine intravenously just before injection of Diodrast.

Certain treatment measures are useful if complications arise. Among these are the application of an icebag to the swelling neck and undertaking tracheotomy in the presence of severe respiratory embarrassment. Administration of papaverine and sympathicolytic drugs and of histamine intravenously is helpful if postangiographic vasospasm is suspected, or stellate block is repeated. Epinephrine or ephedrine is given for urticaria or other allergic manifestations.

DURAL SINUS VENOGRAPHY

Ray and associates have perfected two technics for visualization of the dural venous sinuses. Direct injection of contrast mediums into the sinuses is necessary to be absolutely certain of their patency or occlusion and, in the event of obstruction, to reveal the presence or absence of functioning collateral connections (Fig. 100).

In one method, a catheter is put into the basilic vein of the arm and is threaded upward under fluoroscopic control through the subclavian vein to the superior bulb of the internal jugular. Injection of 25 cc. of 35 per cent Diodrast is made while pressure is being applied to both jugulars, thereby demonstrating the sigmoid and transverse sinus, the torcular, the superior and inferior petrosal and the cavernous sinuses. Lateral films are taken at one-half second exposure.

In the other procedure, a cranial bur hole is made in the midline of the skull just in front of the hair line, or the posterior angle of the open fontanel is pierced in infants. A no. 8 ureteral catheter is inserted through a nick in the wall of the superior sagittal sinus and is passed posteriorly for 3–4 cm. The catheter is kept open with heparin in saline. Then 15 cc. of 35 per cent Diodrast is injected rapidly and anteroposterior and lateral films are made in one-half second exposures. The superior sagittal and transverse sinuses and the internal jugular veins are visualized. In anteroposterior films the relative dominance of the lateral sinuses may be seen. Cerebral veins do not appear unless opened as anastomotic channels when the superior sagittal sinus is occluded by thrombus or tumor.

ELECTROENCEPHALOGRAPHY

Electroencephalography is a simple, painless and absolutely safe diagnostic neurologic technic but is also the least informative and accurate in cerebrovascular disease. However, because of the simplicity and atraumatic nature of the procedure and because repetition is easy and ready, an electrical record should be made in every patient with hemiplegic stroke, intracranial hemorrhage or other variety of vascular processes. Valuable information may be and often is made available, and if findings are negative, nothing has been lost but a little time.

PROCEDURE.—Electrodes are applied to symmetrical points on the frontal, parietal, temporal, anterior temporal and occipital scalp areas. Leads from each ear lobe or mastoid tip are yoked together as an indifferent reference and the patient is grounded. Impulses from the brain are picked up by the electrodes and are transmitted to the electroencephalograph, where manifold amplification is undertaken by a system of vacuum tubes and electrical energy is changed to mechanical energy to deflect a pen writing on a strip of paper which is moving at a controlled speed (Fig. 26, A). The record is taken with the patient's eyes closed. The patient is often encouraged to sleep, or somnolence is induced with barbiturates, and a period of hyperventilation is usual at the end of the recording session. Component waves in a normal waking electroencephalogram, changes in sleep and pathologic frequencies are discussed in Chapter 5.

BIBLIOGRAPHY

Broman, T., and Olsson, O.: Experimental study of contrast media for cerebral angiography, with reference to possible injurious effects on the cerebral blood vessels, Acta radiol. 31: 321-334, 1949.
Ecker, A. D.: The Normal Cerebral Angiogram (Springfield, Ill.: Charles C Thomas, Publisher, 1951).

Foltz, E. L.; Thomas, L. B., and Ward, A. A.: The effects of intracarotid Diodrast, J. Neurosurg. 9:68-82, 1952.

Gross, S. W.: Cerebral arteriography in the dog and man with a rapidly excreted organic iodide, Proc. Soc. Exper. Biol. & Med. 42:258-259, 1939.

Ray, B. S.; Dunbar, H. S., and Dotter, C. T.: Dural sinus venography as aid to diagnosis in intracranial disease, J. Neurosurg. 8:23-37, 1951.

Sugar, O.; Holden, L. B., and Powell, C. B.: Vertebral angiography, Am. J. Roentgenol. 61:166-182, 1949.

Sweet, W. H.; Sarnoff, S. J., and Bakay, L.: A clinical method for recording internal carotid pressure: Significance of changes during carotid occlusion, Surg., Gynec. & Obst. 90:327-334, 1950.

Ziperman, H. H.; Hughes, R. R., and Shumacker, H. B.: The effect of barbiturates and other drugs on mortality from Diodrast in the mouse, Angiology 1:427-431, 1950.

CHAPTER 21

Therapeutic Technics

STELLATE BLOCK

There are many controversial aspects of procaine blockade of the stellate ganglion as a treatment of cerebrovascular disease. However, clinical experience with this procedure for almost two decades indicates that it may be of considerable benefit in relieving neurologic deficit attendant on acute ischemia of the brain. Logically, the use of stellate anesthesia should be restricted to pathologic conditions producing intracranial arterial vasospasm, and benefit from sympathetic nerve block can only mean revival of ganglion cells which are nonfunctioning but not dead. Since one can never know exactly what part angiospasm is playing in an acute cerebrovascular accident, stellate block may be used judiciously in any type of nonhemorrhagic stroke. Direct microscopic observation of the monkey cerebral cortex before and after procaine block of the stellate ganglion reveals increase in cortical capillarity and dilatation of arterioles (Huertas and Forster).

In the performance of stellate block, a local anesthetic solution is injected in the vicinity of the stellate ganglion by an anterior, anterolateral or posterior approach. The most useful agent is 2 per cent procaine (Novocain) hydrochloride in the amount of 5–10 cc. Longer-acting procaine, ammonium or alcohol mixtures in propylene glycol or oil are too irritating and indefinite in their action to be recommended. Xylocaine may be substituted effectively. Smaller amounts of Xylocaine solution (2–5 cc.) may be used and the anesthetic effect is longer lasting. Before injection of procaine near the stellate ganglion, the injecting needle is aspirated. If air (apex of lung), blood (regional veins and arteries) or cerebrospinal fluid (dural sleeve around cervical nerve root) is present in the syringe, the procedure is terminated or the needle is withdrawn and replaced more accurately.

380

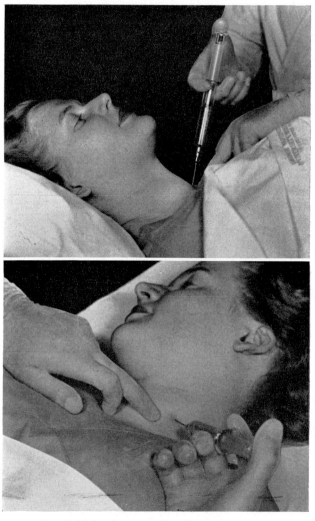

FIG. 124 *(above)*.—Stellate block, anterior method.
FIG. 125 *(below)*.—Stellate block, anterolateral method.

A barbiturate should always be administered orally or by injection one-half hour before stellate or other temporary nerve block to prevent the rare but severe procaine reaction which may be manifested by convulsions or sudden death. Facilities for resuscitation should be available when stellate block is performed on outpatients.

ANTERIOR METHOD.—The neck is extended over a sandbag or pillow and the head is not rotated. The skin is punctured 2 fingerbreadths above the sternoclavicular joint. The trachea is held medially and the great vessels of the neck lie laterally. A 20–22 gauge needle, 5 cm. long, is passed directly in toward the seventh cervical vertebra at right angles to the neck and is directed slightly medially, entering between the sternal and clavicular heads of the sternocleidomastoid muscle (Fig. 124). When bone is encountered, it is the junction of body and transverse process of the seventh cervical vertebra. At this point, if aspiration is negative, 5–10 cc. of 2 per cent procaine or Xylocaine is injected.

ANTEROLATERAL METHOD.—The neck is extended over a pillow which also underlies the shoulder on the side of injection, and the head is rotated so that the patient faces toward the opposite side. A skin wheal is made over the transverse process of the seventh cervical vertebra, which is palpable at the first skin crease above the clavicle (Fig. 125). A 22 gauge needle, 5 cm. long, is inserted until it strikes the tip of the transverse process, along which it slides until the body of the sixth cervical vertebra is contacted. Here aspiration is made, and 10 cc. of 2 per cent procaine is injected. Procaine will reach the stellate ganglion easily by spreading through the soft tissues even from the body of the fifth cervical vertebra (Fig. 126). Introducing the needle over the tip of a finger which depresses the dome of the pleura as it rests on the clavicle will help to avoid pneumothorax.

POSTERIOR METHOD.—The stellate ganglion is reached by puncturing the skin of the back just below the vertebra prominens (seventh cervical) and 1–2 fingerbreadths lateral to the spine of the first thoracic vertebra. The needle point is directed slightly medialward between the transverse processes of these vertebrae to the body of seventh cervical vertebra, where injection is made after aspiration. A narrow-gauge spinal puncture needle is necessary. The posterior approach is least recommended because of the greater possibility of complications.

RESULTS.—Success in the accurate placement of the local anesthetic is evidenced immediately or at least in 15–30 minutes by the appearance of some or all phenomena of the Claude-Bernard-Horner syndrome: ipsilateral drooping of the eyelid, small pupil, enophthalmos, conjunctival and retinal vasodilatation, stuffiness of the nose and warmness and dryness of the ear, face and arm. The full blown syndrome need not be present for therapeutic efficacy. Neurologic signs of cerebral ischemia should begin to regress as soon as Horner's syndrome develops, but delay need not preclude eventual benefit.

COMPLICATIONS.—Reported complications of stellate block include sudden death, particularly in the elderly, due to "pleural shock" (air embolism) or a vagus reflex; tension pneumothorax from perforation of

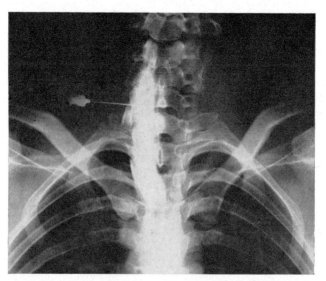

FIG. 126.—Diffusion of injected substance (Diodrast) after anterolateral stellate block. (Courtesy of F. A. D. Alexander and B. K. Lovell.)

the apical pleura and lung; accidental high spinal anesthesia; intra-arterial injection of procaine; acute asthma, and increased intraocular tension with precipitation of glaucoma.

LIGATION OF THE CERVICAL CAROTID ARTERY

Cervical carotid artery ligation is the procedure of choice in the treatment of carotid-cavernous fistula, many bleeding or enlarging congenital arterial aneurysms of the circle of Willis and some types of arteriovenous anomaly of the cerebral hemisphere. The actual technic of ligation is not difficult; what does require care, study and thought is avoidance of crippling or lethal neurologic consequences. The occasion for carotid ligature influences the result; the mortality from common or internal carotid ligation in the course of resection of metastatic malignancy or tumor of the carotid body is at least 50 per cent, whereas carefully planned ligature of the common carotid artery for control of intracranial carotid aneurysm usually is without deleterious sequel.

Whenever carotid ligation is undertaken in the treatment of cerebrovascular disease, the aim is to prevent episodes of bleeding from congenital or acquired arterial or arteriovenous lesions. This is achieved by allowing thrombosis or healing of points of vascular rupture through reduction of intravascular pressure distally, within the skull, but without causing ipsilateral cerebral ischemia at the same time. Fortunately, in most persons the cross-hemispheral circulation through the circle of Willis is not strong enough to defeat attainment of this goal but is sufficient to allow ligation to proceed without serious cerebral anemia on the same side, provided certain factors are understood and precautions taken.

TECHNICS OF LIGATION

EXPOSURE AND IDENTIFICATION OF CAROTIDS.—The common carotid artery is approached through a transverse incision 5 cm. long made in the lower skin crease of the neck, centered on the arterial pulsation felt just medial to the anterior border of the sternocleidomastoid muscle. The internal carotid, particularly if the superior cervical ganglion is also to be visualized, is best reached through a diagonal incision 9–10 cm. in length, beginning at the mastoid tip and extending along the anterior border of the sternocleidomastoid to a point 2 or 3 cm. below the carotid bifurcation at the upper border of the thyroid cartilage. The carotid sheath is reached by blunt dissection toward the pulse, tying off intervening small vessels and avoiding regional nerves. The fibrous sheath is opened, care being exerted to prevent laceration of the internal jugular vein. The vein and vagus nerve are then separated from the carotid artery (Fig. 127).

The carotid sinus reflex should now be depressed by injection of procaine into the adventitia of the carotid bifurcation. Below the bifurcation, the vessel is single; above the sinus there are two large arteries, the internal and external carotids. Three means of distinguishing the internal from the external carotid are provided. (1) The internal carotid is actually external (lateral) and anterior to the external carotid at their mutual origin. (2) There are no cervical branches from the internal carotid, whereas eight branches arise from the external artery, the superior thyroid coming off and down just above the bifurcation and being most easily visible in investigation of this region. (3) Temporary clamping of the external carotid will cause the temporal pulse to disappear, whereas occlusion of the internal carotid does not have such an effect. If all vessels are in spasm, instillation of procaine solution into the field will revive the temporal pulse and allow identification to proceed.

COMPLETE LIGATION IN CONTINUITY.—The usual method of occlusion is double ligation of the carotid with heavy silk suture. The artery is encircled by careful dissection between adventitia and media, surrounding

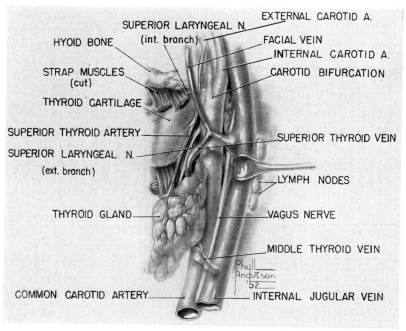

SUPERIOR LARYNGEAL N.
EXTERNAL CAROTID A.
HYOID BONE
(int. branch)
FACIAL VEIN
INTERNAL CAROTID A.
STRAP MUSCLES
(cut)
CAROTID BIFURCATION
THYROID CARTILAGE
SUPERIOR THYROID ARTERY
SUPERIOR THYROID VEIN
SUPERIOR LARYNGEAL N.
(ext. branch)
LYMPH NODES
THYROID GLAND
VAGUS NERVE
MIDDLE THYROID VEIN
COMMON CAROTID ARTERY
INTERNAL JUGULAR VEIN

Fig. 127.—Surgical anatomy of the cervical carotid artery.

fibrous tissue is stripped from a segment of vessel 2 cm. long, and the two ligatures are placed so that there is about 5 mm. of intervening artery. In elderly patients one must be careful to avoid excessive vigor in closing these heavy ligatures; the carotid, when sclerosed, has been torn in half in this manner.

Poppen prefers imbrication of the carotid between two heavy ligatures placed as just described. The arterial segment then looks like a horseshoe in cross-section and intimal damage particularly is avoided. Silk or cotton tape may be used instead of suture material to obviate a possible cutting effect of the latter. Many surgeons have advised the use of strips of fascia, either alone or under silk ligature for protection of the artery. Major arterial vessels can also be occluded with aluminum bands or broad tantalum clips, which may be removed readily if need be.

PARTIAL, PROGRESSIVE OCCLUSION.—If tolerance of preliminary compression is poor or if the patient is elderly, partial occlusion of the common or internal carotid artery is preferable to complete obstruction, or the common carotid may be ligated first and the internal carotid tied off three to seven days later. Krayenbühl estimates the retinal blood pressure after common carotid ligation and, if the systolic reduction is not sufficient, then ligates the internal carotid. A method of progressive partial occlusion which eliminates the need for preliminary compressive build-up of tolerance and promises to be very efficacious consists in placing a screw clamp around the carotid artery at operation, with the turning-shaft of the screw left projecting from the incision. A Hoffman clamp, used to control urologic tubing, may be used as a temporary occlusive device (Swain), or the more complicated Selverstone clamp (Codman and Shurtleff, Inc., Boston) is employed for complete obstruction of the vessel. The artery is shut off 50 per cent at surgery; if this degree of compression is withstood successfully, the clamp is slowly closed completely during the next several days. If signs of cerebral ischemia appear, the clamp is reopened. When complete closure has no untoward effect, the artery is doubly ligated, and the Hoffman clamp is removed or the screw is withdrawn from the Selverstone clamp which remains in place permanently. Penicillin or another antibiotic is administered during the period of progressive closure to prevent infection.

LIGATION AND DIVISION.—Division of the common carotid between ties instead of ligation in continuity is advocated to eliminate the possibility of embolism from thrombosis and to prevent late, fatal erosion at the point of ligature (Rogers). There is, of course, no possibility of removing obstructing ties in the event of hemiplegia.

COMPLICATIONS

Fatal or neurologic complications resulting from unilateral carotid ligation are due to low circulating cerebral blood volume, circulatory stasis in the presence of increased intracranial pressure, inadequate cross-circulation through the circle of Willis or vasospasm in intracranial arteries distal to the point of cervical ligation. Spontaneous peripheral cerebral thrombosis, propagating intracranial thrombosis extending into the circle of Willis from the cervical carotid or into the brain from a thrombosing congenital aneurysmal sac and cerebral embolism from the site of ligature in the neck are other causes of postligation hemiplegia.

A state of shock, cardiac failure, severe anemia, chronic debilitation or uremia absolutely precludes carotid ligation. The chances of fatal or hemiplegic complication under these circumstances of critically inadequate cerebral blood flow are almost 100 per cent. Nor should ligation be undertaken when the patient is in coma due to recent subarachnoid hemorrhage; such "heroic" treatment is mere folly and operative death is almost invariable.

By and large, the incidence of postoperative mortality and neurologic disability is lower after ligation of the common carotid artery, which I prefer, than after ligation of the internal carotid, despite conflicting experimental evidence. The efficacy of proximal ligature of the common carotid artery in reducing intravascular pressures in even very small cerebral vessels has been demonstrated by Bakay and Sweet. Moreover, Rogers points out that a trickle of blood coursing from the external to the internal carotid above the level of occlusion of the common carotid tends to prevent propagating thrombosis headward. Lastly, an indirect arterial supply on the ligated side, although under low pressure, serves to augment the cross-hemispheral collateral willisian circulation on which the ipsilateral hemisphere now depends.

PREVENTION.—Preoperative *carotid compression* not only serves to estimate the collateral potential of the circle of Willis in the presence of unilateral carotid occlusion but also seems, if repeated over a period of several days, actually to stimulate cross-hemispheral blood supply. The patient in whom carotid ligation is to be performed must be able to withstand 20 minutes of complete, temporary occlusion of the cervical carotid without signs of cerebral ischemia developing, such as hemiparesis, hemisensory loss, aphasia or convulsions. The common carotid artery is compressed against the transverse process of the sixth cervical vertebra manually, with a spring clip or lever bar; disappearance of the temporal pulse is used as a criterion of complete external occlusion. It is advantageous to begin compression with a five minute period and to build up to 20 minutes of obstruction gradually, if possible. The surgeon may prefer to use a screw clamp inserted at open operation for progressive partial occlusion instead of preliminary compression.

Temporary ligature at operation before final permanent occlusion serves as a double check of cerebral collateral flow. The exposed carotid, common or internal, is constricted completely with a suture or band for 20 minutes, during which time the patient is questioned and observed with reference to the appearance of neurologic phenomena (contralateral hemiplegia). Use of local anesthesia increases the accuracy of such a period of observation; however, the patient may be allowed to awaken from general anesthesia.

Measurement of systolic pressure in the distal internal carotid artery during proximal occlusion is particularly informative. If pressures above the point of temporary ligature fall to 30 per cent or less of original values, permanent complete ligation will be followed predictably by neurologic complication (Sweet *et al.*), although partial ligation may be tolerated. Intracarotid arterial tension is estimated by inserting a drip of 5 per cent glucose solution into the distal carotid artery and measuring the height in centimeters which the infusion bottle must be raised to oppose systolic thrust. *Electroencephalography* during surgery has been suggested by Rogers. Unfortunately, absence of unilateral slow waves at the time of ligation does not preclude late complication, although early appearance of delta activity reveals cerebral ischemia.

Antispasmodic therapy includes the intramuscular injection of 65 mg. of papaverine every four hours for three or four doses during the immediate postoperative period and continuous procaine blockade of the superior cervical ganglion through a polyethylene catheter inserted in the sheath of the ganglion at operation. Injections of 10 cc. of 2 per cent procaine into the wound are made every four hours during the first two postoperative days.

Thromboembolic complications may be avoided by the systemic use of heparin for three or four days after operation. The patient must not have had a subarachnoid hemorrhage during the preceding three weeks, and protamine sulfate should be available for immediate use if intracranial bleeding recurs. Bed rest for seven to 10 days after surgery and caution against manipulation of the operative area tend to prevent embolism from the site of ligature.

A head-down position, blood transfusion and administration of oxygen are all indicated as emergency measures if *circulatory hypotension* develops after ligation. All precautionary measures cited are doubly in order if the second major carotid artery is to be ligated.

TREATMENT.—Convulsive seizures and hemiplegia developing in the immediate postoperative period herald the appearance of cerebral ischemia. Removal of ligatures or of the clamp is mandatory if not more than four hours have passed since surgery. If neurologic deficit first appears after that time, reopening the artery usually does no good, although Brackett has reported recovery from hemiplegia after removal of an occluding band from the carotid 2½ days after ligation. Inhalation of carbon dioxide-oxygen mixtures in concentrations of 5 per cent and 45 per cent respectively will help to effect intracranial vasodilatation, as will stellate block, papaverine and histamine intravenously (2.75 mg. in 250 cc. of 5 per cent glucose drip). Heparin has no value after hemiplegia has occurred.

LATE SEQUELAE.—Although cerebrovascular resistance is invariably increased after carotid ligation, the cerebral blood flow is maintained at normal levels except when neurologic complications develop (Shenkin *et al.*). Nonetheless, air studies of the brain made some time after ligation of the carotid artery almost always reveal homolateral cerebral atrophy which usually is unaccompanied by neurologic complaints. Rarely, the hyperactive carotid sinus syndrome is a sequel of ligation. Even more unusually, erosion and rupture of the carotid artery at the site of ligature may occur after permanent occlusion. Cervical arteriovenous fistula has been reported.

SUBTEMPORAL DECOMPRESSION

This operation, one of the oldest in neurosurgery, is of value in cerebrovascular disease for the evacuation of an intracerebral blood clot, to tide a patient with thrombosis of a major intracranial sinus through the period of increased intracranial pressure and to preserve vision in occasional patients with malignant hypertension. It is a standard procedure for removal of epidural and subdural hematomas.

Under local or general anesthesia, a linear incision 6–7 cm. long is made from a point just above the ear diagonally to the zygomatic process. The temporalis muscle is split in the line of its fibers and held apart with self-retaining retractors, and a bur hole is made just below or at the suture of the squamotemporal bone. The dura is incised, the subdural space is inspected for hematoma, and the cortex, which is that of the inferior parietal lobe or the superior temporal gyrus, is coagulated. If intracerebral clot is suspected, a ventricular cannula is passed into the cerebral hemisphere, though never to a depth greater than 4 cm., in the direction indicated by the neurologic status of the patient or preoperative roentgen study.

When decompression is to be completed, the temporalis muscle is retracted further and temporal bone is removed as completely as possible with rongeurs, beginning at the bur hole. Craniectomy is extended in all quadrants until a defect roughly 4 × 4 cm. is created. The dura is further incised and opened in stellate fashion. If high-grade increased intracranial

390 CEREBROVASCULAR DISEASE

pressure is to be controlled, exposure of the brain to the floor of the middle fossa is essential.

CRANIOTOMY

Craniotomy is the surgical procedure which permits the complete evacuation of intracerebral hematoma, the intracranial clipping or "trapping" of congenital aneurysm, the radical removal of arteriovenous malformations and the extirpation of hemangioblastomas of the cerebellum or drainage of their cysts. Occasionally, intracranial exploration is the only way to distinguish absolutely between cerebral infarction and brain tumor.

CONTROL OF HEMORRHAGE. The most decisive single factor in the success or failure of definitive surgery of vascular anomalies is the control of operative hemorrhage. Therefore, adequate preparation of the patient demands a good circulating blood volume and properly cross-matched blood in reserve for transfusion. The skill of the surgeon is taxed to the utmost. He must know when to ligate vessels with silk, when to apply silver clips, when and how to coagulate with the Bovie endotherm, when to rely on tampons of gelatin sponge or crushed muscle, and when simple temporary pressure on a bleeding vessel will suffice. Suction must be at hand, and two suction apparatuses may be necessary.

Artificial hypotension.—Specialized methods of induced hypotension which have been developed to deal with the problem of operative hemorrhage now permit greater safety in radical neurosurgical procedures. Not only is bleeding less with a low blood pressure, but release of vasoconstricting substances in a shocklike state may assist hemostasis by controlling small-vessel ooze. Gardner has advocated *preliminary venesection* to the extent of as much as 1,600 cc., with surgery then performed in a dry field. Blood is reinfused rapidly through a peripheral artery if the physiologic situation becomes critical and is reinforced routinely at the end of operation. The heart and brain receive blood preferentially when it is given intra-arterially and under pressure.

Total *spinal anesthesia* and the systemic injection of *hexamethonium* have also been employed successfully to lower blood pressure during surgery. Use of hexamethonium is becoming routine in operations on dangerous vascular anomalies and is the preferred method of inducing surgical hypotension. The anesthetist must be in absolute control at all times and be able to give blood intravenously or intra-arterially at a moment's notice. He keeps the patient well oxygenated and cannot allow depressed physiologic processes to deteriorate below a reversible level.

The application of negative pressure (suction) to the legs will complement the effect of hexamethonium. Arfonad may be preferred as a hypotensive agent.

Complications of induced hypotension have included cerebral infarction, coronary thrombosis, the lower nephron syndrome and thrombotic episodes elsewhere in the body. So frequent and disastrous are these side effects that many anesthetists have abandoned this hemostatic procedure. Use of artificial hypotension definitely involves a calculated risk.

Temporary occlusion of the ipsilateral cervical carotid may be effected

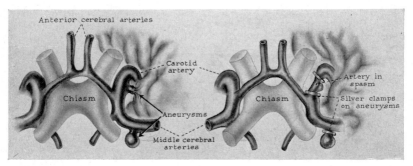

FIG. 128.—Isolation of intracranial aneurysms by application of silver clips. (Courtesy of R. C. Bassett.)

during surgery instead of general hypotension. The artery should be released every 15–20 minutes, and inhalation of 5 per cent carbon dioxide may be instituted to produce cerebral vasodilatation.

INTRACRANIAL ANEURYSM

The usual approach to aneurysm of the circle of Willis, the same as that for exposure of the pituitary gland, is through a frontotemporal craniotomy (Fig. 78). Great care must be exercised in approaching the circle of Willis and in retracting the temporal and frontal lobes, since a recently ruptured arterial sac may be only lightly sealed against adjacent cortex. All arteriographic views are helpful, for the aneurysm may lie below a major vessel or be tucked under the sphenoid wing. Resection of the frontal pole may be necessary to visualize a sac on the anterior communicating or anterior cerebral arteries, and the tip of the temporal lobe should be removed in approaching an aneurysm of the middle cerebral artery.

The fact that aneurysms rupture through a necrotic part of the wall, usually the neck, must be recalled. A tantalum or silver clip is applied to the neck, if it is stout, or the saccule may be isolated between clips on a vessel or vessels or "trapped" between a clip on the intracranial carotid above and the cervically ligated artery below (Figs. 78 and 128). Occasionally, the aneurysm may actually be excised while its parent artery is occluded temporarily in a silk noose, and the ostium of the sac is closed with fine silk (Campbell and Burkland). The surgeon may prefer to pack muscle fragments around the sac, wrap the lesion in cellophane or apply sterile liquid latex to it. It is sensible insurance to have a loop around the exposed cervical carotid, common or internal, if it has not been ligated previously.

ARTERIOVENOUS MALFORMATION

The craniotomy approach corresponds to the location of the lesion, and exposure should be generous (Fig. 86). The dura must be carefully reflected, because surface vessels of the vascular anomaly may communicate with intradural channels. The area is then inspected to decide whether to attempt to excise the tangle of arteries and veins in a radical manner or to leave it entirely alone. Half-way measures are not curative and may lead to disaster. Arteries must be occluded before veins; a reverse approach will only cause severe operative hemorrhage.

Intracerebral malformations are often wedge shaped, with the arterial supply internal in location. Surface anomalies may be gradually reduced in size by stroking the vessels with a low-voltage coagulation or cutting current. A particularly refractory lesion may be grasped with gauze and "wrung out," feeding vessels being tied, clipped or coagulated at the stalk. The middle cerebral artery is the most important vessel in the brain, especially on the dominant (left) side, and cannot be sacrificed.

CEREBELLAR HEMANGIOBLASTOMA

Vascular neoplasms of the cerebellum are approached through a standard suboccipital craniectomy. It is important to remove the arch of the atlas in order to free the cerebellar tonsils, which are often incarcerated, and to expose the transverse sinus above if it is apparent that a hemangioblastoma is superior in location and is draining into the sinus. Preliminary puncture of a lateral ventricle will reduce intracranial pressure and permit easier exploration of the posterior cranial fossa. Visible enlargement and palpable softness of a cerebellar hemisphere indicate a cystic lesion. Such a lesion should be aspirated of xanthochromic fluid before the cortex is transected. When the interior of the cyst is inspected, the mural nodule of tumor must be identified and extirpated (Fig. 81). Cavernous or solid lesions should be shrunk with the coagulating current if possible. Residual neoplastic tissue is treated postoperatively with roentgen radiation.

INTRACEREBRAL HEMATOMA

When it is probable that a hematoma in the brain is solid, in part or whole, evacuation underneath a small bone flap (Fig. 58) is preferable to simple aspiration after making a bur hole or subtemporal decompression. A transcortical incision is made after preliminary suction of liquefied clot through a ventricular needle. The solidified hematoma is removed with suction and irrigation, and the interior of the cavity is then inspected for the source of the bleeding. Small aneurysms may be found and clipped; minute angiomas are coagulated or, if no definite point of hemorrhage can be identified, strips of gelatin sponge may be laid over suspicious areas. A hematoma capsule, if present, should be dissected free and may prove to be angiomatous in nature, as was true in one of my patients. If it is easy to perform a small subtemporal decompression, this should be undertaken to control postoperative edema when a large clot has been evacuated.

BIBLIOGRAPHY

Bakay, L., and Sweet, W. H.: Cervical and intracranial pressures with and without vascular occlusion: Their significance in treatment of aneurysms and neoplasms, Surg., Gynec. & Obst. 65:67-75, 1952.

Brackett, C. E., Jr.: Late sequelae of carotid ligation, Neurology 3:316-318, 1953.

Campbell, E., and Burkland, C. W.: Aneurysms of the middle cerebral artery, Ann. Surg. 137:18-28, 1953.

Gardner, W. J.: The control of bleeding during operation by induced hypotension, J.A.M.A. 132:572-574, 1946.

Huertas, J., and Forster, F.: Pharmacodynamic responses of pial vessels, Fed. Proc. 13:72, 1954.

Krayenbühl, H.: Personal communication.

Poppen, J. L.: Specific treatment of intracranial aneurysms: Experiences with 143 surgically treated patients, J. Neurosurg. 8:75-103, 1951.

Rogers, L.: Carotid ligation for intracranial aneurysm: Report of case studied by electroencephalography, Brit. J. Surg. 32:309-311, 1944-45.

Shenkin, H. A., et al.: Hemodynamic effect of unilateral carotid ligation on cerebral circulation of man, J. Neurosurg. 8:38-45, 1951.

Swain, G.: Personal communication.

Sweet, W. H.; Sarnoff, S. J., and Bakay, L.: A clinical method for recording internal carotid pressure: Significance of changes during carotid occlusion, Surg., Gynec. & Obst. 90:327-334, 1950.

Index

A
Abdomen: examination of, 110
Abscess, brain
from cerebral embolism, 175
complicating sinus thrombosis, 273
from venous thrombosis, 265
Acetylcholine: effect on cerebrovascular resistance, 92
ACTH: effect on cerebrovascular resistance, 90
Adrenalectomy: for hypertensive disease, 285
Air embolism, 172
pathology, 173
symptoms, 175
treatment measures, 178
Airway: maintenance of, in stroke patient, 350
Alcohol
injection in migraine, 337
vapor inhalation, for pulmonary edema, 351
Aminophylline
effect on cerebrovascular resistance, 90
in treatment of stroke, 164
Anatomy
of arteries of brain, 24 ff.
carotid system, 26 ff.
circle of Willis, 24 ff.
of dural sinuses, 51, 56 ff.
microscopic
of arteries, 47
of veins, 64
surgical, of cervical carotid, 385
of veins of brain, 50 ff.
vertebral-basilar system, 36 ff.
Anemia
acute, cerebral complications, 319
cerebral, factors in, 82 f.

nonhemorrhagic infarct and, 141
pernicious, 319 f.
sickle cell, cerebrovascular involvement, 320 f.
Anesthesia
effect on cerebrovascular resistance, 91
spinal, for artificial hypotension, 390
Aneurysm
of aorta, cerebral thrombosis from, 133
carotid-cavernous, 235 ff.
symptoms and signs, 236 f.
treatment, 238 f.
cirsoid, 252 f.
angiography in diagnosis, 257
congenital intracranial
associated anomalies, 207
carotid ligation for, 225 ff., 233, 383
causing subarachnoid hemorrhage, 199 ff.
of circle of Willis, 200 ff.
from embryologic failure, 20
intracranial surgery of, 229 ff., 391 f.
in ophthalmoplegic migraine, 333, 335
prognosis, 234 f.
re-rupture of, 228, 233
ruptured — conservative management, 224 f.
sites of, 18, 206, 207
size of, 207
specific arterial syndromes, 212 ff.
miliary, hypertensive hemorrhage from, 182
multiple, 207, 215
treatment, 232
mycotic and neoplastic, hemorrhage from, 202 f.
Angiography, see Arteriography; Venography

Angioma, see Hemangioma
Angiomatosis, encephalotrigeminal, see
    Sturge-Weber disease
Angioreticuloma, see Hemangioblastoma
Angiospasm, see Vasospasm
Anomalies
  arterial, 45
    developmental, 18 ff.
    predisposing to infarction, 135
  arteriovenous, 242 ff.
    associated lesions, 249
    cerebral hemorrhage from, 182
    diagnosis, 253 ff., 258 f.
    differential diagnosis, 259
    etiology, pathogenesis, 242 f.
    location of, 248
    pathology of, 248 ff.
    physiologic effects, 248
    prognosis, 261
    symptoms and signs, 252 f.
    treatment, 259 f., 392
  cerebrovascular, effect on cerebrovascular
    resistance, 84
  congenital, associated with aneurysm,
    207
  of dural sinuses, 22
Anosognosia, 118
Anoxia
  clinical syndromes, 96
  EEG effects, 100
  effect on brain, 94 f.
Anticoagulant therapy
  after carotid ligation, 388
  in cerebral embolism, 177 f.
  in cerebral thrombosis, 164
  in thrombophlebitis, 273
Aorta
  aneurysm of, and cerebral thrombosis,
    133
  coarctation
    with cerebral aneurysm, 207
    and hypertension, 277
Aphasia, 116
  treatment of, 363
Apresoline, see Hydrazinophthalazine
Arsenic: vascular poisoning from, 328 f.
Arterial pressure, see also Hypertension;
    Intracranial pressure
  in carotid system, 77 f.
  measurement, 388
  and cerebral blood flow, 80, 81
  and cerebrospinal fluid tension, 92
  in cerebrovascular accidents, 108

  after cervical carotid ligation, 227
  effects on congenital aneurysms, 202
  effects of gravitational stress, 78 f.
Arteries of brain
  see also specific arteries and conditions
  anastomoses between
    and collateral circulation, 45 ff.
    and extent of thrombosis, 143
    surface, and infarction, 135
  anatomy of, 24 ff.
    microscopic, 47 ff.
    variations in, 45
  anomalies, 45
    causes, 20
    sites of, 18
  autonomic innervation of, 67 ff.
  changes in, during migraine, 333 f.
  direction of flow of blood, 75
  embryologic development, 17 ff.
  stenosis of, causing infarction, 139
  supplying visual system, 114
  surface, 29, 147
  susceptibility to sclerosis, 288
  tissue layers of, 47 f.
Arteriography
  of aneurysm (intracranial), 220 f.
  carotid, 372 ff.
    anesthesia for, 372
    open method, 372 f.
    percutaneous method, 373 f.
    sites of puncture, 27
    taking of films, 374 f.
  carotid-vertebral, 376
  in cerebral arteriosclerosis, 300
  in cerebral embolism, 176
  in cerebral hemorrhage, 193
  in cerebral thrombosis, 158 f.
  complications of, 376 f.
  in hypertensive brain disease, 281
  indications and contraindications, 371
  materials for, 371 f.
  in vascular tumors, malformations, 257
  in venous thrombosis, 272
  vertebral
    open method, 375
    percutaneous method, 376
    sites of puncture, 27, 36
Arteriosclerosis, cerebral, 287 ff.
  cerebral vasospasm and, 124
  cerebrovascular resistance in, 83, 84
  diagnosis, 297 ff., 300 f.
  differential diagnosis, 301
  etiology, pathogenesis, 287 ff.

in infancy, 288
management of patient, 301 ff.
neurologic syndromes of, 295 ff.
pathologic changes in, 289 ff.
pathophysiology, 292
prognosis, 303
symptoms and signs, 292 ff.
thrombosis from, 131
Arteriovenous malformations, see Anomalies, arteriovenous
Arteritis, see also Periarteritis nodosa
rheumatic cerebral, 311
temporal, 313 f.
Aspirin
antipyretic use, 354
for migraine, 336
Atelectasis: treatment, 350, 351
Atherosclerosis
pathogenesis of, 288
pathologic changes in, 131
Auditory artery: distribution, 40
Avellis' syndrome, 155

B

Babinski-Nageotte syndrome, 155
Babinski's sign, 117
Barbiturates: for sedation, 358
Barognosis, 118
Basilar artery
anatomy, 37
aneurysm of, 216, 218
treatment, 232
thrombosis, 152 f.
Bedsores: prevention and treatment, 353 f.
Benedikt's syndrome, 151
Binswanger's disease, 295
Bistrium, see Hexamethonium
Blood
loss (severe), causing cerebral infarction, 140 f.
studies, in diagnosis, 119
sugar level, regulation of, 97
transfusions, for shock, 82
viscosity
and cerebrovascular resistance, 84
in venous thromboses, 270
Blood-brain barrier, 48 f., 102
Blood dyscrasias: cerebrovascular complications, 134, 263, 319 ff.
Blood flow, cerebral, 73 ff.
in arteriosclerosis, 292
with arteriovenous malformation, 248

blood pressure and, 80, 81
carbon dioxide as regulator, 85
cardiac output and, 80
carotid compression and, 78
cerebrovascular resistance, 82 ff.
through circle of Willis, 24
circulation time, 74
direction of
arterial, 75
venous, 50, 76 f.
hormonal effects, 98
intracranial pressure and, 92 ff.
measures to increase, 366
methods of measurement, 73 f.
normal values, 74
peripheral resistance and, 80 f.
in pernicious anemia, 320
Blood pressure, see Arterial pressure
Blood vessels, intracranial
anatomy of, 24 ff., 50 ff.
changes as source of headache, 66 f.
development after birth, 23
embryology of, 17 ff.
late histologic changes, 22 f.
nerve supply of, 65 ff.
roentgen visualization, 370 ff.
supernumerary, 20
Bowel evacuation: in stroke patients, 353
Brain
arteries of, 24 ff.
embryologic development, 17 ff.
internal, 32
surface, 29, 147
arteriovenous malformations of, 242 ff.
atrophy (arteriosclerotic), 290, 298 f.
blood flow, direction, 75 ff.
capillary bed of, 48
circulation
collateral, 45 ff.
physiology of, 73 ff.
cortical localization maps, 147
edema (acute hypertensive), 279 f.
electroencephalography, 99 ff.
extracranial venous drainage of, 62 ff.
hypertensive disease of, 275 ff.
nerve supply to, 65 ff.
oxygen supply of, 73
roentgenography of, 370 ff.
supporting structures, 26
vascular tumors of, 242 ff.
veins of, 50 ff.
embryologic development, 17, 21 f.
waves, 99

Bruit, cranial
  in arteriovenous malformation, 252
  with carotid-cavernous fistula, 237
  in subarachnoid hemorrhage, 212
Buerger's disease, 133, 316 f.

C

Caffeine: effect on cerebrovascular resistance, 90
Carbon dioxide
  -oxygen therapy
    in arteriosclerosis, 302
    for carbon monoxide poisoning, 327
    in cerebral thrombosis, 164
    in cerebral vasospasm, 127
    regulation of cerebrovascular resistance, 85 f.
  tension, effect on EEG, 100
Carbon disulfide: vascular poisoning from, 328
Carbon monoxide: brain lesions from, 326 f.
Carotid arteries
  anastomoses (external and internal), 27, 45 f.
  anatomy of, 26
    surgical, 385
  aneurysms
    cavernous sinus, 213, 235 ff.
    supracavernous, 213 f.
  anomalies of, 45
  autonomic innervation, 68, 70 f.
  calcification, in arteriosclerosis, 297 f.
  compression
    for carotid-cavernous fistula, 239
    effect on collateral flow, 78
    preoperative, technic, 387
  divisions of
    common, 386
    internal, 28 ff.
    internal, in embryo, 21
  exposure and identification of, 384
  ligation, see Carotid ligation
  pressures in, 77 f.
  resection of, for thrombosis, 166
  sinus, 26, 88
    see also Reflex, carotid sinus
  thrombosis of, 143 ff.
    EEG in, 161
    emboli from, 172
    syndromes of, 144 f.
  visualized by angiography, 372 ff.
Carotid ligation, 383 ff.

for aneurysm, 225 ff., 233
  vs. intracranial clipping, 226
  with intracranial surgery, 230, 233
  in specific locations, 230 ff.
for arteriovenous malformations, 260
for carotid-cavernous fistula, 238
complications, 228, 386 ff.
  prevention, 387 f.
  treatment, 388
indications for, 383
technics (cervical), 384 ff.
  in continuity, 385
  partial, progressive, 386
  temporary, 387 f.
Carotid siphon, 27, 59
  aneurysm of, 214
  intracavernous, rupture of, 235 ff.
Cerebellar arteries
  anatomy of
    anterior inferior, 40 ff.
    middle (Foix), 40
    posterior inferior, 42 f.
    superior, 39 f.
  aneurysms of, 219
    treatment, 232
  thrombosis of, 153 f.
Cerebral arteries
  anatomy of
    anterior, 28 ff.
    middle, 31 ff.
    posterior, 38 f.
  aneurysm of
    anterior, 217
    middle, 214, 215 f.
    posterior, 216, 217 f.
    treatment, 231 f.
  thrombosis of
    anterior, 145 f.
    EEG in, 161 f.
    middle, 146
    posterior, 149
Cerebrospinal fluid
  in arteriosclerosis, 297
  bloody
    causes of, 203
    traumatic tap differentiated from hemorrhage, 369
  in cerebral embolism, 176
  in cerebral hemorrhage, 191
  in cerebral thrombosis, 156 f.
  examination, in differential diagnosis, 119 f.
  formation and reabsorption, 101 f.

in hypertensive disease, 280
pressure, see also Intracranial pressure
    measurement, 368 f.
    in subarachnoid hemorrhage, 219 f.
    with vascular tumors, 253
    in venous disease, 270 f.
    and venous pressure equilibrium, 92 f.
    withdrawal, headache from, 67
Cerebrovascular accident, see also specific
    causes
    comparison with other intracranial dis-
    ease, 107
    diagnosis
        general physical examination in, 106
        ff.
        neurologic examination, 111 ff.
        special technics, 368 ff.
    differential diagnosis, 121, Table 1
    general management of patient, 345 ff.
        nutrition, 355 f.
        physical therapy, 359 ff.
        position in bed, 349 f.
        psychiatric treatment, 364 ff.
        respiration, 349 f.
        restraints, 357
        sedation, 357 f.
    therapeutic technics, 380 ff.
Cerebrovascular resistance, 83 ff.
    blood viscosity and, 84
    metabolic regulation of, 85 ff.
    neuroregulation, 87 ff.
Cestan-Chenais syndrome, 155
Chloral hydrate: for sedation, 358, 365
Cholesterol
    in diet, restriction in arteriosclerosis, 302
    formation in atherosclerosis, 288
Choroidal arteries, 44
    anatomy (anterior), 35 f., 39
    aneurysm of, 217
    thrombosis of
        anterior, 146
        posterior, 151
Circle of Willis
    aneurysms of, causing subarachnoid
        hemorrhage, 199 ff.
    anomalies predisposing to infarction,
        135
    blood flow through, 24, 75
    and collateral blood supply to brain, 45
    embryologic development, 18, 20 f.
    functions of, 24 ff.
    structure of, 24
        anatomic variations, 45

Circulation
    of brain
        collateral, 45 ff.
        deficiency, and infarction, 139
        physiology of, 73 ff.
        time, 74 f.
        support of, in cerebrovascular accident,
            163, 348
Claude-Bernard-Horner complex, see Horn-
    er's syndrome
Claude's syndrome, 152
Clipping, intracranial
    of aneurysm, 229, 391 f.
        vs. carotid ligation, 226
        with carotid ligation, 230, 233
    for carotid-cavernous fistula, 238
Coagulation
    of aneurysm, 229
    of surface arteriovenous anomalies, 392
Codeine: in subarachnoid hemorrhage
    therapy, 225
Collagen diseases, 310 ff.
Communicating arteries
    anatomy, 36, 39
    aneurysms of
        anterior, 216, 231
        posterior, 217, 232
    thrombosis of, 149
Consciousness: signs of, 111
Contrast mediums: for angiography, 371 f.
Convulsive seizures, 111 f.
    anticonvulsant drugs for, 358 f.
    cerebral vasospasm initiating, 124
    relation to migraine, 335
    in subarachnoid hemorrhage, 211
    types of, 112
Co-ordination: testing of, 117
Craniectomy, suboccipital: in hemangio-
    blastoma, 259
Craniotomy, 390 ff.
    see also Surgery, intracranial
Cushing's law, 93
Cushing's syndrome: hypertension and,
    276

D

Decompression, subtemporal
    in hypertensive encephalopathy, 283
    indications for, 389
    in sinus occlusion, 273
    technic, 389 f.
Dehydration: in stroke patient, manage-
    ment, 355 f.

Déjerine-Roussy: thalamic syndrome of, 150
Dexamyl: for sedation in psychotic patient, 365
Diet
in migraine therapy, 337
restrictions, in arteriosclerosis, 301 f.
tube-feeding of stroke patient, 356
Dihydroergotamine: for migraine, 336
Dilantin: for convulsive seizures, 358
Diodrast
for angiography, 372
toxic effects, avoidance, 377
Diuretics: to control intracranial pressure, 348
Dura mater: arteries of, 44

E

Eclampsia
cerebral hemorrhage in, 183
cerebrovascular resistance in, 83
hypertensive changes in, 277
Edema
angioneurotic, 315
of brain (acute hypertensive), 279 f.
pulmonary, treatment, 351
Electric shock therapy: in psychotic patients, 365 f.
Electrocardiogram: in diagnosis, 120
Electroencephalogram, 99 ff., 378
alpha, beta and delta waves in, 99
during alterations in carbon dioxide tension, 86
in cerebral arteriosclerosis, 300
in cerebral embolism, 176
in cerebral hemorrhage, 193
in cerebral thrombosis, infarction, 159 ff.
in chronic anoxia, 100
in differential diagnosis, 120
frequency of, factors altering, 99
in hypertensive brain disease, 281
in lupus erythematosus disseminatus, 315
in migraine, 335
normal, 100
in prediction of carotid ligature results, 223
in sleep, 99
in subarachnoid hemorrhage, 221 f.
in vascular tumor, malformation, 257 f.
Embolism, cerebral, 171 ff.
air, 172, 173
diagnosis, 175 ff.

differential diagnosis, 176 f.
etiology, pathogenesis, 171 ff.
fat, 172
mycotic, producing aneurysm, 202
pathology, 173 f.
prognosis, 178
symptoms and signs, 174 f.
treatment, 177 f.
vasospasm in, 124
from venous emboli, 172, 265
Embryology: of intracranial vessels, 17 ff.
Encephalitis
cerebral thrombosis in, 133
hemorrhagic, 305
Encephalography
in arteriovenous malformation, 257
in cerebral arteriosclerosis, 298
in cerebral embolism, 176
in cerebral hemorrhage, 193
in subarachnoid hemorrhage, 220
technic, 370
Encephalopathy
hemorrhagic, from arsenic, 328
hypertensive, see Hypertensive brain disease
lead, 327 f.
Endarteriectomy: for thrombosis, 166
Endarteritis obliterans: pathologic process of, 289
Endocarditis: cerebral embolism with, 171, 173 f.
Enemas: for stroke patients, 353
Enzymes, respiratory: in cerebral metabolism, 98
Epileptic attack, see Convulsive seizures
Epinephrine: effect on cerebral blood flow, 89
Ergot poisoning, 328
Ergotamine
effect on cerebral vessels, 89, 328
tartrate, for headache, 336, 338, 341
Erythroblastosis fetalis, 325 f.
intracranial bleeding in, 183 f.
État lacunaire, 149
in arteriosclerotic brain, 290, 292
Ethyl chloride spray: for hiccough, 352
Exophthalmos
with carotid-cavernous fistula, 236
in subarachnoid hemorrhage, 212
Extremities
examination, 108, 111
regaining function, in hemiplegia, 362, 363 f.

Eye
  examination, 109, 113, 115
  signs
    of carotid-cavernous fistula, 236
    in cavernous aneurysm, 213
    in cerebral arteriosclerosis, 293, 294
    in cerebral hemorrhage, 193
    in von Hippel-Lindau disease, 251
    in hypertensive disease, 279
    in subarachnoid hemorrhage, 210 f.
  source of headache, 342

F

Fat embolism
  causes, 172
  pathology, 173
  symptoms, 175
Fever
  in cerebrovascular disease, 106, 210, 354
    treatment, 354 f.
  effect on cerebral metabolic rate, 97
Fistula
  arteriovenous, 243
  carotid-cavernous, see Aneurysm, carotid-
    cavernous
Fits, see also Convulsive seizures
  hysterical, 112
Fluids
  hypertonic, to reduce intracranial pres-
    sure, 347
  in therapy of stroke patient, 355 f.
Foville's syndrome, 152

G

Gait: testing of, in diagnosis, 117
Ganglions
  parasympathetic, 68, 71
  sympathetic, 67 ff.
Gastromalacia: in cerebrovascular accident,
    352
Glucose
  hypertonic, to control intracranial pres-
    sure, 347
  utilization by brain, 97
Gravity: and intravascular pressures, 78 f.

H

Head
  examination of, in cerebral accidents,
    109 f.
  injury
    cerebral hemorrhage from, 184
    differential diagnosis in, 195
    sinus thrombosis from, 265

Headache, 330 ff.
  differential diagnosis, 332
  histamine, 337 f.
  hypertensive, 341
    in hypertensive brain disease, 278 f.
    treatment, 284
  of intracranial vascular source, 66 f.
  measures to relieve, 357
  mechanisms of, 331
  migraine, 331 ff.
  of muscular origin, 343
  physiology of, 330 f.
  post-traumatic, 340 f.
  referred, 342 f.
  spinal puncture, 342
  of subarachnoid hemorrhage, 209, 225
  tension, 343
Heart
  disease
    cerebral embolism with, 171 ff., 178
    cerebral infarction with, 139
    congenital, and cerebral thrombosis,
      134
  failure, venous or sinus thrombosis in,
    264
  output, and cerebral blood flow, 80
  status, in cerebrovascular accident, 110,
    348
Hemangioblastoma
  cerebellar
    in polycythemia, 324
    surgical approach to, 392 f.
  etiology, 242
  pathology, 243
  prognosis, 260
  surgical treatment, 259
  symptoms and signs, 251
Hemangioma
  arteriovenous, with aneurysm, 207
  cerebral hemorrhage from, 183, 252
  from developmental arrest, 19, 21
  EEG in diagnosis, 257
  etiology, 242
  pathology, 246 f.
  prognosis, 261
  symptoms and signs, 251 f.
  treatment, 260
Hematoma
  chronic
    from injury, 184
    pathology, 186
  from ruptured aneurysm, 204
  surgical removal, 393

Hemiballismus syndrome, 150
Hemiplegia
  acute, prevention of deformities, 360
  basis of recovery in, 363 f.
  facial paralysis in, 115
  formation of bedsores in, prevention and
    treatment, 353 f.
  physical therapy in
    during acute stage, 359 f.
    during chronic stage, 362 f.
  signs of, 116
  sympathicolytic drugs in, 127 f.
Hemogram: in diagnosis, 119
Hemophilia, 321
Hemorrhage, cerebral, 180 ff.
  bloody spinal tap differentiated from,
    369
  complicating vascular disease, 182 f.
  diagnosis, 190 ff., 193 ff.
  differential diagnosis, 194
  etiology, pathogenesis, 180 ff.
  in hemorrhagic disease of newborn, 183,
    325
  location of, 185
  medical therapy, 195
  pathology, 185 f.
  prognosis, 196 f.
  surgical therapy, indications for, 195 f.
  symptoms and signs, 187 ff.
  in thrombocytopenic purpura, 321
Hemorrhage, subarachnoid, 199 ff.
  see also Aneurysm, intracranial
  diagnosis, 219 ff., 223 ff.
  differential diagnosis, 223 f.
  etiology, pathogenesis, 199 ff., 203
  pathology, 203 ff.
  prognosis, 234 f.
  symptoms and signs
    acute episode, 209 ff.
    aneurysmal syndromes, 212 ff.
  treatment
    conservative management, 224 f.
    surgery in, 225 ff., 230 ff.
    use of morphine in, 225, 358
Herpes simplex: in subarachnoid hemor-
    rhage, 212
Hexamethonium
  for artificial hypotension, 390
  in cerebral vasospasm, 127
  effect on cerebrovascular resistance, 92
  for hypertension, 283 f.
Hiccough: control of, 352

von Hippel-Lindau disease, 244, 251
Histamine
  desensitization program, 338
  effect on cerebrovascular resistance, 90
  headache, 337 f.
  therapy
    in cerebral embolism, 177
    in cerebral thrombosis, 164
    in cerebral vasospasm, 127
Hoffmann's sign, 117
Hormones
  effect on cerebral metabolism, 94, 98
  role in hypertension, 276
  sex, use in arteriosclerosis, 302
Horner's syndrome, 152
  signs of, 118
Hospitalization
  of psychotic patient, 365
  of stroke patients, 345
Hydrazinophthalazine
  in cerebral vasospasm, 127
  effect on cerebrovascular resistance, 92
  for hypertension, 283 f.
Hydrocephalus
  with arteriovenous malformations, 248
  ex vacuo, 290, 298
  with hemangioma, 251
  otitic, 269
Hypertension, arterial
  cerebral hemorrhage and, 180 ff., 191
  cerebral vasospasm in, 123 f.
  cerebrovascular resistance in, 83, 84
  clinical conditions associated with, 276 f.
  etiology, pathogenesis, 275 ff.
  medical management, 283 f.
  prognosis, 285
  surgical therapy, 284 f.
Hypertensive brain disease, 275 ff.
  diagnosis, 280 ff.
  differential diagnosis, 282
  etiology, pathogenesis, 275 ff.
  pathology, 277 f.
  symptoms and signs, 278 ff.
  treatment, 283
Hypoglycemia: signs of, 97
Hypotension
  artificial, 230, 390 f.
    complications of, 140, 391
    after carotid ligation, treatment, 388
  systemic
    neurologic sequelae, 140
    supportive measures, 163, 348

I

Infarction, cerebral, 131 ff.
  see also Thrombosis, arterial
  after carotid ligation for aneurysm, 228
  collateral circulation modifying, 135, 138
  diagnosis, 156 ff., 162
  differential diagnosis, 162
    radioactive studies in, 159
  hypertensive hemorrhage from, 181
  medical therapy, 163 f.
  pathology, 136 f., 142
    red, 137 f.
    white, 136
  physiotherapy in, 166
  prognosis, 167
  without thrombosis, 138 ff.
    etiology, pathogenesis, 138 ff.
    prodromal symptoms, 142
Infections
  bacterial (pyogenic), 305 ff.
    soft tissue, 264
    treatment, 307
  mycotic, 310
  rickettsial, 307 f.
  spirochetal, 309 f.
  virus, 310
Insect stings: cerebral thrombosis from, 133
Intracranial pressure
  and cerebral blood flow, 92 ff.
  increased
    in cerebrovascular accident, 346
    and hypertension, 277
    management, 346 ff.
    physiologic effects, 93 f.
  variations, 93
Iodide
  potassium, in arteriosclerosis, 303
  in treatment of stroke, 164

J

Jaundice, infectious, 310

K

Ketosis: cerebral metabolic rate in, 98
Kidney
  disease, hypertension and, 275 f., 277
  polycystic, with cerebral aneurysm, 207
Korsakoff's syndrome
  in subarachnoid hemorrhage, 212
  in Wernicke's disease, 326

L

Laboratory examinations: in diagnosis of cerebrovascular accident, 119 f.
Lead: vascular poisoning from, 277, 327 f.
Leptospirosis, 310
Leukemia: cerebral complications, 322 f.
Ligation, see Carotid ligation
Lindau's disease, 244 f.
Lung
  edema of, treatment, 351
  examination, 110
  function, supportive measures, 348 ff.
  inflammatory processes of, reaching brain, 265
  x-rays, in diagnosis, 119
Lupus erythematosus disseminatus, 314 f.
Lymph nodes: examination, 108

M

Magnesium sulfate
  for hypertensive crisis, 283
  proctoclysis, to control intracranial pressure, 347 f.
Manganese poisoning, 328
Mastoiditis: sinus thrombosis in, 269
Medulla oblongata
  arterial supply of, 42 f.
  venous drainage of, 56
Meningeal arteries: anatomy, 44
Meninges: signs of irritation, 111
Meningitis, 306 f.
Mental status
  with cerebral arteriosclerosis, 293
  estimation, in diagnosis, 113
Mercurialism, 328
Mesencephalon
  arterial supply, 39
  hemorrhage in, 186, 189 f.
  infarctions in, 151
  veins of, 56
Metabolic processes: and cerebral blood flow, 85 ff.
Metabolism, cerebral, 94 ff.
  in arteriosclerosis, 292
  changes in, causing syncope, 81
  depression of, 98
Migraine, 331 ff.
  cerebral vasospasm in, 123
  epileptic, 335
  medical treatment, 336
  ocular palsies in, 333, 335
  ophthalmoplegic, cavernous aneurysm diagnosed as, 213

Migraine *(cont.)*
  surgical therapy in, 337
  symptoms and signs, 334 f.
  vascular changes in, 333 f.
Millard-Gubler syndrome, 152
Mönckeberg's sclerosis, 289
Monro-Kellie doctrine, 74
Morphine
  to reduce fever, 354
  in subarachnoid hemorrhage, 225, 358
Mouth: examination, in cerebral accidents, 109
Myopexy: for infarction, 166

N

Neck: examination of, in cerebral accidents, 110, 111
Nephrectomy: in malignant hypertension, 285
Nerve block
  in atypical facial neuralgia, 340
  of cervical ganglion after carotid ligation, 388
  of stellate ganglion, 380 ff.
    anterior method, 382
    anterolateral method, 382
    in cerebral embolism, 177
    in cerebral thrombosis, 164 f.
    in cerebral vasospasm, 128 f.
    complications, 383
    posterior method, 382
    for pulmonary edema, 351
    for thalamic pain, 358
Nerves
  carotid, 68, 70
  cranial
    examination of, 113 ff.
    lower—distribution, 66
    paralysis of, 115, 294
    relation to circle of Willis, 25
    signs in subarachnoid hemorrhage, 211
  facial, 71, 115
  glossopharyngeal, 66, 72, 115 f.
  of Hering, 88
  optic, 113
    in hypertensive disease, 279
    in subarachnoid hemorrhage, 211
  petrosal, 68, 71
  trigeminal, 65 f., 115
  upper cervical, distribution, 66
  vagus, 66, 72, 115 f.
  vasomotor, 67 ff.

  parasympathetic, 71 f.
  regulating cerebrovascular resistance, 87 ff.
  sympathetic, 67 ff.
  vasosensory, 65 ff.
  vertebral, 68, 69
Nervous system
  autonomic, 67 ff.
    syndromes, in cerebrovascular disease, 118
  findings, in arteriosclerosis, 293 f.
Neuralgia
  atypical facial, 339 f.
  trigeminal
    arteriosclerosis causing, 295
    vs. atypical facial neuralgia, 339 f.
Nevus
  cutaneous, with arteriovenous malformation, 252
  flammeus, in Sturge-Weber disease, 249 f., 253
Nicotinic acid
  in cerebral thrombosis, 164
  effect on cerebrovascular irrigation, 90
  in psychoses of senility, 366
  for vasospasm, 127
Nitrates: effect on cerebrovascular resistance, 90
Nitrite, amyl
  for cerebral embolism, 177
  for cerebral thrombosis, 164
  for cerebral vasospasm, 127
L-Nor-epinephrine: effect on cerebrovascular resistance, 90
Nutrition
  maintenance, in stroke patient, 355 f.
  in psychotic patients, 365
Nystagmus: in diagnosis, 115

O

Obstetric delivery: venous or sinus thrombosis after, 264 f.
Occupational therapy, 365
Ophthalmic artery, 28
  aneurysm of, 214
Oxygen
  deprivation, effect on brain, 95
  poisoning, 97, 349
  supply
    of brain, 73, 94
    and cerebrovascular resistance, 86
    effect on EEG, 100
  therapy, *see also* Carbon dioxide-oxygen
    for stroke patients, 349

P

Pain
  conduction, 71
  sensation, testing of, 118
  -sensitive structures in cranium, 330
  thalamic, control of, 358
Papaverine
  for cerebral embolism, 177
  for cerebral thrombosis, 164
  use after carotid ligation, 388
  for vasospasm, 127
Paraldehyde: for sedation, 358, 365
Paralysis, see also Hemiplegia
  agitans, 295 f.
  cranial nerve, 115, 294 f.
  pseudobulbar, 296
  treatment, 303
Paramedian arteries, 42 f.
Parasites: as intracranial emboli, 173 f.
Parkinsonism, arteriosclerotic, 295 f.
  differentiated from degenerative form, 296
  medical therapy for, 303
  x-ray changes in (skull), 298
Pelvis: examination of, in cerebral accidents, 111
Periarteritis nodosa, 311 f.
Peripheral resistance: and cerebral blood flow, 80 f.
Pheochromocytoma
  cerebral hemorrhage in, 183
  hypertension from, 276
Phlebitis
  systemic, cerebral involvement in, 265
  venous and sinus
    diagnosis, 272 f.
    pathology, 265, 267
    prognosis, 273
    symptoms and signs, 267 f.
    treatment, 273
Physical therapy
  for hemiplegia, 166, 359 ff.
  in acute stage, 359 f.
  in chronic stage, 362 f.
Physiology
  of headache, 330 f.
  of intracranial circulation, 73 ff.
Pia-glial membrane, 48, 102
Plexus
  basilar, 61
  choroid, 44
  nerve
    carotid, 70

  vertebral, 69
  of vessels, in embryologic development, 17 f.
Pneumoencephalography, see Encephalography
Poisons, cerebrovascular, 326 ff.
  vasospasm from, 125
Polycythemia vera: cerebrovascular involvement, 324
Pons
  arterial supply of, 41
  hemorrhage into, 189
  infarctions in, 152
  veins of, 56
Pontile arteries, 40
Porphyria, 310
Potassium
  in cerebral metabolism, 98
  chloride, for vertigo, 302
  deficiency, therapy for, 356
  iodide, in arteriosclerosis, 303
Priscoline
  effect on cerebrovascular resistance, 92
  in hemiplegia, 128
  in hypertensive crisis, 283
Procaine
  block, see Nerve block
  and cerebrovascular resistance, 92
  periarterial infiltration, for headache, 337, 341
Proctoclysis: magnesium sulfate, method, 347 f.
Psychoses
  arteriosclerotic, causation and symptoms, 296 f.
  after cerebrovascular disease, management, 364 ff.
  Korsakoff syndrome, 326
  with subarachnoid hemorrhage, 212
Psychotherapy
  for atypical facial neuralgia, 340
  in cerebrovascular disease, 364 ff.
  for migraine patients, 336
  for tension headache, 343
"Pulseless disease," 134
Pulse rate: in cerebrovascular accidents, 106
Purpura, thrombocytopenic, 321

R

Raynaud's disease: cerebral vasospasm in, 123
Rectum: examination of, 111

Reflexes
  carotid sinus
    conditions increasing, 88
    depression of, during carotid ligation, 384
    hyperactive, treatment, 163
    testing of, 116
  in cerebral arteriosclerosis, 293
  in cerebral hemorrhage, 188
  examination, in cerebrovascular accident, 117
Rehabilitation: of hemiplegic patient, 359 ff.
Relapsing fever, 309
Respiration
  measures to improve, 349 f.
  type and rate, in cerebrovascular accidents, 108
Restlessness: control of, 225, 358
Restraints: for stroke patient, 357
Rheumatic fever: cerebral involvement in, 133, 311
Rocky Mountain spotted fever, 308 f.
Roentgenography, see also specific methods
  in arteriovenous malformation, 253 f.
  in cerebral arteriosclerosis, 297
  in cerebral hemorrhage, 191 f.
  in cerebral thrombosis, 157 f.
  in differential diagnosis, 119
  in hemangioma, 253 f.
  in hypertensive brain disease, 280
  in subarachnoid hemorrhage, 220 f.
  in vascular tumors and malformations, 253 ff.
  in venous disease, 270
Roentgen rays: effect on cerebral vessels, 328
Roentgen therapy: for vascular anomalies, 259

S

Salt
  restriction, in migraine, 337
  retention, 355 f.
  -wasting syndrome, 356
Schmidt's syndrome, 155
Scopolamine hydrobromide: for pseudobulbar palsy, 303
Scurvy, 324
Sedation
  to control vomiting, 352
  in psychotic patient, 365
  for restlessness, 358

in subarachnoid hemorrhage, 225
Senility: psychoses of, management, 364 ff.
Sensation: testing of, 117 f.
Serum albumin: to reduce intracranial pressure, 348
Serum sickness, 315
Shock: from hemorrhage or trauma, 82
Sicklemia: brain involvement in, 320 f.
Simmond's disease: from cavernous aneurysm, 213
Sinuses, see under Carotid artery; Venous sinuses
Skin
  care of, in stroke patient, 353 f.
  examination, 108
Skull
  examination, in cerebral accidents, 109 f.
  injury, see Head injury
  x-rays, see Roentgenography
Spasticity: control of, 360
Speech
  disturbances, in cerebral accidents, 116
  therapy in aphasia, 363
Spinal arteries, 43 f.
  thrombosis of, 155
Spinal puncture
  to control increased intracranial pressure, 346
  in differential diagnosis, 119 f.
  headache, 342
  in hypertensive encephalopathy, 283
  procedure, 368 f.
  in subarachnoid hemorrhage, 225
Status epilepticus: treatment, 359
Stellate block, see under Nerve block
Stereognosis, 118
Stress
  in migraine, 333
  syndrome in hypertensive disease, 275
Stroke, see Cerebrovascular accident; specific conditions
"Strokelets," 140, 152 f.
Sturge-Weber disease
  capillary sclerosis in, 290
  clinical triad of, 253, 259
  etiology, 243
  pathologic changes in, 249 f.
  skull x-rays in, 253 f.
  surgical treatment, 260
Sucrose: hypertonic, for control of intracranial pressure, 347

Surgery, intracranial
of aneurysms, 229 ff., 391 f.
prognosis after, 235
control of hemorrhage in, 390 f.
of hemangioblastoma, 392
indications for, 390
of intracerebral hematoma, 393
for vascular anomalies, 259 f., 392
Sympathectomy
in arteriosclerosis, 302
in cerebral thrombosis, 165
in cerebral vasospasm, 129
for hypertensive disease, 284
Sympathicolytic agents
in cerebral thrombosis, 164
in cerebral vasospasm, 127 f.
effect on cerebrovascular resistance, 92
for hypertension, 283 f.
Syncope
causes, 81, 83
in "little strokes," 140
Syphilis
cerebral thrombosis from, 133
cerebrovascular, 309

T

Takayasu's syndrome, 134
Tela choroidea, 44
Telangiectasia, 19, 248
pial, 243
in Sturge-Weber disease, 249, 250
Tetraethyl ammonium nitrite: effect on
cerebrovascular resistance, 92
Thiamine deficiency, 326
Thorotrast: in angiography, 371 f.
Thromboangiitis obliterans, 133, 316 f.
Thrombosis, arterial, 131 ff.
see also Infarction, cerebral
in Buerger's disease, 316
carotid, emboli from, 172
after carotid ligation, 228
diagnosis, 156 f., 162
differential diagnosis, 162 f.
from brain tumor, 159, 161, 163
EEG in, 159 ff.
etiology, pathogenesis, 131 ff.
febrile, 133, 306
life management after, 166
medical therapy, 163 f.
in midbrain, 151
pathology, 136 ff.
predisposition to, 134 f.
prognosis, 167

surgical therapy, 164 ff.
symptoms and signs, 142 ff.
syndromes for specific arteries, 142 ff.
Thrombosis, venous and sinus
diagnosis, 270 ff.
differential diagnosis, 272 f.
etiology, pathogenesis, 263 ff.
marantic, 263, 268
pathology, 265 ff.
prognosis in, 273
symptoms and signs, 267 ff.
treatment, 273
Tic douloureux, see Neuralgia, trigeminal
Topognosis, 118
Tracheotomy: in stroke patient, 350
Trauma
causing carotid-cavernous fistula, 236
cerebral hemorrhage from, 184
cerebral thrombosis from, 133
sinus thrombosis from, 265
Trypsin: in treatment of stroke, 164
Tumor
brain
cerebral hemorrhage with, 183
differentiated from hypertensive disease, 282
differentiated from thrombosis, 159,
161, 163
headache from, 342
vascular, 242 ff.
vascular—differential diagnosis, 259
emboli in cerebral vessels, 173, 203, 236
pathology, 174
symptoms, 175
Typhus fever, 307 f.

U

Ulcer
decubitus, prevention and treatment,
353 f.
neurogenic, in cerebrovascular accident,
352
Urinalysis: in diagnosis, 119
Urinary tract: drainage, in stroke patient,
351

V

Vascular disease
arterial, cerebrovascular resistance in, 83
cerebral hemorrhage in, 182 f.
cerebral thrombophlebitis from, 265
collagenous, 310 ff.
inflammatory, 305 ff.
cerebral thrombosis in, 133

Vasoconstrictor drugs: effect on cerebrovascular resistance, 89 f.
Vasodilator drugs, *see also* specific drugs
in cerebral arteriosclerosis, 302
in cerebral thrombosis, infarction, 164
for cerebral vasospasm, 127
effect on cerebrovascular resistance, 90
Vasospasm, cerebral, 122 ff.
after carotid ligation, 228
differential diagnosis, 126 f.
diseases accompanied by, 123 f.
etiology, pathogenesis, 122 ff.
prognosis, 129
symptoms and signs, 125 f.
treatment measures, 127 f.
Veins
jugular, 62 f.
thrombosis of, 270
systemic, emboli from, 172
vertebral, 62, 63 f.
Veins of brain, 50 ff.
anastomoses among, 54 ff.
anastomotic
of Labbé, 52
of Trolard, 52
basal, 54
of Rosenthal, 54
of brain stem, 56
cerebellar, 56
cerebral
external, 50 ff.
internal, 53 ff.
obstruction, effect on cerebrovascular
resistance, 85
direction of blood flow through, 76
embryologic development, 17, 21 f.
emissary, 62 ff.
galenic system, 53 f.
microscopic anatomy, 64
petrosal, 56
phlebitis of, 267 ff.
terminal, 53, 55
thrombosis of, 263 ff.
transverse caudate, 55
Vena cava, superior: thrombosis of, 270
Venesection
for heart failure in stroke, 348
for hypertensive crisis, 283
to induce hypotension (surgical), 390
Venography
dural sinus, method, 377
indications and contraindications, 371

Venous disease, *see* Phlebitis; Thrombosis
Venous pressure, 79 f.
and cerebrospinal fluid tension, 92 f.
Venous sinuses, dural
anatomy, 51, 56 ff.
cavernous, 59
-carotid artery fistula, 235 ff.
circular, 60
embryologic development, 21 f.
occipital, 59
petrosal, 60 f.
phlebitis of, 268 f.
sagittal, 57 f.
sigmoid, 61
sphenoparietal, 59
straight, 58
tentorial, 56
thrombosis of, 263 ff.
transverse, 61
Ventriculography, 370
in cerebral hemorrhage, 193
in cerebral thrombosis, 157
in hemangioblastoma, 257
in hypertensive brain disease, 280
in sinus thrombosis, 271
Vernet's complex, 155
Vertebral arteries
anatomy, 27, 36 f.
aneurysm of, 216, 218 f.
treatment, 232
anomalies of, 45
autonomic innervation of, 68, 69
paramedian, 42
thrombosis of, 155
visualized by angiography, 375 f.
Villaret's syndrome, 155
Virchow-Robin space, 48
Virus diseases: of brain, 310
Visual system
arterial supply, 114
examination of, 113
Vitamin deficiencies: cerebrovascular complications, 324 ff.
Vomiting: control of, 352

W

Walking: relearning process, in hemi-
plegia, 362
Wallenberg syndrome, 41, 154
Weber's syndrome, 151
Weil's disease, 310
Wernicke's disease, 326
Winiwarter-Buerger disease, 133, 316 f.